A Hospital
for Ashe County

CONTRIBUTIONS TO SOUTHERN APPALACHIAN STUDIES

A Hospital for Ashe County

*Four Generations of Appalachian
Community Health Care*

Janet C. Pittard

Contributions to Southern Appalachian Studies, 38

McFarland & Company, Inc., Publishers
Jefferson, North Carolina

ALSO OF INTEREST

Stephen Shoemaker: The Paintings and Their Stories
(Stephen Shoemaker and Janet Pittard, 2013)

The present work is a reprint of the illustrated case bound edition of A Hospital for Ashe County: Four Generations of Appalachian Community Health Care, *first published in 2016 by McFarland.*

LIBRARY OF CONGRESS CATALOGUING-IN-PUBLICATION DATA [new form]

Names: Pittard, Janet, 1950–, author.
Title: A hospital for Ashe County : four generations of
Appalachian community health care / Janet C. Pittard.
Other titles: Contributions to southern Appalachian studies ; 38.
Description: Jefferson, North Carolina : McFarland & Company, Inc., 2016. |
Series: Contributions to southern Appalachian studies ; 38 |
Includes bibliographical references and index.
Identifiers: LCCN 2015036639 | ISBN 9781476668000
(softcover : acid free paper) ∞
Subjects: | MESH: Ashe Memorial Hospital. | Ashe County Memorial
Hospital. | Hospitals, Community—History—North Carolina. |
Physicians—North Carolina—Interviews. | History, 19th Century—
North Carolina. | History, 20th Century—North Carolina.
Classification: LCC RA981.N82 | NLM WX 28 AN8 |
DDC 362.1109756/835—dc23
LC record available at http://lccn.loc.gov/2015036639

BRITISH LIBRARY CATALOGUING DATA ARE AVAILABLE

ISBN (print) 978-1-4766-6800-0
ISBN (ebook) 978-1-4766-2414-3

Edited by Robert Franklin
Typeset by Phyllis Efford

Printed in the United States of America

*McFarland & Company, Inc., Publishers
Box 611, Jefferson, North Carolina 28640
www.mcfarlandpub.com*

To the community of Ashe County,
who gave of themselves to build a hospital to serve their own
and created a health care legacy spanning generations.

Acknowledgments

Many people have assisted and encouraged me over the past year and a half, suggesting people to interview, relating anecdotes, searching their attics for photographs and news clippings, and helping me to accurately weave together the story of Ashe Memorial Hospital and four generations of Appalachian community health care. To all those who shared with me their time, their memories, and their hearts, thank you for making it possible for me to tell this story. I am indebted to Doris Oliver for identifying people for me to interview and answering my many questions about the old hospital and its staff; to David VanHoy for sharing his wealth of knowledge of the area and its people; to Anne Shoemaker McGuire for her guidance and encouragement in researching the local landscape; and, especially, to my dear friend Evelyn Jones, for introducing me to the many delightful and interesting people she persuaded to be interviewed for this book and for being my navigator on the back roads of Ashe County. I will remember the many hours we spent together with gratitude and affection.

My brother, David Chiswell, is my ace when it comes to finding a needle in a haystack of historical information. An archivist by trade, he provided me with invaluable research, sought out pertinent reference books, photographs, microfilmed copies of newspapers, and manuscripts from Special Collections at Appalachian State University, the North Carolina Department of Cultural Resources, and the Louis Round Wilson Special Collections Library at the University of North Carolina at Chapel Hill.

The images reproduced in this volume are an important part of telling the story, and I am grateful to McFarland & Company, Inc., Publishers, not only for their interest in this project, but for their help with scanning and preparing the images for publication. Special thanks go to artist Stephen Shoemaker for allowing his painting of Ashe County Memorial Hospital to be used as the cover.

Finally, this book could not have been completed without the support of my husband, Louis. Thank you for always being there to share my dreams.

Table of Contents

The Old Ashe County Memorial Hospital—A Legacy

It is a stately edifice, despite the broken windows and scraggly lawn,
This place where people came to be healed, to give birth, to die.
Its halls are empty now,
No longer filled with the clatter of gurneys and nurses scurrying to answer calls.
A few ghosts linger, of course, as they often do, guarding the past.
They remind us to be respectful of who and what has gone before us,
Those who tended to the sick and injured,
Held the hands of mothers in labor,
Comforted those at the end of a long hard life,
And those not ready to see their loved ones leave.
They dried the tears of joy and sorrow and pain and tried to make it better.
Sometimes they succeeded and were repaid with a smile, a thank you,
Or maybe a sack of potatoes from the garden.
Sometimes they failed and bore the news of their defeat to the ones who waited.
Those lost were not anonymous folk, but neighbors, friends, and kin,
Making that walk down the hall longer and sadder and that embrace more dear.
Next door, the nurses' quarters is alive with the squeals and laughter of children.
Converted to a daycare, it reminds us life rumbles on,
Better for those who came before.
That is the legacy of this place,
That its presence made a difference in the lives of those it served.
That the community that conceived and supported this great endeavor still lives
In the hearts and memories of those who witnessed these events firsthand or
In the pardonable pride of later generations,
Mindful of their achievements.

Janet Chiswell Pittard

Preface

On May 23, 2014, I was invited to the home of Evelyn Price Jones, widow of Dr. Dean C. Jones, Jr., to meet with Evelyn and her son, Dr. Charles Jones. Referred to me by Henry Doss and Chris Arvidson, patients of Dr. Charles, the doctor and his mother were pitching an idea for a book about the history of Ashe Memorial Hospital in Jefferson, North Carolina, the community that willed the hospital into being, and the four generations of doctors in the Jones family, who served the region for the last one hundred plus years and played a major role in the hospital's evolution. I was not sure I wanted to take on a project of this magnitude, but I was willing to listen.

Looking out the window from where I sat at Evelyn's kitchen table, I could make out the back of the old Ashe County Memorial Hospital on McConnell Street, where I was told Charles's grandparents, Dr. Dean Jones, Sr., and his wife, Lettie, worked and lived, and Charles's father, Dr. Dean C. Jones, Jr., grew up and met Evelyn. The hospital building is vacant now, replaced in 1971 by the larger, more modern facility, renamed Ashe Memorial Hospital (AMH), a few miles down the road. But this story, as it was beginning to unfold in the conversation around the table, was not about the hospital building; it was about the people who saw the need for it, dreamed it, planned it, built it, worked in it, were treated and cared for in it, and continue to support it. These people included natives of the area whose families went back to before the American Revolution and relative newcomers, who, while "not from around here," joined the community and tried to make a contribution, without mucking up what drew them here in the first place. The people were the well-to-do and the poor and those in-between. They were the sick and the healed and the healthy-as-a-horse. They were the newborn and the unborn and the aged. At one time or another, they probably all had occasion to be in the hospital, either as a patient or a visitor or a caregiver. This was about an Appalachian community, a community that looked after its own and did what was necessary to accomplish that, in spite of the obstacles they confronted.

A hospital for Ashe County was the life goal of Dr. Dean Jones, Sr., explained grandson Charles, and when it first opened in 1941, as Ashe County Memorial Hospital, Inc., Dr. Jones, Sr., was the resident physician and surgeon in the hospital and did his own lab work and x-rays. The history of the hospital was intertwined with that of the Jones family, as well as the community and its leaders. These people came together with the Works Progress Administration (WPA) during the hard times of the Great Depression, to build a hospital and an Appalachian health care legacy. Like the old lantern on Evelyn's living room mantel, the story of how this vision became a reality was part of the Jones family heritage. The lantern is thought to have been carried in the early 1900s by the first generation of Jones family doctors, Charles's great-grandfather Dr. Arthur Lee "Bud" Jones, lighting his way as he made his house calls, traveling on horseback along the rough roads and footpaths of Ashe County, North Carolina, and Grayson County, Virginia.

As we talked, Evelyn held a box of newspaper clippings and photographs in front of her, treasured relics, chronicling the history of the Jones family and the hospital. On top was a copy of the *Ashe Memorial Hospital Monitor, Fall, 1997*, reporting the return to Ashe County of her son Charles, to practice medicine as a general and vascular surgeon at Ashe Memorial Hospital. When Dr. Charles Jones started his practice at Ashe Memorial July 14, 1997, he was following in the footsteps of his father, grandfather, and great-grandfather, who joined other dedicated medical professionals in providing health care for this Appalachian community during a span of time that saw two world wars, the Great Depression, and multiple local natural disasters, including catastrophic floods and extreme snow events. There was a story here, and I wanted to tell it.

Having decided to take on the project, I wanted the story to reflect the variety of people who influenced the progress of community health care in Appalachia, with Ashe County and the surrounding area as my primary focus and with Dr. Bud Jones and his descendants as my common thread. But I didn't want to restrict my narrative to physicians and surgeons and nurses—they were a big part of the story, but they were not the whole story. I wanted to include the contributions of as many people as possible—maintenance people, administrators, bookkeepers, office workers, security, volunteers—anybody who had anything to do with making the hospital run. I wanted to give the story an accurate context, historically and culturally, to represent those who provided various forms of health care–related services for the community before there were doctors and surgeons and hospitals to be had—healers and midwives and grannies with potions and poultices for every ailment. I wanted to talk about the sicknesses and diseases and injuries with which mountain families had to contend. I wanted to represent the diversity of people who helped take an Ashe County hospital from a dream to a reality—farmers, businessmen, Rotary, ministers, educators, woman's clubs, children and young people who participated in the fundraising, and local doctors and other medical professionals, who dedicated their lives to taking care of a community of friends and neighbors. I also wanted to reflect the development of community health care, the expansion of hospital services, and present day changes in hospital management, not in detail, but enough to capture the contrast with the early days of Ashe County Memorial.

My research drew on local resources, such as publications produced by or associated with the Ashe County Historical Society, especially *The Heritage of Ashe County, Volumes I and II*, archived materials at the Museum of Ashe County History and Special Collections in the Belk Library at Appalachian State University, and microfilmed local newspapers from the Ashe County Library. My researcher, David Chiswell, relied heavily on microfilm copies of *The Skyland Post* from the State Archives in the North Carolina Department of Cultural Resources in Raleigh, especially to establish the chronology of events relating to Ashe

County Memorial Hospital and other health care resources in the area. Many of the photographs came from collections on file at the Department of Cultural Resources. David and I also reviewed the papers of Congressman Robert L. Doughton at the Wilson Library on the campus of the University of North Carolina at Chapel Hill. This provided valuable insight into the role of the Congressman in obtaining the WPA funding for the construction of Ashe County Memorial Hospital. The original ledger of Ashe County Memorial Hospital, Inc., loaned to me by AMH, provided the minutes of board meetings, shareholder meetings, and executive committee meetings, from the first meeting of shareholders in the Superior Court Room in the Ashe County Courthouse, December 12, 1939, through the early 1950s. Zetta Barker Hamby's *Memoirs of Grassy Creek: Growing Up in the Mountains on the Virginia–North Carolina Line* was my primary source for early health care and remedies common to the area, and *Crossings: Memoirs of a Mountain Medical Doctor*, by Elam S. Kurtz, M.D., and Michael D. Kurtz, provided me information specific to the contributions of Dr. Elam Kurtz and others.

My most important sources of information, however, were the people of Ashe County. I talked to as many as I could to capture the diversity of those involved in the development of community health care in the region and the grand endeavor of building a hospital. From July 2014 through July 2015, I conducted a hundred interviews. People were generous with their time and honest with their comments. They trusted me with their treasured family photographs and other mementos of the past. Where I needed background on people who were gone, I talked to descendants. I looked for personal impressions and anecdotes that would help me know these people of another time and what motivated their interest and support of community health care. One lady I talked to was 100 years old. Many were well into their nineties and had to search into the long ago for bits and pieces of recollection. Those interviews were some of the most precious and revealing. This is their story, told as they remember it, not as a textbook history, but as a scrapbook of memories. I have set their story against the backdrop of community health care in Appalachia, as it evolved over the generations, because I believe this account of the hospital in Ashe and a community taking care of its own has been replayed many times in the greater Appalachian community. And I believe what Ashe County achieved at a point in time when people had yet to recover from the Great Depression, stood on the brink of World War II, and were taxed with flooding and snows, was nothing short of amazing.

Introduction

The road up to the cemetery was steep and rough, but my passengers were game, so I put my Jeep Wrangler in four-wheel drive, and we made it up there—Evelyn Jones, Nell Jones Taylor, granddaughter of Dr. Arthur Lee "Bud" Jones, and Nell's husband, Tom Taylor. It was worth the trek. There is something about an old cemetery that evokes a connection with those whose remains lie there, even for those of us who did not have the privilege to know them personally. I could almost hear the gruff voice of Dr. Bud and feel his tall presence in that quiet place, overlooking the land and the people for whom he cared so long ago. I wonder, does he know the legacy he started?

Four generations ago, when Dr. Bud Jones made his house calls on horseback, community health care in Appalachia was a story of courage and perseverance and caring. It still is. That story is epitomized in the community of Ashe County, where Dr. Bud practiced. Located in the northwestern corner of North Carolina, in a section of the Appalachian Mountains known as the Blue Ridge, the county is bordered by Tennessee to the west, Virginia to the north, and Watauga County, North Carolina, to the south. The area is called the High Country, where the North and South Forks of the New River snake through the landscape, join just south of the Virginia state line, and flow north into Virginia. Like most Appalachian communities, Ashe County was and still is sparsely populated; according to the Ashe County Chamber of Commerce, the estimated population in 2015 was 27,755. Like the rest of the country, its people struggled during the Great Depression, to put food on the table, to educate their children, and to take care of one another in sickness. Descended from a fiercely proud and independent pool of immigrants to the New World, including Scots and Scotch-Irish, Germans, Dutch, Swedes, and French Huguenots, these mountain people were not of a mind to wait for somebody else to solve their problems, least of all anybody representing the government. They were more likely to resist this last resource, to relocate to avoid it, as some of their ancestors had, or to take matters into their own hands, as they did during the American Revolution, when British Army Major Patrick Ferguson threatened to invade and lay waste to their land. They did not wait for General George Washington and the Continental Army to come to the rescue; these folks picked up their rifles, rode out with their own horses, food, clothing, and gun powder, with no promise of pay, and made their way to Kings Mountain, South Carolina, where they defeated the British. Some went on to fight at Cowpens, but eventually most simply returned home to their families and farms and resumed tending to their own business. They were called the Overmountain Men, and they did not wait for history to happen to them, they made their own history and helped set the course for American independence.[1]

I see that same do-it-yourself spirit of the Overmountain Men in the more recent history of Appalachia, especially where I live now in Ashe County. Of course times have changed, but I do not think people have abandoned the self reliance and determination that marks their heritage. I think when the challenge or opportunity presents itself, the people here, like their ancestors, are capable of marshaling their resources and making things happen. The evidence of this is in the exceptional state ranking achieved by the Ashe County public schools, the popularity and support of the Ashe County Library, the vitality and diversity of the Ashe County Arts Council, the success of the Florence Thomas Art School, the continued growth of the Museum of Ashe County History, the active Chamber of Commerce, the involvement of business in the welfare of the community, the outreach efforts of local churches, and the continued support for Ashe Memorial Hospital.

1

Horseback Doctors

During the nineteenth and early twentieth centuries, a wide variety of people, with a wide range of qualifications and education, formal, informal, and nonexistent, practiced some form of medicine. They included healers, practitioners, midwives, physicians, and surgeons. The quality of care they provided ran the gamut from superior to better-than-nothing to outright quackery. Whatever their preparation, these people faced huge challenges: diseases that were not wholly understood in terms of cause and treatment; surgeries performed on kitchen tables or outdoors; payment for service that was sporadic at best and often took the form of barter; and transportation.[1] In this time before paved roads and four-wheel drive vehicles, getting to a patient in rural western North Carolina was a major obstacle to providing medical care. And then there were the winters, snow and ice, worse in the old days than now, say the locals. Physicians were scarce, but a few from the very early days stand out in regional histories and personal recollections of natives to the region and form a representative sample of those who came to be known as "horseback doctors."[2]

Many young men who wanted to become doctors in the early 1800s, and it was typically men and not women in those days, had no medical degree from an accredited medical college. Instead they arranged to "read medicine" in the office of an established physician. Aras Bishop Cox started reading medicine at age 25. Born in Floyd County, Virginia, January 25, 1816, he pursued numerous careers besides medicine, including farmer, teacher, elected official, merchant, military commander, writer, and preacher in the Methodist Episcopal Church. By 1842 he was teaching school in Grayson County, Virginia. He married Phoebe Edwards in 1845 and settled in the Stratford Community, in what is now Alleghany County. In 1849, he was elected Clerk of Superior Court of Ashe County, an office he maintained for eight years. He and his wife moved to a farm in Nathans Creek in 1852, where he opened a store. Today the old homeplace is on the National Register of Historic Places. He served in the Confederate Army during the Civil War, not as a physician or surgeon, but as a captain commanding infantry and later as a chaplain. In 1869, Dr. Cox moved his family away from Ashe County and lived in several places before settling in Nebraska. He continued to practice medicine and preach, and in 1900, while visiting in Ashe County, finished his book *Foot Prints on the Sands of Time*, a history of southwestern Virginia and northwestern North Carolina. Dr. Cox died January 30, 1907.[3]

Dr. Edmund Franklin Foster honed his skills as a surgeon in the Confederate Army

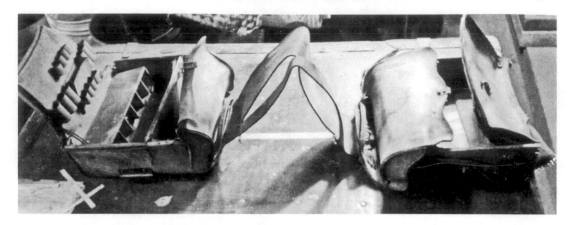

In the days before automobiles and paved roads, horseback doctors braved the rugged terrain and extreme cold of Appalachia to make their house calls. Saddlebags like these belonging to Drs. Thomas Jones and Lester Jones were used to carry medications and medical instruments (courtesy C. B. Jones and family).

during the Civil War. Born January 2, 1829, in Wilkes County, he set up his medical practice in Jefferson in the 1850s, after receiving his degree from medical school in Richmond, Virginia. Once in Ashe County, he met and married Ellen Coreen Murchison, whose father had moved the family from Salem, North Carolina, to set up a law practice in Ashe County. Dr. Foster was discharged from his post in the Confederate Army for health reasons and returned to Ashe County to practice medicine.[4]

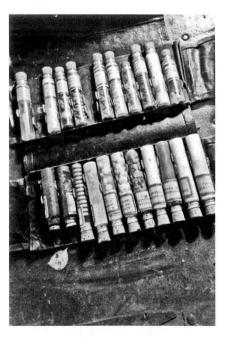

This carrying case was designed to safely transport vials of medicine. Some doctors made their own pills (courtesy C. B. Jones and family).

Ninth generation Ashe County native and author of *Memoirs of Grassy Creek*, Zetta Barker Hamby (1907–1997), writes the first doctor she ever ran across was Dr. Alfred W. Wagg. Dr. Wagg served as a surgeon in the Confederacy during the Civil War and was experienced in trauma cases, important in the rural mountain area he served, where hard work and severe injuries went together with unfortunate regularity. Later in his career, in 1880, he was employed by the Board of County Commissioners as the county physician, but when Hamby met him, he kept an office in the back of a store he owned and operated in Grassy Creek with his son, Charlie Wagg.[5] Hamby's daughter, Gayle Winston, recalls the story of how her grandfather, Zetta's father, Charlie Barker, was thrown from his wagon when his team of mules took off on a fast-paced, unauthorized excursion. He dislocated his shoulder in the resulting melee, and Dr. Wagg was summoned. As the patient was experiencing severe pain, Wagg administered chloroform as an anesthetic. Chloroform was known to have some unfortunate side effects, causing people to talk out of their heads and other unseemly behaviors. When the doctor pulled Barker's arm back in the socket, Barker, no longer in his right mind, spat in the doctor's face. Wagg took offense and stalked to the door. Barker's wife, no doubt in a panic at being left with an irate husband whose arm was only partially repaired, managed to smooth things over and persuade the doctor to return and complete the task at hand. For the rest of his life Barker had to sleep with a cloth strap securing his arm to his side, for fear of reinjuring the arm.[6]

A close friend of Dr. Wagg, Dr. Burgess "Cox" Waddell, practiced in the Grassy Creek area as well and, as reflected in hospital records, eventually served on the medical staff at Ashe County Memorial Hospital. Waddell, the elder of the two, reportedly walked with a distinctive bouncy stride, as though he were bow legged, prompting locals to joke about the two doctors, "one came a waggin' and one came a waddelling." Born February 28, 1869, in Alleghany County, North Carolina, to Houston and Martha Jones Waddell, Cox Waddell began his education in a one-room school house, near Piney Creek in Alleghany County. Robert Lee Doughton, later Con-

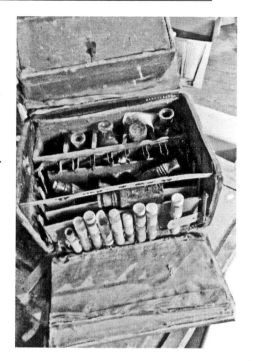

Drs. Thomas and Lester Jones of Lansing used this medicine bag for house calls in the late 1800s to early 1900s (courtesy C. B. Jones and family).

gressman Doughton, was one of his teachers, and the two became lifelong friends. Waddell attended Baltimore School of Medicine, graduating with honors two years later, and came home to practice in Scottville, on the Ashe–Alleghany line. Soon he relocated to Grassy Creek, more convenient to the Fields Mills, a large textile operation, which offered the doctor incentives to treat its workers. He purchased Oak Shade Farm and eventually moved his office out of his home and built a clinic on his property, near the Grassy Creek Post Office and Gordon Sturgill's General Store.[7]

After he replaced his trusty gray mare with a Model "T" Ford, he established clinics at Grant, Troutdale, and Konnarock, Virginia, and Sturgills in North Carolina. He travelled to each on a regular basis, much like modern doctors who maintain practices in multiple locations. Kemp Nye, who wrote a biography of Dr. Waddell, assisted the doctor in his practice and drove his car for him. According to local historian David VanHoy, since telephone service had yet to come to many in the region, families requiring the doctor's services tied a white cloth on their mailbox, so he knew to stop when he passed through on his rounds. To break the monotony of their long drives to see patients, Kemp called out words for Waddell to spell. The wordsmith was well-versed in Latin too, and students in Grassy Creek sought out the doctor for help with their Latin.[8]

Dr. Waddell knew what everybody needed in the way of medications and carried a supply with him, but if he was out of stock, he was not averse to using a tried and true home remedy instead. Nye relates that if he ran out of aspirin, Waddell used an old Cherokee remedy he had learned from the Indians around Mount Rogers: "Strip some bark from a willow sapling and chew it, then take a swig of vinegar." As was the norm for rural doctors of his day, he did everything from routine treatment to emergency surgeries. If he encountered an injury which taxed his trauma skills, he called for assistance from his friend Dr. Wagg.[9] Dr. Waddell died August 29, 1946, and is buried in the Grassy Creek Community Cemetery.[10]

Dr. Joseph Orrin Wilcox operated his own medical school at his homeplace on the North Fork of the New River, near Creston in Ashe County. The school provided an affordable alternative to aspiring physicians unable to attend a medical college. Born December 2, 1844, Wilcox was a graduate of what was later known as Johns Hopkins University in Baltimore, Maryland.[11] Pat McNeill's grandfather on her mother's side, Augustus Franklin Wilcox (1849–1906) was brother to Dr. J. O. Wilcox. Pat hunted through papers belonging to her mother Ruby Carrington Wilcox Hudler and found notes her mother made regarding the Wilcox genealogy, including biographical notes about Dr. J. O. Wilcox, her grandfather Augustus Franklin Wilcox, and other family members. These notes were the basis for her contribution on the subject to the Ashe County Historical Society's publication entitled *The Heritage of Ashe County North Carolina, Volume II, 1994.*[12] Augustus Franklin and his brother Joseph Orrin, both farmers, owned a considerable tract of land together in Pond Mountain, Horse Creek, Grassy Creek, and Staggs Creek, estimated to cover a six mile radius.[13]

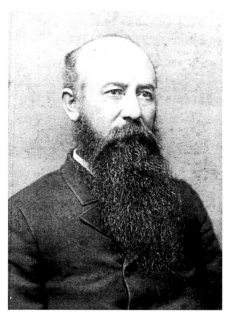

In the early days of community health care in Appalachia, not everyone who aspired to practice medicine had the means to attend a big city medical college. An alternative was offered by Dr. Joseph Orrin Wilcox, who operated a medical school in the late 1800s at his homeplace on the North Fork of the New River near Creston (courtesy Ashe County Historical Society).

Dr. Wilcox is believed to have been the only doctor for the North Fork of the New River and had a good reputation as a physician, with a large practice. As part of his lesson plan at his medical school, Wilcox assigned his medical students to retrace his steps, visiting his patients and making diagnoses.[14] Many graduated from his school and became successful practitioners, a testament to this teaching methodology.[15]

According to research done by Betsy Barber Hawkins of Florida, great-granddaughter of Dr. Wilcox, the Wilcox family came to Ashe County by way of Grayson County, Virginia, but Joseph Orrin was born in Hamptonville in piedmont North Carolina, where his father, Miles, shared a mercantile business with the Cowles family from Connecticut in the early 1800s. Dr. Wilcox married Civil War widow Marticia (or Martitia) Worth Wagner, daughter of David and Elizabeth Worth of Creston. (It is her daughter, Mariana Martitia Wilcox Barber, who is grandmother to Betsy Barber Hawkins.) Marticia Wilcox died shortly after the birth of her daughter, and Dr. Wilcox married Margaret Henry of Raleigh, whose acquaintance he made while serving in the North Carolina State Legislature.[16] Dr. Wilcox died of typhoid fever September 4, 1898, at age 53, and is buried in the Wilcox Cemetery on the hill in front of and across from the home constructed after the original, built by Wilcox in the 1860s, burned in the early 1900s. The back parlor of the original home was used as a morgue during Wilcox's lifetime.[17]

Dr. Manley Blevins practiced medicine in Ashe County for 57 years and was a familiar sight to many, travelling on horseback or driving a horse and buggy to see his patients. He reportedly never refused to make a house call, regardless of the weather or the patient's ability to pay. Wylene Blevins Barker, was only a youngster when Dr. Blevins died, but she remembers he was her grandmother's doctor and delivered all ten of her children at the family's home. After ten deliveries the doctor must have known the family well, but he was not kin, despite having the same last name. Born April 11, 1859, to Dr. Daniel and Emeline Edwards Blevins at what later became known as Scott Place, in the Phoenix Creek section of Ashe County, Manley Blevins read medicine at a young age with his father and then with Dr. J. O. Wilcox. He pursued his education at the Baltimore School of Medicine and began his practice in 1882. He was licensed in 1885 and admitted to the North Carolina State Medical Society in 1905.[18] He was considered to be especially skilled in the treatment of typhoid and pneumonia and in pediatrics, drawing on a combination of the old and new ways in health care. He was the county physician for two years, served during World War I in the Volunteer Medical Service Corps, and attempted to establish a hospital in West Jefferson around 1926 but was unsuccessful. Although in poor health, he continued to practice medicine until a few days before he died, December 9, 1939, at 80 years old. His funeral reportedly was attended by one of the largest crowds ever present for a burial in Ashe County.[19]

In the days before the Civil War, the few physicians serving in Appalachia ranged significantly in level of expertise. Some took advantage of regional medical schools like that of Dr. J. O. Wilcox or a medical college, if one was within reach, geographically and financially, and then pursued their clinical experience in an urban hospital. But sometimes medical training was limited to attendance at a few medical lectures and an apprenticeship or preceptorship arrangement with an experienced physician or surgeon. Others simply worked with an established physician and never received any formal medical education. In years to come, laws would be set up to define and upgrade the status of physicians. Legislative efforts to regulate medical licensing were postponed with the onset of the Civil War but resurfaced when the war ended, with the establishment of legal guidelines and the founding of state medical societies and state medical boards. Many successful doctors did not qualify under the new laws and lost their licenses or ended up with limited licenses.[20] It is important to note that the term "physician" is sometimes preferred by scholars when referring to someone who possesses an M.D., rather than the term "doctor." For purposes of this book, I have chosen to use the terms interchangeably.[21]

The tough conditions encountered by physicians in Appalachia, starting with the horseback doctors and continuing to more modern times, made heroes and legends out of some who met the challenges. The close relationships they formed with their patients and patients' families, staying in homes, waiting days for fevers to break or some other danger to pass, gained them an important place in the community, and many babies were named after the local doctor who delivered them.[22] These early physicians were among the most educated men in the communities they served and often assumed other leadership roles, particularly in education and politics, but they were not perfect. It is important to acknowledge that the stress of being a physician then, as now, could be overwhelming at times. Some were able to cope, and some were not, seeking solace in alcohol or drugs or simply giving up. Because communities were indebted to them for their care and held them in high esteem and affection as neighbors and friends and leaders, their foibles most often were overlooked, and they were protected by the people they served.[23] Rather than devote time to their faults, I have concentrated on the perseverance and care demonstrated by these physicians and surgeons, which, after all, is the story most worth remembering.

2

Early Health Care Resources

During those early years when physicians were few and far between in rural Appalachia, the population managed its health care with a healthy or sometimes unhealthy dose of homemade remedies to treat illness or injury. Mountain people relied on folklore passed from one generation to another, some with origins in the old country and some learned from Native Americans, especially the use of medicinal herbs, roots, barks and leaves, readily accessible in the woods around them.[1]

In her book *Memoirs of Grassy Creek*, Zetta Barker Hamby describes a variety of common illnesses and the remedies applied in her day. The daughter of Charlie Columbus Barker (born 1877) and Minnie Lena Spencer Barker (born 1877), Zetta was born and raised in the community of Grassy Creek on the Virginia–North Carolina line. Once, when she was a child, she had croup, an inflammation of the throat and windpipe, causing difficulty in breathing. On the advice of her grandmother, she was treated with a spoonful of lamp oil. "I could just feel the choking going away," she reports.[2]

Lamp oil was also used to swab the throat in cases of diphtheria, a highly infectious disease, characterized by fever, weakness and the formation of membranes or blisters in the throat, which caused difficulty in breathing. Outbreaks of diphtheria sometimes killed several in the same family in only a few days.[3] Gayle Winston, Hamby's daughter and a tenth generation Ashe County native, relates to me a story her mother told about a girl who had diphtheria. She craved cornbread but was told the hard crust would hurt her blistered throat. Her parents finally gave in to her craving, afraid she was going to die, deprived of the one thing she wanted to eat. Apparently the cornbread raked off the blisters on the way down, and she recovered.

Whooping cough, characterized by coughing and trouble breathing, was another disease afflicting children that was typically treated with home remedies, such as a simmered mixture of equal parts of honey, sweet oil and vinegar.[4] Scarlet fever seemed to hit children more than adults, often causing permanent damage to the eyes, ears, heart and kidneys of those who survived. Usually starting out with fever, headaches and sore throat, the disease then progressed to a red rash on the chest and throat. When diagnosed in the patient's home, the family was immediately quarantined. Isolation was also prescribed for consumption or tuberculosis, which could strike as early as the teens and early twenties. Patients were either relegated to sleeping porches or sent to sanitariums. Children sometimes died from flux or diarrhea, an illness which usually occurred in the summer months. Hamby's three year old sister was very ill with this disease, and after home remedies and a doctor's initial treatment resulted in no improvement, the doctor suggested fat mutton. This was duly prepared and fed to the child, and she began to improve. Some patients drank a concoction of water and mud, used as mortar in field rock chimneys, or water mixed with pulverized charcoal. Influenza hit the Grassy Creek area with a vengeance in 1918, Hamby recounts, taking many lives. Five in her family were in bed with the flu at the same time. Her father, not a smoker, believed that smoking a pipe would prevent the flu and lit up accordingly.[5] Hamby's husband, Gwyn, was a smoker, and Gayle Winston says when she had earaches, he would blow smoke into her ears, and it would give her some relief.[6]

Typhoid fever, scarlet fever, tuberculosis, smallpox and other contagious diseases took their toll on the region, wiping out entire families.[7] With no hospitals, patients had to stay at home with their families. In some cases, like the highly contagious typhoid fever, a room not accessible from inside the house was constructed off the porch for the patient.[8] In later years, heart disease would replace these epidemics as a leading cause of death in Appalachia.[9]

As not much importance was given to hand washing or the proper cleaning of minor injuries, infections were not uncommon for people working on their farms, splitting wood, mending fences and tending to livestock. Blood poisoning could develop from a splinter left untended for too long, and amputations could result. Tobacco chewers sometimes took a wad of tobacco out of their mouths to put on a wound.[10] Gayle Winston remembers her mother putting bacon on a splinter to draw it out and taking a spoonful of sugar with kerosene for a cold. Two or three doses of sulfur and molasses were prescribed for the entire family as a spring tonic.[11] Preventive concoctions were regularly administered to all ages. Ashe County native Calvin Miller claims his mother was a great believer in cod liver oil, and he drank gallons of the stuff.[12] Whiskey, not the store bought kind, but homemade, adds Winston, was prescribed for colds, and most recipes for spring tonics included a hefty dose of the medicinal libation.[13]

People had definite ideas about what was healthy and what was not. Stephen Shoemaker's grandmother on his father's side, Lilly Dell Walker Shoemaker (1872–1966) was a no-nonsense little woman with no shortage of advice on almost everything, from making biscuits to sin and damnation. She dipped snuff but would not drink the juice of boiled cabbage, claiming it was poison and would kill you.[14]

Notions abounded regarding the cause of disease. Cornetta Price, sister-in-law to Evelyn Jones, says when her Grandmother Young was diagnosed with breast cancer, she was convinced the cancer was caused by somebody throwing an ear of corn and hitting her in the chest when she was working in the corn patch. Her surgery was successful, and she lived for many more years.[15] Various birth defects were attributed to something the mother had seen or touched when she was pregnant.[16]

Mountain people have always had a reputation for hardiness, accepting illness, like extreme weather conditions, as part of what life throws at you, but that does not mean they did not take advantage of available health care resources. It was a long time before there were enough doctors to take care of the sick and deliver babies in Appalachia or for people to have the means to get to a doctor's office, if there was one to be had. People sometimes turned to healers or faith healers, self-professed and otherwise, who called on prayer to relieve the suffering of the afflicted or simply had a curative gift. Midwives did most of the deliveries in the early days, and midwifery continued to be a trusted choice for deliveries for many years before the advent of laws regulating medical licensing. Usually the midwife was not a stranger to the patient but a relative or neighbor, fetched by the husband or an older child to walk or ride the distance to the home of the patient. She charged either a very modest fee or none at all. Her skills probably were learned from another midwife, or she drew on her own child birthing experience. Formal training for this profession did not come until much later.[17] Sometimes this worked out fine for the mother and sometimes not. One practice that sounded particularly scary was called "snuffing the mother," where the midwife held tobacco snuff or black or red pepper under the mother's nose to make her sneeze, supposedly inducing labor.[18] Unsanitary conditions and superstitious practices associated with obstetrical procedures were identified by country doctor Dr. Benjamin Earle Washburn, in his book *A Country Doctor in the South Mountains,* as a leading source of ill-health among the mountain women in the early 1900s.[19]

In his address at the dedication of Ashe County Memorial Hospital in November 1941, Dr. W. S. Rankin of the Duke Endowment, indicated that 475 babies were born each year in Ashe County, and one third of the mothers received no professional medical care, instead relying on midwives.[20] From 1925 until 1950, there were still more midwives than physicians in Ashe County, and midwives formed a vital part of community health care in Appalachia well into the twentieth century.[21] The gradual increase in availability of physicians would eventually result in a decline in the practice. In 1940, midwives were used in 14.3 percent of births in Appalachia, but by 1956, this rate had dropped to 3.2 percent.[22] With regulation of the practice of midwifery sought and obtained, and passage of such legislation as the Sheppard-Towner Maternity and Infancy Protection Act of 1921 and the North Carolina Midwifery Act of 1935, oversight of the practice was initiated, and the district health department, established in 1938, dispatched public health personnel to monitor practices accordingly.[23] Mrs. H. P. Guffy of the children's and infants' division of the N.C. Health Department spent the month of August 1941 conducting schools for midwives in the various communities of Ashe County, and Dr. Robert King, director of the district health department, issued a reminder that attendance at the schools was required by law for midwives.[24] At the time there were an estimated 75 midwives in the county, although some of these were not fully qualified under the new law.[25]

Although sometimes referred to as a midwife, Mrs. Cora Reeves, of the Grassy Creek area, provided services extending far beyond delivering babies. Well known for her ability to diagnose and treat various illnesses, as well as her midwifery skills, Mrs. Reeves included in her repertoire of prescriptions, instructions to "scrape raw beet and bind on the foot when one has stept on a nail or for blood poison." An alternative for treating rusty nail wounds was to "bind a raw, mashed onion on after soaking it in wood lye."[26]

Mrs. Reeves recorded her various remedies and treatments in a "commonplace book," which I first heard about from David VanHoy. As Evelyn Jones and I settle in the back parlor of VanHoy's old farmhouse in Grayson County, Virginia, in early February 2015, I ask our host if he knows of Mrs. Cora Reeves, as I have been unable to locate anyone who remembers

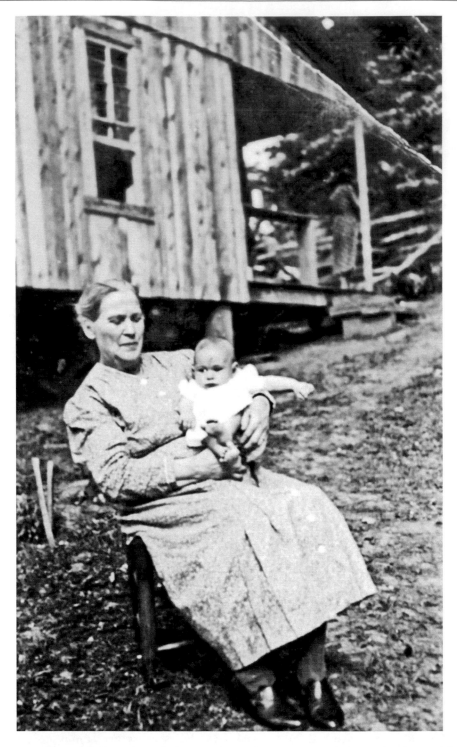

Doctors were few and far between in the late 1800s to mid–1900s in Appalachia, and midwives delivered most of the babies. Midwife and healer Mrs. Cora Ennis Reeves (1867–1947) of Grassy Creek delivered more than 500 babies in her career and is pictured here with Ralph Carter, the last baby she delivered (photograph, circa 1941-1942, courtesy David VanHoy).

her. "You're sitting in the room where she died," he responds. It is soon apparent I have stumbled onto the mother lode of information on Mrs. Reeves and pretty much everybody and everything else that had to do with the area. VanHoy produces an old photograph of Cora Reeves holding the last baby she delivered and explains he refers to Cora Reeves as "Mama," because he grew up in her house, helping out Miss Ruby, one of the five children of Cora and Billy Reeves. Since he heard everyone else calling her "Mama," he followed suit.

It is not known how much formal education Cora Reeves received, but she and her husband put great stock in education, and that included educating their three girls—Hazel, Ruby and Myrtle, all of whom graduated from Trinity College, now known as Duke University. Unlike many midwives of her day, Mrs. Reeves did receive some training and became licensed in midwifery, thanks largely to the efforts of Dr. Cox Waddell, who organized a licensure program for midwives and encouraged her to pursue the official designation, after Virginia enacted legislation in the early 1900s requiring such.[27] I found no other record of formal training or any claims to that effect. Apparently Mrs. Reeves's talent came naturally—a gift. She pulled aching teeth and treated babies for "thresh," sometimes called "thrash" or "thrush," a condition of the mouth and gums, which made it difficult for the baby to nurse. And she took the time to record her remedies in her commonplace book for others to use. Her knowledge about food preservation and drying animal skins and a host of other things was shared freely with her neighbors, much like a home extension agent. She managed to do all this and look after her home and family and see to the college education of her three daughters.[28]

Cora Ennis Reeves was born September 10, 1867. She married Charles William "Billy" Floyd Reeves December 31, 1884, and moved to the small farmhouse in Grayson County, on the North Carolina border, in 1885. She bore two sons and three daughters, delivered more than 500 babies, and helped countless others with their health related issues. "When Mama would have a baby to die, she would bring the dead baby home, and her husband would build a small casket and bury the baby in the yard," says VanHoy. "People had an acceptance of death," he adds by way of explanation of this service provided by Cora Reeves and her husband. "One third of the babies in 1925 died."

Mrs. Reeves rode out to her calls all hours of the day and night, traveling for miles on a horse outfitted with a side saddle. How did her family manage in her absence? VanHoy responds, "Miss Ruby was making biscuits when she was four years old." Mrs. Reeves regularly conferred with doctors on the appropriate treatment for various injuries and illnesses, and VanHoy shows me a box of those letters and the responses she received. Cora Reeves died of heart disease June 12, 1947, at age 79. Her obituary, written by her daughter Ruby, states, "She was a devoted wife, a kind and loving mother and a good friend and neighbor to those living around and about her." Her work as a midwife and health advisor was not viewed as a profession, which might have been construed as unseemly in her day. Her service to her community was simply being "a good friend and neighbor." Like most people who performed these services, there often was no remuneration or expectation of such. This was the mountain way.

People did not completely abandon the old ways after physicians and a hospital were available. Gene Hafer shares this personal experience in an interview in August 2014. He was around eight or nine years old when his father Lem Hafer took him to the big Ashe County Memorial Hospital for Dr. Dean Jones, Sr., to look at the plantar warts on the bottoms of his feet. "We can put some acid on them and burn them off," Gene heard the doctor tell his father. Gene shouted, "No!" So a few days later his father took him to see Amos Graybeal, who lived between West Jefferson and Jefferson. They met Mr. Graybeal on his front porch and talked over the problem. The man took Gene's foot in his hand, counted the warts, went into the house, came back in a bit and said, "They'll go away now." There was no secret charm in evidence, no magic words, no rubbing with castor oil, chicken gizzard, or stump water. Concluding his story, Gene reports, "In a few weeks, the warts went away and never came back."

The day Gene Hafer got his foot tended, a young girl watched the proceedings from the old glider on the porch. The girl was Elizabeth "Lib" Graybeal, granddaughter of Amos Graybeal and daughter of Hessie Reeves and Bernard Graybeal, owner of the Ford dealership in downtown West Jefferson (where the movie theater is now). Gene put me in touch with Lib Graybeal McRimmon shortly after his interview, and Evelyn and I visited with her on that same front porch to talk about her grandfather and her recollections of that day.

McRimmon, her parents, and siblings lived with her grandparents, Amos and Daisy Burkett Graybeal, in the home passed down through Daisy Burkett's father Christian Burkett. The Burkett's moved to the area in the 1800s, before the town of West Jefferson existed. There was only one other house in the valley then, so Lib reckons the ancestral home is one of the oldest within the West Jefferson city limits. Her Grandfather Amos was a farmer and had no medical training of any kind, but he must have had a reputation for being able to cure warts for Lem Hafer to have sought him out. "He sat right there on this porch," Lib recalls. She watched her grandfather take the boy's foot in his hand. "He rubbed it with his thumb this way and that," she demonstrates. "That was all he did." Apparently her grandfather did not advertise his special gift, nor is Lib aware of any fee being charged. "I never heard him talk about it," she reflects. The only other time she witnessed her grandfather doing anything like this was once when she and her father took Amos somewhere up beyond Lansing to see a farmer who requested his assistance with a similar case. "As far as I know, that was the only medical thing he did."

When I talk with Ashe County native John K. Reeves, Lib's first cousin, he confirms Amos Graybeal's reputation for curing warts. Reeves's sister claimed Mr. Graybeal "rubbed off" a wart on her finger. Reeves and his family spent considerable time at the Graybeal home. Since he had no grandparents left, Amos and his wife Daisy became surrogate grandparents. "I remember he (Amos) had a big full mustache, and he loved to tell ghost stories. He scared us kids to death." Lib adds a distinguishing feature she remembered about Amos Graybeal—he had wens (i.e., bumps) on his head, which were surgically removed later in his life. I have never heard of such a thing and make a note to ask Dr. Charles Jones about wens. Amos Graybeal lived in the same house until his death August 31, 1961, at the age of 93.

"My grandmother knew of a man who could relieve the pain of burns," recalls Gene Hafer. "He didn't take away a scar, but he could take away the pain." People with the ability to treat burns were referred to as "burn doctors" or sometimes as "fire doctors."[29] In *Memoirs of Grassy Creek*, Zetta Hamby mentions "nose-bleed stoppers," people reputed to be able to stop severe nosebleeds.[30] The details of how these cures were accomplished, whether by prayer or reading a certain passage from the Bible or some more secular means, may be known only by those who practiced them, if indeed by them. Nevertheless, this kind of "alternative" medicine was not uncommon in early days, and although dismissed by some as hocus pocus, sometimes, for whatever reason, it seems to have worked.

Stephen Shoemaker tells a story about home doctoring, handed down on his Pappy Brown's side of the family. Pappy Brown's mother, Shoemaker's great-grandmother Brown and her husband owned property in Watauga County that would become part of the Cone Manor estate. One of her younger children accidentally got hit in the head with a double sided axe when he walked behind his brother, who was chopping wood. The blow cracked open his skull so bad the brain matter was exposed. There was no doctor near, so the mother cleaned the wound, put the piece of skull back in place, covered it with a sticky potion, the consistency of tar, and wrapped up the child's head. He survived his mother's do-it-yourself brain surgery and made a full recovery—no infection, no mental or physical impairment, just a scar on his scalp.

Mountain people continued to make use of whatever information was available to them with regard to health, blending the old with the new. Dr. Edward J. Miller, born and raised in Nathans Creek, in Ashe County, remembers his mother consulting *Blum's Almanac,* regarding the appropriate time to address certain medical-related matters. The popular almanac, which is still around, was first printed in Old Salem, North Carolina, more than a hundred years ago. The publication included a section on signs of the zodiac, and many followed this guidance faithfully.[31] "There is something to be said for the placebo effect," Dr. Miller acknowledges with a chuckle. "I'm all for it." Calvin Miller says "I think most everybody had *Blum's Almanac;* that and the Bible were the two books found in homes, and people probably read it as much as their Bible."[32] Evelyn Jones recollects Dr. Dean C. Jones, Jr., scheduled surgery for a patient once, and, hearing the date appointed, the patient protested, "Oh, no! You can't do that—the signs aren't right!" The doctor rescheduled the surgery. "He always maintained that patients bled more under certain signs."[33] Retired nurse Doris Oliver adds, "More babies are born with a new moon or a full moon."[34] Besides the almanac, a popular medical reference guide in some parts of Appalachia was Dr. John C. Gunn's *Domestic Medicine or Poor Man's Friend in the Hours of Affliction, Pain and Sickness,* published in Knoxville, Tennessee, in 1830. But tried and true home remedies most often were recorded on scraps of paper and passed down in families like recipes for squirrel stew and stack cake.[35]

While the people of Appalachia held onto their home remedies, the arrival of peddlers and other itinerant vendors made patent medicines more readily available, and an assortment of concoctions found their way into the modest storehouse of affordable medical treatments for families.[36] All manner of claims were made as to the origins and miraculous curing powers of these products. In an effort to establish credibility, some manufacturers purported to rely on secret Native American botanical formulas, but most of the time these tonics and elixirs contained more alcohol or opium than bona fide herbal ingredients.[37] Some were moderately helpful, some were downright dangerous, and some did nothing whatsoever one way or the other. Zetta Hamby lists a cupboard full of home medications in use during her day, including such store bought ingredients as sulfur (also called brimstone), Epsom salts, castor oil, alum, camphor, calomel, turpentine, lamp oil, baking soda, Castoria, Rosebud and Cloverine salves, and Watkins and Rawleigh liniments.[38]

In the late 1800s and early 1900s, the J. R. Watkins Medical Company, based in Winona, Minnesota, and the W. T. Rawleigh Company, of Freeport, Illinois, offered enterprising folks looking for an alternative to farm life, the opportunity to sell its medicinal products.[39] Gayle Winston, remembers the Rawleigh man, who made regular calls, peddling his products. There were liniments for aches and pains—for people and their horses—and salve in thin little tins and clove oil for tooth aches.[40] Anne McGuire's grandfather, Pappy Brown, was a Rawleigh man and worked Ashe County and the surrounding area. He swore by his medicated ointment, and Anne claims some local doctors recommended it for hemorrhoids.[41] Rawleigh is still in business, and Evelyn Jones pulled out a kitchen drawer and handed me a tin of medicated ointment to prove it—"Famous Old-Fashioned Formula."

The patent medicines were readily used in combination with the old standards of honey, molasses, charcoal, burnt clay from rock chimneys, teas made from elder bloom, mint, sassafras bark and roots, boneset tea, penny royal, burdock roots, and salves from Balmgilead buds. The buds came from the *populus balsamifera* plant, and the salve made from the buds was used primarily to treat burns, cuts, and dry skin. Evelyn Jones recalls she and her brothers used to gather Balmgilead, also called Balm of Gilead or bammy (or bama) gilly buds, to sell. "The trees grew close to the creek where I grew up." Zetta Hamby also mentions asafetida, a gum resin, sometimes tied up in small cloth bags and hung around the necks of children to ward off sickness. Evelyn Jones's mother made poultices for Evelyn and her brothers. Evelyn does not know if it worked, but vows it sure did stink. "It was awful!" Her mother kept a supply of asafetida in a drawer in the dining room buffet. It came in a block or a cake. "We didn't even want to open that drawer, it smelled so bad."[42] When Evelyn and I interview 100-year-old Ruby Ashley in November 2014, she comments on the use of home remedies, and apparently asafetida had made a lasting impression on her as well. Boneset tea, used for fever, was another remedy with which she was well acquainted. At age six or eight years old, Ruby had typhoid fever—twice. "I was real sick," she recalls. "I thought snakes were crawling down from the mantle over the fire. That typhoid fever was pretty rough stuff."

I escaped castor oil and asafetida, but my mother frequently used paregoric for a multitude of ailments. She mixed it with a spoonful of sugar and a little water. It was still terrible. I was horrified to discover this stuff was camphorated tincture of opium, available over the counter in drugstores at the time.[43]

Mineral springs became popular for medicinal purposes in the United States around the early 1800s, although Native Americans had discovered the curative powers of springs long before whites ever set foot on their land, as had the Romans and those who came before them, a continent away. Ashe County is home to a number of mineral springs, including Plummer Mineral Springs, owned by Professor Robert E. Lee Plummer, an educator and founder of Healing Springs High School, who was instrumental in marshaling support for the Ashe County Memorial Hospital. Plummer shipped his water for sale, but his spring was not developed as a resort, nor were nearby Foster Springs and Eureka Springs. Healing Springs or Bromide Arsenic Springs Hotel and Shatley Springs did become vacation spots. The healing properties of the Bromide Arsenic Springs Hotel were widely touted in the late 1880s, and *The Virginia Medical Journal* added credibility to the claims by reporting successful results relayed by doctors and patients. In the April 9, 1949, edition of *The State Magazine,* an article entitled "Things of Interest in Ashe County," by Ira T. Johnston, speculated Healing Springs was destined to become a hospital and full-fledged health resort. But interest in the springs came and went, and in 1962, the Healing Springs Hotel was destroyed by fire.[44] People still fill up their water bottles at the springs. The cabins, spring house and grounds are now listed on the National Register of Historic Places, and recently the cabins were restored.[45]

Martin Shatley discovered the healing properties of a spring on his land when he washed his face and hands in the water one summer day in 1890. Shatley was plagued with a skin disease and noticed a significant improvement in his condition a short time after being exposed to the spring's water. He tried bathing in the spring for awhile, and his skin was healed. Word spread, and a resort with cabins and dining developed around the spring.[46] Today Shatley Springs is a destination restaurant and a regular stop for tour buses, and people continue to fill up gallon plastic jugs with the water to take home.

3

The Jones Memorial Infirmary at Lansing

Sometimes referred to as Ashe County's first hospital, the Jones Memorial Infirmary was built in 1882 by Dr. Thomas Jefferson Jones, no kin to Dr. Bud Jones as far as anybody can tell. C. B. Jones, a physician's assistant (P.A.) at Ashe Memorial Hospital, is the great-grandson of Dr. Thomas Jones and says he wishes he had a dollar for every time somebody asked him if he was related to the doctors Dean Jones, Sr. and Jr. In September 2014 I visited C. B. Jones at his home in Jefferson, North Carolina, where he had gathered his two sisters, Betsy Little and Geneva Coffey and Betsy's husband, James Little, to help recall the family genealogy and the story of the Jones Memorial Infirmary. We sat on the back porch amidst a treasure trove of old photographs and memories and talked until supper time.

As the mountains gradually produced more physicians from within its own communities, and others "not from around here" made their way to the mountains to practice medicine, the local population adapted to the opportunity for a more advanced form of health care, developing the trust to turn to doctors in times of sickness and adding the trained professional as a health care option. But hospitals were for big cities, and even the word "hospital" was unfamiliar to some in the far reaches of Appalachia. A place where sick people went for rest and treatment was more likely referred to as an infirmary.[1]

C. B. Jones and his sisters are the seventh generation of the Jones family to live in Ashe County. John McSeoin Jones, born in 1768 in Belfast, Ireland, was the first generation of the family to come to the county. The first doctors to surface in this line were two sons of Alexander Jones and Charlotte Faw Jones, who made their home in Copeland, just above Clifton in Ashe County. One of these sons, Dr. William Jones, moved to Cumberland Gap, Virginia with his family, but his brother, Thomas Jefferson Jones (1855–1932), great-grandfather of C. B. Jones, Betsy Little, and Geneva Coffey, stayed in Ashe County. He started out as a teacher in Piney Creek and later attended the Medical College of Baltimore in 1879. He completed his residency at the University of Tennessee, specializing in pediatrics and women's diseases. Apparently, "obstetrics" was not a term readily used during that time, as when Thomas Jones was licensed to practice medicine in 1882, his license listed his specialty as "pediatrics and women's diseases." He practiced in Grant, Virginia, early in his career but moved back to Lansing in Ashe County around 1882, perhaps maintaining a

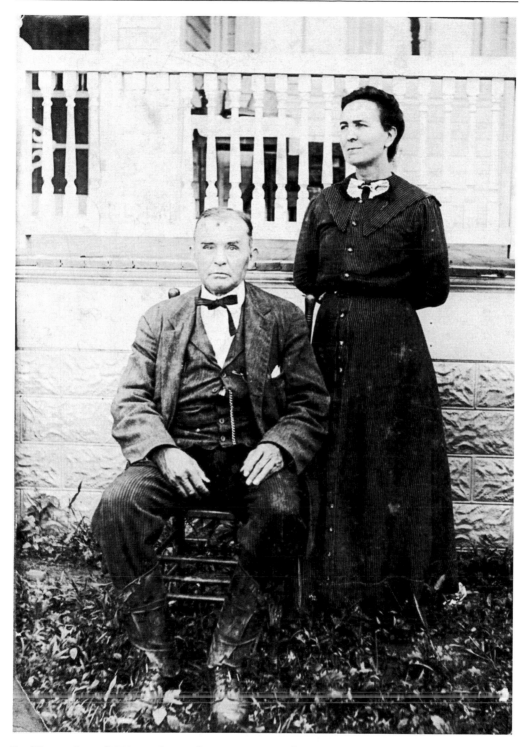

Dr. Thomas Jones (1855–1932) moved to Lansing around 1882 and built a two room office, known as the Lansing Infirmary. He married Rebecca Elizabeth Graybeal Jones, who operated the local switchboard from their home. Their son, Dr. Lester Jones (1884–1938), practiced with his father in the Lansing Infirmary for twenty years (courtesy C. B. Jones and family).

branch office near the Virginia line. In Lansing he built a house and a separate two room office next door to treat his patients. This office building became known as the Lansing Infirmary. The Rev. William A. Patton, known to the family as "Preacher Patton," a friend of Dr. Jones from his days in Grant, Virginia, settled in Ashe County around the same time as Jones came back and built the doctor's home and office.

Like Dr. Bud Jones, the great-grandfather of Dr. Charles Jones (the other, unrelated set of Joneses), Dr. Thomas Jones found he needed to make house calls to reach many of his patients. He went on horseback in those early days, and the family still has his saddle and the saddle bags which carried his medical tools and medicine vials. Geneva Coffey remembers her grandmother telling how she had to boil water on the stove to pour on her husband's boots, frozen to his stirrups from long treks to check on his patients during the tough Ashe County winters. He eventually purchased a car, but that was before the days of four-wheel drive, and its usefulness was limited according to the road conditions. Dr. Thomas Jones's wife, Rebecca Elizabeth Graybeal (1851–1931), daughter of Joseph and Clarissa Faw Graybeal, was the switchboard operator for the community, and the switchboard was located in their home. People called the switchboard to report their ailments and medical needs to the doctor. Dr. Jones joined the Ashe County Medical Society in 1888, serving in several different capacities, including the offices of secretary, president and treasurer. He joined the North Carolina Medical Society in 1904.

The couple had two children, Thomas Lester and Effie Charlotte Jones. Thomas Lester Jones (1884–1938) spent his childhood making calls with his father, so his choice to follow in his father's footsteps was a natural one. He attended the Medical College of Virginia in Richmond and joined his father in the practice in Lansing. Father and son practiced together in the one-story infirmary for about twenty years. Preacher Patton built a home for Dr. Lester Jones, near that of his parents. Jones took this opportunity to have Preacher Patton make significant renovations to his father's two room office, adding a second level and enlarging the office of the elder Jones, including the distinctive lattice-trimmed balcony, also used on the home of Dr. Thomas Jones and helpful in dating the building in old photographs. The father and son team worked together until 1932, when Dr. Thomas Jones passed away. The newly renovated infirmary was not yet fully equipped and operational at the time, and Dr. Lester Jones named the finished building "the Jones Memorial Infirmary," in honor of his late father.

In 1903, Lester Jones married Bessie Dean Dougherty of Clifton, daughter of Joseph and Elizabeth Latham Dougherty and first cousin to brothers B. B. and D. D. Dougherty, who started Appalachian State University in Boone as a teachers college in 1899. The couple had three children, one of whom was Charles "Bernard" Jones, born in 1909, the father of C. B. Jones, Geneva Coffey and Betsy Little. Bernard Jones accompanied his father on his house calls and became known in the community as "Little Doc," a nickname that stuck through his adulthood, although he did not become a doctor. Dr. Lester Jones was one of the first in the county to get an automobile, and part of Bernard's job on the calls was changing the tires, a frequent necessity on the rough back roads of the county.

Bernard was in the first graduating class of Lansing High School in May 1927 and attended Appalachian State University from 1928 to 1932, earning his B.S. in science and

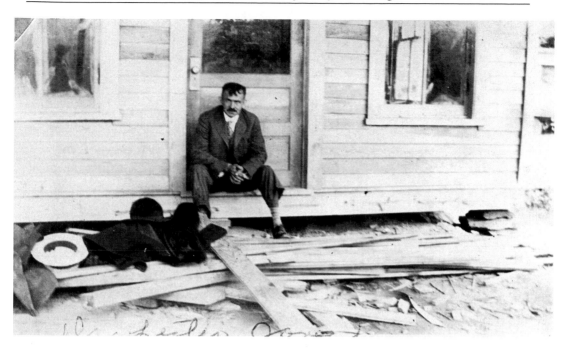

Dr. Lester Jones renovated and expanded the two room Lansing Infirmary, renaming it the Jones Memorial Infirmary in honor of his father, Dr. Thomas Jones (courtesy C. B. Jones and family).

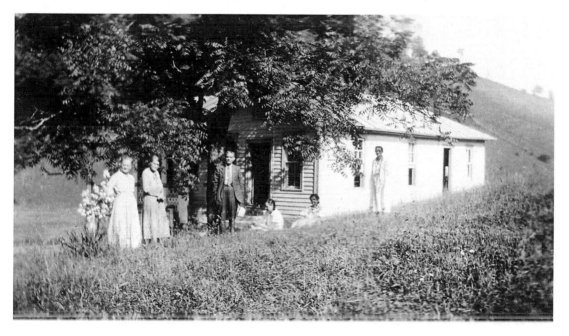

A second story was added in the renovations to the infirmary, as seen here from the rear (photograph, circa 1882, courtesy C. B. Jones and family).

mathematics. He wanted to become a doctor, majoring in chemistry and biology, and was on his way to Duke Medical School when his father died. It was the Depression, and his father had raised him to believe that as the man of the family, it was his responsibility to take care of everybody else. He abandoned his plans for medical school and returned home

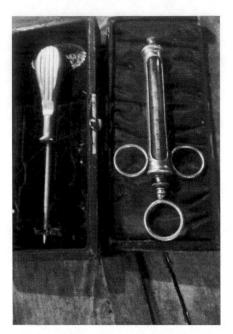

to do his duty. Bernard taught for ten years at various schools in the county, and, while working at Fleetwood High school, met his bride to be, Geneva Divers, a graduate of Radford College in Virginia, who taught home economics at Fleetwood. Geneva Divers was the daughter of Alfred and Mary Bessie Divers of Roanoke, Virginia. Alfred Divers was an engineer for the Norfolk & Western Railway and was moved to Fleetwood for a job on the Virginia Creeper line. The family lived in a

Left: **These medical tools belonged to Drs. Thomas and Lester Jones, left: ronsur trephine, used to take bone marrow; right: syringe, with interchangeable needles, used for pulling fluid from the chest and lungs and for transfusions.** *Below:* **These surgical instruments from the late 1800s to early 1900s, probably were used in the Lansing Infirmary by Drs. Thomas and Lester Jones. The third instrument from the left is a burr hole, and the other tools are believed to have been used as handles for leveraging. A burr hole was used to drill a hole in the skull to let the pressure off the brain (both photographs courtesy C. B. Jones and family).**

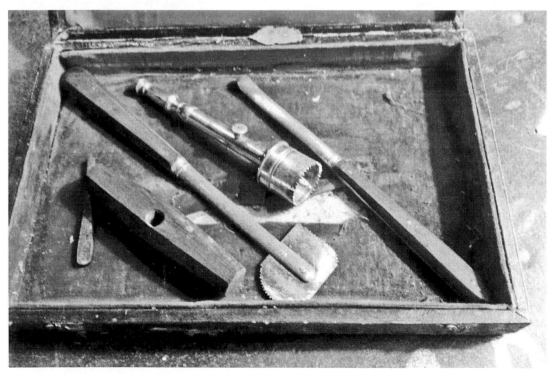

Right, top: **This machine is believed to have been used to cauterize wounds with electricity, and may have had other medical uses. The meter controlled the intensity of the voltage.** *Bottom:* **Dr. Lester Jones stands in the Jones Memorial Infirmary sometime after the 1932 death of his father, Dr. Thomas Jones, who died before the newly renovated infirmary was fully equipped (photograph, circa 1934-35, both courtesy C. B. Jones and family).**

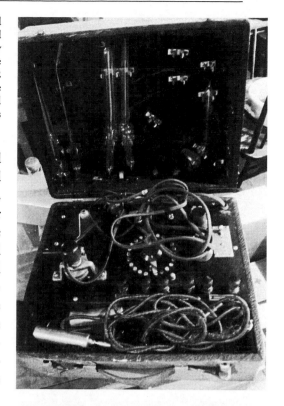

caboose during their time there. Bernard and Geneva eloped to Independence, Virginia, and were married at the courthouse there in 1936. They had to keep their marriage a secret for awhile, as they could not teach in the same school if they were married. The couple moved into the home of Bernard's parents, Lester and Bessie, taking the upstairs, while the older couple lived downstairs. When the United States entered World War II, Bernard was deferred due to an old injury. He worked as a chemical supervisor in Elkton, Maryland, for Triumph Explosives and returned home to Lansing with the Radford Division of the Norfolk & Western, where he stayed until his retirement in 1974.

Bernard's mother-in-law, Mary Bessie Divers, was a registered nurse, and when it came time for her daughter Geneva to deliver each of her three children, Mary Elizabeth (Betsy), Charles Bernard (C. B.), Jr., and Helen "Geneva," she insisted her grandchildren be born in the big Jefferson Memorial Hospital in Roanoke, Virginia, where she lived and could keep an eye on things. So, although their parents lived in Lansing, C. B., Betsy and Geneva were born in Roanoke. They grew up in the home shared by their parents and grandparents near the Jones Memorial Infirmary. According to the three siblings, their grandfather

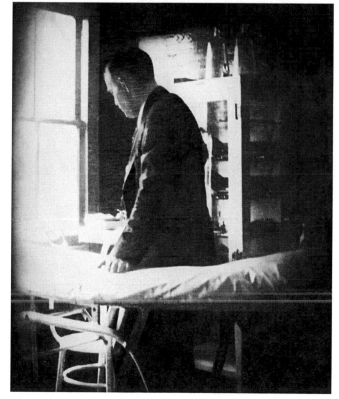

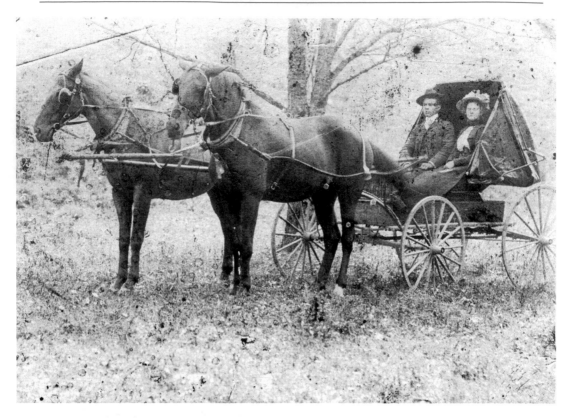

Dr. Lester Jones married Bessie Dean Dougherty in 1903. The couple had four children, including Bernard Jones, father of AMH Physician's Assistant C. B. Jones and Geneva Coffey and Betsy Little (courtesy C. B. Jones and family).

Dr. Lester Jones was known as a perfectionist, and his intensity was reflected in his eyes, as evidenced in old family photographs of him.

It was a young Dr. Dean C. Jones, Sr., who treated Lester Jones for a bowel obstruction toward the end of his life. Ashe County Memorial Hospital was not built at the time, and the only choice for hospitalization was in Wilkesboro. There were no antibiotics at the time, and Lester knew the surgery would result in death. He opted not to make the trip to Wilkesboro and died at his home. With his death in 1938, the infirmary closed, and much of the equipment and furniture was donated to the new Ashe County Memorial Hospital when it opened in Jefferson in 1941.

Growing up in the multigenerational household of the Dr. Lester Jones and Bernard Jones families, there was a heavy emphasis on education by both parents and grandparents. There was never any discussion about "if" the children would go to college, only "where." "Daddy bugged us all about being a doctor," recalls Geneva Coffey, "and then he started on the grandchildren." His son, C. B., Jr., brought the medical tradition back to the family. C. B. first got the "bug" to pursue a career in the medical field and received his first medical training in the Air Force Medical Corps 1967–1971, stationed in Myrtle Beach, South Carolina, and then Korea. In 1973, he graduated from the Wake Forest University Physician's Assistant Program.

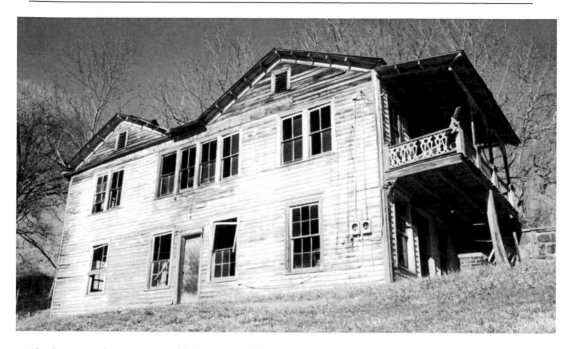

The distinctive lattice trimmed balcony was added to the Lansing Infirmary with the second story, when Dr. Lester Jones renamed it the Jones Memorial Infirmary (photograph taken November 20, 2010, by Joe R. Blevins;).

C. B. Jones soon returned home to Ashe County to be a P.A. in the emergency department at Ashe Memorial Hospital. He admits he never thought he would live in his home county when he grew up. "I wanted to live somewhere where I didn't have to explain where I came from." Another generation has taken up the medical mantle, as well. Dr. Charles Stuart Coffey, son of Thomas Stuart Coffey III and Geneva Jones Coffey of Morganton, North Carolina, currently works at the Medical University of San Diego. He is a cancer surgeon, and his wife, Christanne Hoffman Coffey, is an emergency medical specialist in outdoor wilderness medicine, a good example of the level of specialization available today.

I decided to take a look at the old Lansing Infirmary, and my husband Louis volunteered to drive me out N.C. Highway 194 past the old Lansing School, where we found a faded sign for "Jones Memorial Infirmary." The family still owns the building. Dr. Lester Jones's rare Queen Anne style home is owned by Geneva Coffey, and the nearby home of Dr. Thomas Jones is owned by C. B. Jones. The buildings are part of the county's rich history and an important part of the story of health care in the region.[2]

4

Dr. Arthur Lee "Bud" Jones: First Generation of a Family Legacy

While many doctors around the turn of the last century were still learning their medical skills by interning with an established doctor, the founder of the Jones family tradition of doctoring, Dr. Arthur Lee "Bud" Jones, was not among them. In 1901, at age 28, he graduated from the Medical College of Virginia. Later he studied surgery at the University of Pennsylvania Medical School, graduating in 1907, at the age of 34. A surgical residency followed, in a hospital associated with the University of Pennsylvania. I interviewed Nell Jones Taylor, granddaughter of Dr. Bud, in the summer of 2014, at the family's cabin in Helton Creek. Taylor, an amateur genealogist, was my primary source for Dr. Bud and his wife Fannie.

Family records indicate Bud was born to William Cicero Jones (1848–1914) and Mary Senter Jones (1851–1922) and raised on a farm in Silas Creek, in Ashe County. William Cicero Jones was a farmer and owned about 300 acres. Apparently a man of many talents, he also was a blacksmith, a carpenter, and co-owner of a sawmill and a water mill with his brother Winfield Jones, grinding wheat and corn for the community. William Cicero's sons, Arthur Lee "Bud" and Felix, did the thrashing for the community. Mary Senter's father was John Senter, a cabinetmaker in Ashe County. Her great-grandfather is believed to be Asa Senter, an officer in the American Revolution. Senter Church, near the old Nathans Creek Post Office site, was named for John

Dr. Arthur Lee "Bud" Jones (1872–1952) was the first generation in the Jones family to become a doctor. For the majority of his career, he practiced in Ashe County and the surrounding area and in Chilhowie, Virginia (courtesy Evelyn Jones).

30

Senter's ancestors, a line heavily populated with ministers, which extended into Grayson County, Virginia. Mary and William Cicero married around 1868 and lived at Silas Creek. The couple had eight children: Arthur Lee, John Edgar, Walter Winfield, William Edwin, Etta Jane, Margaret Ida, Minnie Ann, and Rebecca Alafair. Education was important in the family, and four of these children became teachers in the public schools of Ashe County. Bud married Melvina Frances "Fannie" Kirby on November 4, 1901, shortly after graduating from medical college. Fannie, described as a tiny woman, especially compared to Dr. Bud, was born in Helton Creek on September 26, 1881, the daughter of Millard Filmore Kirby (1854–1925) and Ida Ruth Goodman (1862–1921). Taylor speculates the couple knew each other from school or church, as they both grew up in the close-knit Helton community.

After receiving his medical degree, Dr. Bud returned home and practiced in Brandon, North Carolina, for a few years. When the house in Brandon burned to the ground in 1905, Dr. Bud moved his family to the home of his father-in-law, Millard Filmore Kirby, in nearby Helton, North Carolina. The house stood off N.C. Highway 194 at Helton Creek but burned down in the 1920s. The foundation is visible behind the home which took its place on the property, built by Nell Taylor's Uncle Bryan Kirby. A natural spring was worked into the foundation of the original house, providing water inside. Millard Filmore Kirby built a house for his large family "up the holler" and sold his old house and a part of the farm to Dr. Bud.

During Dr. Bud's years at the University of Pennsylvania Medical School, Fannie stayed at home in Helton with their two boys, Hunter and Dean. According to Taylor, her mother's brother, Ed Perkins, helped remodel the old Millard Filmore Kirby home to include an operating room on the second floor, and the home served as an office and clinic for Dr. Bud's practice. By 1924, the family had grown to five children. Taylor's father was the oldest of the five: Hunter McGuire (1902–1996); Dean Cicero (1904–1984); Myrtle Ruth (1913–2003); Ethel Hope (1917–1980); and Frances Kirby (1924–1991). Hoping Hunter would become a doctor, Dr. Bud named him for noted surgeon and educator Dr. Hunter Holmes McGuire, General Stonewall Jackson's surgeon during the Civil War.[1] Dr. Bud named his next son Dean Cicero, after his father William Cicero Jones, and in hopes he would become a lawyer, like Cicero, the famous lawyer, philosopher and politician of Ancient Rome. This plan came to an unceremonious end when Dr. Bud invited Hunter to witness an arm amputation he was to perform. "My daddy passed out," laughs Taylor. Hunter returned home and declared he did not want to become a doctor. In an interesting twist of fate, Hunter became a lawyer, and Dean Cicero became a doctor. In keeping with Dr. Bud's philosophy of sleeping outside to maintain good health, Taylor says, Hunter and Dean slept year round in a screened room on the back of their father's house. When she asked her father if they got cold, he just laughed.

Dr. Bud trained his wife Fannie to assist him in his medical practice, serving as his nurse. This was her only medical training. Sometimes a neighboring physician would help with the anesthesia, but more often it was Fannie who acted as anesthetist for Dr. Bud's surgeries. Emergency surgeries for acute appendicitis, bowel obstruction, skull fractures, and amputations were among the operations performed. Fannie sterilized the instruments and sheets, heating the sheets in a dry oven; the surgical instruments were boiled. As there was

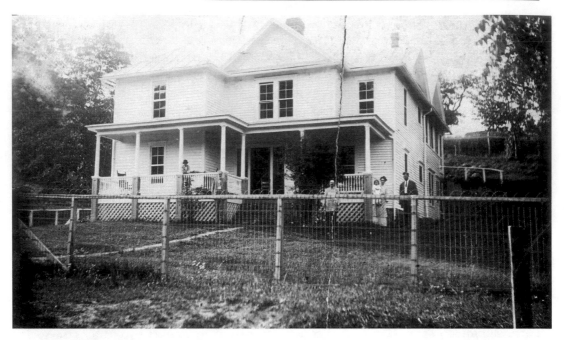

Above: **Dr. Bud Jones and his family lived in this home in Helton, and he used the second floor for his medical clinic, office and operating room (courtesy Evelyn Jones).** *Below:* **Early in their marriage, Dr. Bud Jones trained his wife Fannie to assist him in his surgeries (courtesy Evelyn Jones).**

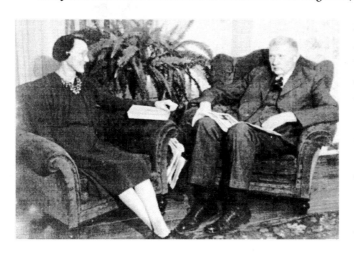

no hospital in the area, if a patient needed more complex surgery than Dr. Bud could perform in his office, the patient probably took the train to Abingdon, Virginia. People could flag down the train, nicknamed the Virginia Creeper, anywhere along its route from Elkland (now Todd), North Carolina, to Abingdon, where it turned around for the return trip. According to Dr. Charles Jones, families often put their ailing loved ones on the train, not knowing if they would ever see them again.[2]

Lonnie Jones, Museum of Ashe County History board president and member of the Ashe Historical Society board of directors, passed along this tale about one of Dr. Bud's surgeries. "Hamilton Howell was my grandmother's uncle," Lonnie begins, "and he had to have his leg amputated by Dr. Bud." After the surgery, Dr. Bud told Howell's sons to bury the leg. They buried it in the Ham Howell Cemetery off North Fork New River Road, about half a mile from the Howell homestead. Although the surgery went fine, after awhile Howell began to complain that his leg hurt—the one that was gone. Dr. Bud called on Howell to see how he was doing, and Howell told him about the pain in his missing leg. Dr. Bud

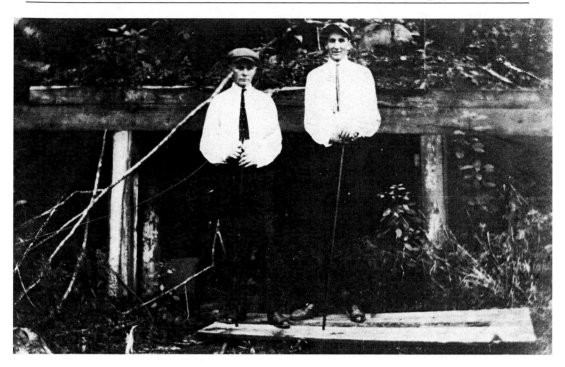

Dr. Bud Jones hoped his first son, Hunter McGuire (right), would become a surgeon and his second son, Dean Cicero Jones (left), would become a lawyer, so he named Hunter after a famous surgeon and Dean after a famous lawyer, hoping to steer them in the right direction. Things did not turn out exactly as planned (courtesy Evelyn Jones).

directed the sons to dig up the leg and turn it around. The boys dug up the leg, turned it around, and reburied it. Hamilton Howell never complained about the pain in his leg again.[3] When Lonnie told me this story, I suspected he was pulling my leg, but local historian and undertaker David VanHoy assures me burying amputated limbs was common practice in the old days. Custom also dictated that the limb be buried in familiar ground so the wound would heal and facing east to cut the pain. VanHoy claims he has built caskets for limbs on request and has followed strict instructions as to the burial in familiar ground and the placement of the limb facing east.[4]

The Jones family archive contains a letter postmarked in Helton July 12, 1907, written by Dr. Bud to Mr. R. L. Ballou. "I wish to buy a good saddle horse and have been informed you have one to sell," the doctor writes. "A good saddle horse" was key to doing the business of doctoring. Travel was difficult in those days, and most people could not get to Dr. Bud's office, so he went to them. Most babies were delivered in the patient's home. If somebody spotted the doctor on his way to a house call, relates Dr. Charles Jones, word quickly spread, and folks waited on the side of the road to catch him on the way back to treat their ailments. Dr. Bud was known to pull a tooth for a quarter, while his patient sat on the road bank.[5]

Family lore has it that one time, up around Mud Creek (now called School House Road) in Grayson County, Virginia, Dr. Bud performed an emergency appendectomy on a dining room table in the patient's house. The patient was Evelyn Jones's great uncle Adolphus "Doc" Price. Sometimes when the doctor performed these on-site surgeries, folks would get wind of the event and show up with their blankets and picnic baskets and camp out in the yard, waiting to hear whether or not the patient made it. Fannie had the tougher job, Dr. Bud always declared. She dripped the ether to put the patient to sleep, and while Dr. Bud performed the operation and then headed back home, Fannie moved in with the family to nurse the patient until he or she got better.[6]

In Dr. Bud's time, not much could be done for some sicknesses. Not long ago, a woman told Evelyn Jones she remembered when Dr. Bud was called to her family's home to tend to her mother, who had pneumonia. "We can't fix that," the doctor told the family sadly, when he gave his diagnosis.[7] Nell tells a story about her mother, Mattie Perkins Jones's side of the family. Mattie's youngest sister, Alta, suffered from osteomyelitis, a bone infection which can cut off part or all of the supply of blood to the bone, causing the bone to die. Dr. Bud, their family's physician, recommended Alta be sent to Johns Hopkins Hospital in Baltimore, Maryland, for treatment, as there was nothing more he could do. The oldest sister in the family, Stella, was given the responsibility of taking her baby sister to Baltimore on the train, admitting her to the hospital there and staying with her for the duration of her treatment. Stella was eighteen years old; Alta was three. It was not usual for young women to travel alone on a train in the early 1900s, but people did what they had to do. Alta recovered but with a short leg, as was often the case with this terrible disease, in the days before antibiotics.

Dr. Bud suffered a stroke around 1914, which left him with a marked tremor and a stutter. As a result, his words came out in bursts, making him sound curt and gruff. "I was terrified of him, as a kid," admits Taylor. "Once, when I was taken to Granddaddy's office in Lansing for a shot, I was so scared of him coming at me with that shaking needle, I broke away and ran down the streets of Lansing with my family chasing me. I was taken back to the office and got my shot." Evelyn Jones remembers being taken to see Dr. Bud at the Lansing office, when she was a little girl and had a skinned knee. She couldn't understand his stuttering, raspy voice and had to get her father to interpret the doctor's instructions. Apparently, that gruff voice, coupled with his size, was off-putting to more than one person.[8] Cornetta Price, Evelyn's sister-in-law, recalls her father taking her to see Dr. Bud at his office in Helton. "I was a little scared," she admits, calling to mind the strange room with its brown jugs with stoppers, holding the liquid medicines, the shelves with his books and supplies, the doctor's chair, and examining table. "I didn't see any other patients, just a few men sitting on the front porch. I'd just as soon not have gone." Despite his impairments, Dr. Bud continued his medical practice, and his patients reportedly loved him.[9]

According to Emmett Barker, who grew up in the area near Lansing served by Dr. Bud, the doctor saved the empty brown jugs and medicine bottles from his practice for the local moonshiners, an early effort to recycle, born of hard times. Since there were no pharmacies, and it was a long way to go to get medicine, Dr. Bud tried to keep a supply of medicines to meet the needs of his patients. "When I went into town to sell eggs," recalls Barker, "the neighbors asked me to pick up their medicine at Dr. Bud's office. If you came to pick up medicine, you had to wait if he was operating." There was no front desk with a receptionist or a nurse to assist.[10]

Initially, Dr. Bud rode horseback to make his calls. By all accounts, he was a big man for his time, about six feet three inches tall and 220 pounds, with reddish hair, which continues to show up in the Jones family gene pool. The doctor must have cut an impressive figure astride his horse on the mountain roads. "Dr. Bud rode so much on his rounds, his horse knew where to go as good as he did," declares Barker. This was fortunate as the doctor could get "right dozey" on the long ride home from a late call. "He rode as far as Whitetop, which was about four hours on horseback. He could be out half the night. Sometimes his feet would freeze in his stirrups. He was that tough!" Appalachia had an abundance of transportation challenges, explains Barker, and Ashe County had some of everything, including a swing bridge on Deep Ford and parts of Horse Creek and Stagg Creek where a pole boat was required to get across. "There were not many bridges, so everybody had a pole boat. Even in later years, some kids had to take a pole boat to catch the school bus." If Dr. Bud was too far away to answer a call from another patient, Dr. Lester Jones, also of Lansing, sometimes went in his place.[11]

Later Dr. Bud owned a car, and after his stroke, patients most likely came to his office, or someone drove him to make his calls. If somebody needed him, though, he was determined to get there. Barker remembers once when Dr. Bud was unable to get down a steep embankment to a patient's house, and he suffered the indignity of being carried piggyback down the bank by a friend.[12] This difficulty with getting around, explains Nell, was one of the determining factors in Dr. Bud and Fannie's 1918 move to Chilhowie in Smyth County, Virginia, where Dr. Bud had a small office beside his home. The community of Chilhowie was located in a valley, making it easier for Dr. Bud to get to where he needed to go. Visible from Whitetop Mountain, Chilhowie was about an hour from Lansing in those days. Sons Hunter and Dean were charged with the task of driving the family's cattle from Helton over Whitetop Mountain to the new home in Chilhowie.

Besides its more manageable terrain, Taylor continues, Chilhowie was a more prosperous area, and, with the education of his children to consider, this was another factor in the decision to move. Both Hunter and Dean were sent to Emory and Henry College in Emory, Virginia, close to Chilhowie. Hunter then went to Harvard Law School and Dean to the University of Pennsylvania Medical School. To help finance these advanced learning endeavors, Dr. Bud left his family in Chilhowie and traveled to southwest Virginia to practice medicine in the coal fields for several years. His speech difficulties became too much of an impediment to his work there, and he returned to Chilhowie. Probably with some help from sons Hunter and Dean, Dr. Bud and Fannie also managed to send their three daughters to college.

For much of his time in Chilhowie, Dr. Bud maintained an office in Lansing, as well as the office beside his home, dedicating certain days a week to his patients in Lansing. He had a room above his Lansing office where he stayed while he was working. In 1937, he commuted to Lansing to take over his son's practice there, while Dr. Dean Jones, Sr., was involved in the establishment of the Ashe County Memorial Hospital in Jefferson. Dr. Bud's office in Lansing was across from the hardware store downtown, near where the U.S. Post Office is now. "He was really a gentle and kind man," Taylor says of her grandfather, "but he was very strict—no alcohol, no smoking, and no cussing." Dr. Bud practiced in Lansing for several years, but, eventually, a heart ailment resulted in increasing disability, and he returned to his home in Chilhowie.

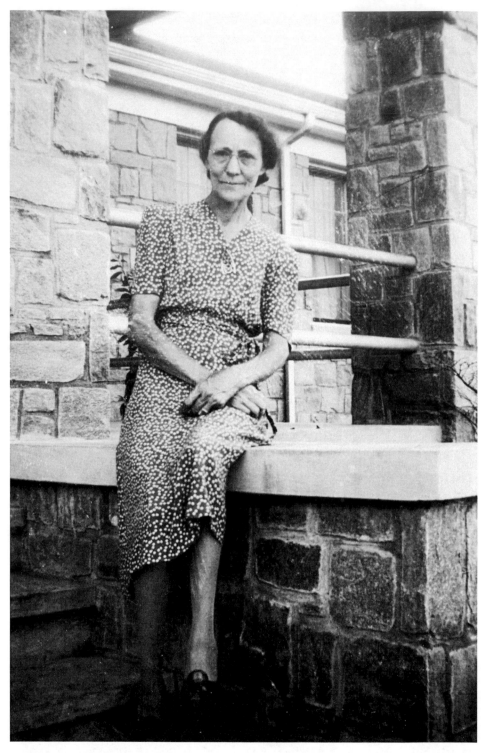

Dr. Bud and Fannie Jones lived to see the completion of the first Ashe County Memorial Hospital. Fannie, pictured sitting on the front stoop of the hospital, died there September 4, 1961 (courtesy Evelyn Jones).

Taylor remembers going to stay with her grandparents when they lived in Chilhowie. The elder Dr. Dean's son, Dean C., Jr., spent time in Chilhowie too, often visiting at the same time as his cousin Nell. Nell and Dean C. were both visiting in Chilhowie during the height of the polio epidemic. Dr. Dean and his wife Lettie sent word to Dr. Bud and Fannie not to let Dean C. and Nell come home, because there were so many cases of polio in West Jefferson. The public schools started back late that year, because of the epidemic, not opening until October.

Toward the end of Dr. Bud's life, a horse fell on his leg and crushed it, further impairing his mobility. By then he had retired from his medical practice, but his physical disability prevented him from enjoying fishing and other leisurely pastimes. He died in Chilhowie, July 24, 1952, at the age of 79, just a week before his eightieth birthday. He is buried at Helton Methodist Church Cemetery, on a hill behind the Helton Methodist Church on Highway 194.

Fannie died nine years later, September 4, 1961, in Ashe County Memorial Hospital. It is known that she was in an oxygen tent at the time, but it is not known for how long. She had lived for a number of years with her daughter Frances and her husband Marion Pool in Charlotte. Marion told Taylor (his niece) he remembered driving in the car to the train station in Charlotte with Hunter Jones and Fannie in 1953. They were involved in a car accident, and Fannie suffered a broken pelvis. Pool said the mishap probably extended Fannie's life, because when she was taken to the hospital, it was discovered she had cancer, and she was able to get treatment. Taylor suspects when it was clear Fannie did not have long to live, she was taken back to Ashe County, so Dr. Dean could take care of her.

On that beautiful Ashe County summer day when I interviewed Nell Taylor, Evelyn Jones and I and Nell and her husband, Tom Taylor, visited the gravesite Dr. Bud shares with his beloved wife Fannie. Both lived to see their son, Dr. Dean Jones, Sr., realize the dream of a hospital for Ashe County, but community health care in Appalachia had a long way to go before that dream would come true.

5

Medical Help from the Outside

A few medical professionals ventured into the Appalachian community from the outside, offering their services to a populace gradually coming to terms with the benefits offered by modern medicine. I wrote the following story about two such outsiders for the January 2008 issue of *Our State Magazine*. The story was recounted by Dr. Mary T. Martin Sloop with LeGette Blythe in Sloop's award-winning autobiography, *Miracle in the Hills*.[1]

It was around the early 1900s, when Dr. Mary Martin Sloop tackled her first surgical emergency. She and her husband, Dr. Eustace H. Sloop, were still new to their mountain home in the community of Plumtree in Avery County, when a dozen or so men arrived at the shack the doctors used for their joint practice. The men bore a young blacksmith on a stretcher, the son of the old man leading the party. Eustace was up the river tending to a patient, but the diagnosis was obvious to Mary—a ruptured appendix and almost certain death if not treated immediately.

Mary left the patient in the care of his companions and set off on foot, across the river, to the store on the other side—her objective, the procurement of a fifty-pound lard can and a ten-cent tin pan to use as a sterilizer. By the time she returned, her husband was back. Together they punched holes in the bottom and top of the lard can and put water in the pan to heat on the oil stove. They placed a thermometer in the top of the makeshift sterilizer, and Mary spent most of the night preparing the dressings and placing them in the sterilizer one at a time. They pulled out gowns and masks, leftover from their college days, and moved their patient to a nearby building still under construction. The structure had a roof but no walls. They put down boards for flooring and fashioned their operating room. Kerosene lamps provided light.

By now it was morning, and folks started to gather around, many toting their shotguns and rifles, as was common in those days. Some argued the new doctors would kill the young man, but the patient's father saw the Sloops as the only chance for his son. He insisted the operation proceed, and Mary warily eyed the firearms as they made ready for surgery. They opened up their patient, and the abdomen was as bad as they feared. It was touch and go for awhile, but, thankfully, the operation was a success. The blacksmith healed quickly and soon returned to work. Word of the surgery spread and helped win the trust and respect of the Appalachian community the Drs. Sloop would spend their lifetimes serving. In true pioneer spirit, they continued to improvise, setting up operating rooms under the shade of large trees, using kitchen tables or boards laid across sawhorses. Maybe the mountain air contributed to their recovery rate or the sturdiness of the mountain people, but despite inadequate equipment and sanitation, the people fared well in their care, and the Drs. Sloop made a difference, not just in community health care, but in education, preservation of mountain heritage crafts, founding and operating the Crossnore School, and building a church and Sloop Memorial Hospital.

Dr. Heinz Meyer (1899–1987) is another outsider offering insight into the diversity of people who influenced health care in Appalachia. Meyer, a physician, was a German Jew interned in the Buchenwald Concentration Camp in the early days of the Nazi regime. Fortunately, he escaped his imprisonment and made it to the United States with his family in 1938. His arrival roughly coincided with an appeal from the United Lutheran Church of America (ULCA) for physicians to help with their Mountain Mission, and Dr. Meyer responded. He traveled in Appalachia with Pastor Kenneth Gordon Killinger, a native of the area, known throughout the ULCA as the "Mountain Missionary." Killinger's ministry was a comprehensive one, encompassing the health, educational, and economic needs of

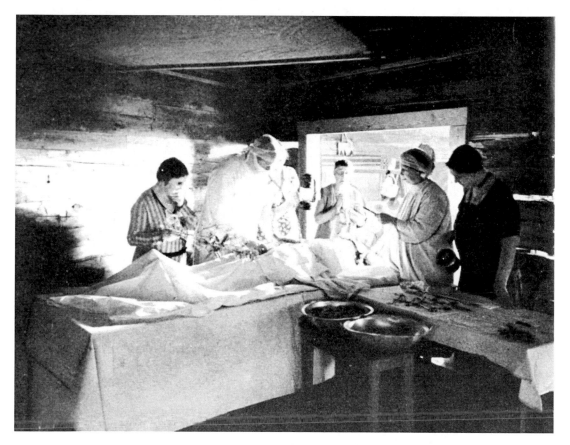

Dr. Mary Martin Sloop (1873–1962) and her husband Dr. Eustace Sloop (1878–1961) were among those who came to Appalachia to offer their services and made significant contributions to the improvement of community health care in the region. In this photograph published in the autobiographical work *Miracle in the Hills*, the couple performs surgery in a mountain cabin (photograph, circa 1917, courtesy N.C. Department of Cultural Resources).

his flock, as well as the spiritual. Meyer and his wife, a nurse, moved to Konnarock, Virginia, to help with a newly opened medical center, where the couple would live. Although an outsider, Meyer quickly gained a reputation for his skill and compassion. If people were too sick to get to the center, he visited them in their homes, bringing modern medicines not common in Appalachia up to that time and treating a variety of diseases and ailments, including whooping cough, dysentery and rickets. Ahead of his time in his emphasis on preventive health care, he instructed patients and their families in better nutrition, prenatal care, and the importance of isolating the sick and maintaining good health.[2]

Dr. Meyer was the doctor for the Konnarock Girl's Training School, where Evelyn Price Jones went to school as a girl. During her stay there, Evelyn was designated the school nurse for the girl's dormitory. She had no formal training for the post, but the job seemed to come naturally to her. She recalls taking temperatures and getting her supplies from the medicine cabinet, basically a first aid kit, in the principal's office. If one of the girls came to her with a complaint she thought warranted Dr. Meyer's attention, she alerted the principal, who put in a call for the doctor on the old crank phone in her office, and he came the short distance from the medical center to the school. "I liked him and respected him," Evelyn says of Dr. Meyer. When a terrible stomach flu made the rounds at the school, Evelyn stayed well while the other girls got sick, probably owing to her aversion to Dr. Meyer's standard treatment for the malady—a buttermilk diet. "I hated buttermilk," Evelyn confesses. She finally got the flu after everyone else was over it but somehow avoided the dreaded buttermilk diet.[3]

Evelyn's sister-in-law Cornetta Price was the unofficial taxi service for taking patients to Dr. Meyer's office. She was one of the few in the community who owned a car, and that was sufficient qualification for the community to tap her for the job. This sometimes put Cornetta in the position of deciding who was sick enough to warrant a trip to the doctor and who was not. Her experience laid the groundwork for her work in later years in the office of Dr. Jan Gable, who took Dr. Meyer's place when he retired.[4]

The Tennessee Valley Authority recognized Dr. Meyer's efforts for health and nutrition with an appropriation for a five year study of the effects of diet on health. After 13 years of working at the center, the Lutheran Church rewarded Dr. and Mrs. Meyer for their dedication, by building them a home, and Dr. Meyer lived in Konnarock for the rest of his life. The medical advances he brought to his adopted home, so far away from his homeland, would benefit generations to come and help forge the legacy of community health care in Appalachia.[5]

The Lutheran ministry brought in another major contributor to the health care of the region, Sister Sophia Moeller (1904–1987), who came to the Whitetop community as a deaconess nurse in the Lutheran Church. She employed a no-nonsense approach in her medical ministry, not hesitating to speak her mind. A caring person, she was dedicated to serving people and bringing good health care to those off the beaten path, sometimes traveling to them on horseback.[6]

Originally from a farm in South Carolina, Sister Sophie, encouraged by her father's stories of the deaconesses in Germany, entered the deaconate in Philadelphia. Despite not having a high school diploma, she managed to get into nursing school, taking an equivalency exam and passing with flying colors. She graduated as a registered nurse (R.N.) and spent some time working in Pennsylvania before the church came looking for medically trained staff for the newly opened Konnarock and Cabin Creek health care facilities in the mountains of Virginia. By 1938, she was working out of the Helton Health Center on Cabin Creek, another of Pastor Killinger's projects, and working with Dr. Meyer. The part of Appalachia she served was isolated, with dirt roads and few cars, no electricity, running water or telephones. There are many stories of Sister Sophie being rousted from her bed in the middle of the night to drive in heavy snow as far as her old Plymouth would go and then walking the rest of the way to tend to a patient or deliver a baby.[7] Sister Sophie also provided transportation to the doctor, dentist and the hospital, if required. Evelyn Jones tells a story about when she was a little girl, living in Whitetop. "I was helping Uncle Kyle reset tobacco. The day was hot, and the work made it hotter." Evelyn began to feel sick. In retrospect, she was probably having a heat stroke. She told her uncle she didn't feel well and got under a sweet apple tree. As Evelyn was not one for malingering, her uncle was concerned. By the time Evelyn's mother saw her, Evelyn's face was almost purple. "She called Sister Sophie to take me to Dr. Bunch, who had an office near Sturgills, a community in Ashe County, not far out of Lansing."[8]

Sister Sophie sat up with the sick and the dying and helped families in any way she could through trials, both physical and spiritual, and the plain everyday struggles of surviving in a world not given to easy living. A licensed nurse-midwife, she delivered more than 300 babies during her forty-year career.[9] Doris Oliver, a retired R.N. from Ashe Memorial Hospital, remembers Sister Sophie delivering babies around the time she (Doris) first started work at the hospital. "Unlike the self-taught midwives, Sister was a trained nurse practitioner. If Sister suspected there would be problems with a delivery, she would accompany her patient to Ashe County Memorial Hospital, where she would often assist with the delivery."[10] Both Dr. Elam Kurtz and Dr. Dean Jones, Sr., at Ashe County Memorial held her professional judgment as a mountain midwife in high regard. Evelyn Jones recalls when she had her appendix and tonsils taken out by Dr. Dean Jones, Sr., it was Sister Sophie who administered the ether. "I was fighting going to sleep," relates Evelyn, "and they kept saying, 'Evelyn, breathe deep, breathe deep, or we're going to go to sleep before you do.'"[11] Dr. Elam S. Kurtz paid tribute to Sister Sophie at the homecoming at Faith Lutheran Church July 5, 1987. "To have known Sister Sophie is to have known a great chapter in the history of our mountains."[12]

By 1960, Sister Sophie was 56 years old and had been caring for her beloved mountain people for 21 years, birthing babies, patching wounds, nursing sick children and adults, holding the hands of the sick, and praying over the dying. Faith Lutheran Church at Whitetop proclaimed "Sister Sophie Day." Sister Sophie died February 25, 1987. Dr. Heinz Meyer, with whom she had worked for many years, died a week later. Missions like those of Sister Sophie and Dr. Meyer brought attention to the particular health care needs of the mountain region and helped lay the groundwork for the state and federal government assistance which would one day follow.[13] Meanwhile, the people of Appalachia would do as they had always done—look after their own, as best they could.

6

Dr. Dean Jones, Sr.:
Second Generation of a Family Legacy

If there is a hero in the story of how Ashe County Memorial Hospital came to be, I would have to pick Dr. Dean Jones, Sr., the second generation of the Jones family legacy of doctoring. He would decline the accolade, of course, as by all accounts he was a modest man, prone to award others credit. There were many others who played a big part in the dream of a hospital in Ashe County, but Dr. Dean, as he came to be called, was certainly the driving force behind the project. He was connected with the hospital from the beginning, raising money for its construction, recruiting workers to finish the project, and then serving as resident physician, surgeon, and superintendent. Ashe County Memorial Hospital was his life's work.[1]

Born February 8, 1904, in Brandon in Ashe County, Dean Cicero Jones was the second of the five children of Dr. Arthur Lee "Bud" Jones and Fannie Kirby. Thanks to the hard work of his parents, he was able to pursue his higher education earlier in life than his father, attending Emory and Henry (E & H) Preparatory Academy 1918–1920 and Emory and Henry College 1920–1923. Dean Jones received his M.D. from the University of Pennsylvania Medical School in 1927 at the age of 23, served a two year rotating internship at the University of Pennsylvania Hospital and a three month residency at Seaside Hospital in Staten Island, New York, and started practice in Charlotte in 1930. He practiced in Robeson County, North Carolina, a short time and then came home to Ashe County and practiced in Lansing. In the late 1930s, Dr. Jones approached Dr. Fred Hubbard of Wilkes Hospital for advice on pursuing surgery as a specialty. The two arranged for Jones to assist Hubbard with surgeries at Wilkes on certain, designated days of the week. In 1938-1939, Jones went back to the University of Pennsylvania for a postgraduate course in surgery, followed by a three month residency in surgery at St. Joseph's Hospital in Lancaster, Pennsylvania. In the meantime, Drs. Jones and Hubbard began discussing the possibility of a hospital in Ashe County. A dream was taking shape.[2]

Partner to Jones in life and work, Lettie Wagoner was his sweetheart in the seventh grade in the community of Helton. Lettie was born October 1, 1903, to Jacob David Wagoner and Nora Goss Wagoner of Tuckerdale in Ashe County. When the train known as the Virginia Creeper came to the area, it was routed through where the Wagoners' house had been in Tuckerdale, and they moved to Helton. Lettie and her family moved from Helton to Quarryville, Pennsylvania, but she and Dean stayed in touch. The two married May 21, 1930, and had one child, Dean C. Jones, Jr., born in Charlotte, February 12, 1931. By the late 1930s, Dr. Dean and Lettie were back living and practicing medicine in Lansing. Lettie accompanied the doctor on house calls, especially deliveries, acting as his nurse and taking care of the new babies, while her husband took care of the mothers. The family rented the Maw Miller house in Lansing, and Dr. Dean had a thriving practice at his office in downtown Lansing. Dean C., Jr., started school there, and Lettie walked with him to school every day.[3] Emmett Barker, who grew up near Lansing, recalls, "A lot of parents walked their kids to school then." I asked Emmett how far it was from the Maw Miller house to the Lansing School. "It was about a half mile, but it was a long half."[4]

The family was back in Ashe County for good, and folks found their way to Dr. Dean all hours of the day. One evening, relates Evelyn Jones, a rowdy group of men, who had been fighting among themselves, brought a fellow shot in the scuffle to the

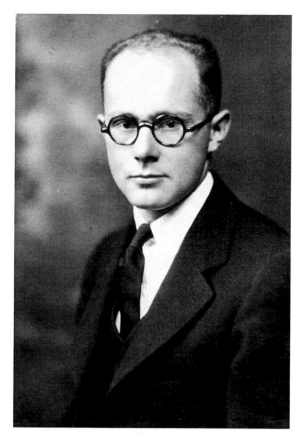

Dr. Dean C. Jones, Sr. (1904–1984), the second generation in the Dr. Bud Jones family to become a doctor/surgeon, became the superintendent and resident physician/surgeon of the new Ashe County Memorial Hospital, which opened in November 1941 (courtesy Evelyn Jones).

doctor's door. In the course of explaining what had happened, they got into another fight, and the man who had been shot hid in a ditch, afraid he was going to be killed. Dr. Dean had to settle the ruckus before he could treat the patient.[5]

When Dr. Jones was named superintendent and resident physician and surgeon of the new Ashe County Memorial Hospital in 1941, he turned over the office in Lansing to his father Dr. Bud, and he and Lettie and Dean C., Jr., moved from Lansing to Jefferson, where they lived in the hospital for the next fifteen years. Dr. Jones was the only physician on staff when the hospital first opened and assisted Dr. Fred Hubbard, the head of surgery for the new hospital, until Hubbard entered military service, and Jones assumed full responsibility for the surgical duties at Ashe County Memorial.[6] The kinds of surgeries performed in the small hospital ranged from the ordinary to the out of the ordinary. Dr. Jacqueline DuSold says Dr. Jones was known to have performed a surgical procedure called a burr hole, where a hole was drilled in the patient's skull to relieve pressure in the brain against the skull, a surgery more commonly performed by a neurosurgeon in a big city hospital.[7] During the

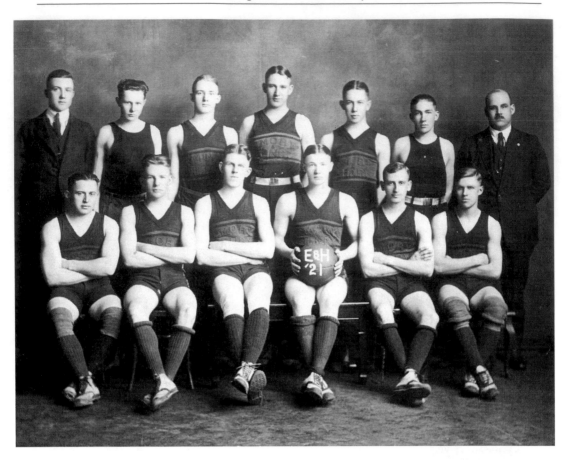

A good athlete and avid sports fan, Dean Jones, Sr., second from the left on the back row, participated in varsity baseball and basketball at Emory and Henry College. The basketball games were so rough in those days, claims Dean Sr.'s grandson Charles, that Dean Sr. lost a tooth on one defensive play, and no foul was called (photograph, circa 1921, courtesy Evelyn Jones).

first ten years of the hospital's development, Dr. Dean was primarily responsible for its financing and growth, as well as the medical staffing. Before his retirement in 1979, he would take the hospital from its modest beginning to a modern, multimillion dollar medical complex.[8]

Lettie joined her husband in the hospital venture from the start, active in the project's fundraising and a public relations wonder woman before and after the facility's opening. Besides touting the hospital's services to the public, she created a homelike atmosphere for patients and staff. "Lettie was the matriarch of the hospital," says Nell Taylor, a description echoed by many I interviewed about Lettie.[9] The doctor's wife worked alongside Langdon Scott, who was appointed the hospital's business manager shortly after its opening.[10] Lettie took no payment for her efforts in those early years, says Nurse Ruby Lum, but eventually received a small salary. Staff was limited when the hospital became operational, and Nurse Doris Oliver remembers when Lettie headed out the door with her husband, she would call to the nurse on duty, "If anybody comes in wanting to pay on a bill, take the money and put it in the narcotics box."[11]

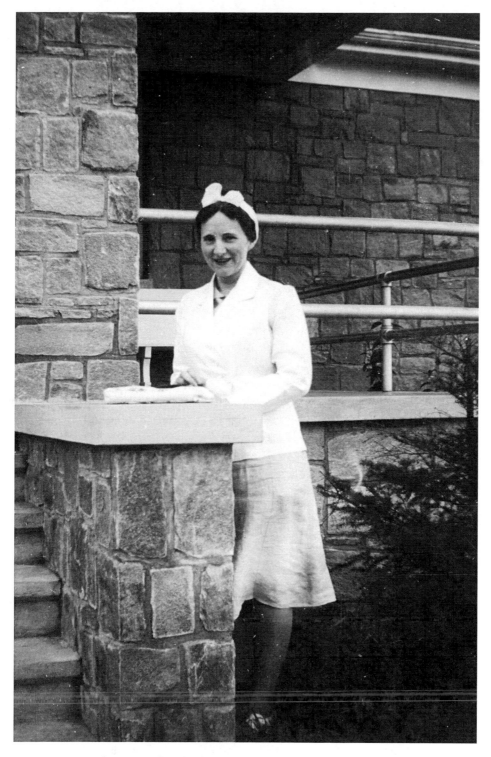

Lettie Wagoner Jones (1903–1983), wife of Dr. Dean Jones, Sr., was born in Tuckerdale in Ashe County. She helped manage the business end of the hospital in the first years of its operation, while her husband ran the medical side (courtesy Evelyn Jones).

Lettie helped everybody, recalls her daughter-in-law Evelyn Jones. If somebody needed a coat, she found them a coat; if somebody needed a blanket, she got them a blanket; if they had no transportation to get to the hospital, she arranged for somebody to pick them up. She brought the patients flowers in pretty little vases to cheer them. But Lettie, though quiet like her husband, was no shrinking violet, assures Betty Avery, who grew up knowing the couple. "She spoke her piece."[12]

While Lettie made the hospital feel like a home for staff and patients, it *was* home for her and her husband and son. The family had a bedroom and a sitting room, with a connecting bath. Dean C. slept on a couch in the sitting room. Anne Shoemaker McGuire remembers going with her mother, Evelyn Shoemaker, to visit Lettie in the Jones's rooms at the hospital. Dean C. was away at school by then. "Mrs. Jones and Mother were real good friends," says Anne. Anne was not comfortable at the hospital, though, "I thought that was the creepiest place! I didn't wander around. I stuck close to Mother."[13]

Living in the hospital meant Dr. Dean was on call constantly. Staff took advantage of the doctor's close proximity, and Ruby Lum recalls, "If something happened to a baby in the nursery, we just grabbed the baby and ran down the hall to Dr. Dean's room, and he treated the child there." Dr. Dean did all his own lab work and x-rays until Henry Lum joined the hospital and assumed these responsibilities. His morning hours were dedicated to surgeries, and the afternoon and evening hours were for office visits, approximately twenty to thirty outpatients a day. No appointments were scheduled for the outpatients; it was first come, first served. The process or lack thereof seemed to work, says Ruby Lum. Dr. Dean did not send anybody home untreated; he simply kept working until the last patient was seen, sometimes into the late evening. Mornings and evenings, Dr. Dean made his rounds to visit his patients in the hospital, and he checked in on the patients of other doctors as well. Doris Oliver remembers Dr. Dean regularly visiting her father, J. E. Oliver, a patient of Dr. Keys, when he made his rounds. A doctor visit in the 1940s to early 1950s usually cost two to three dollars, and nine months' worth of pregnancy care, including delivery, ran about 75 dollars. In the early days of the hospital's existence, Dr. Dean reportedly treated hospital employees for free.[14]

Dr. Dean and Lettie were dedicated to the hospital and to providing health care to the region. The doctor maintained, "Work was his greatest hobby." The overworked Dr. Dean was famous for falling asleep at family dinners, even when the family was eating at a restaurant. His brother Hunter would remind the children not to bother the doctor, "Let him sleep; he works so hard." Years later, Hunter's daughter, Nell Taylor, recalls, Dr. Dean C., Jr., would doze off the same way. When Dr. Dean could catch a little personal time, he enjoyed sports, especially basketball, an interest he would pass along to his son. Later, father and son played together on a community basketball team. Dean C. claimed his father had the sharpest elbows of anybody he knew. Dr. Dean, Sr., liked football too, especially, says Evelyn Jones, if the University of North Carolina at Chapel Hill was playing. But getting a few hours of relaxation was tough while running a hospital. The staff tried to arrange the schedule so Dr. Dean could be off on Wednesdays, but this effort met with mixed success, relates Dr. E. J. Miller. A patient came into the hospital on a Wednesday; the staff explained it was the doctor's day off, and the patient responded, "I know. I thought he wouldn't be as

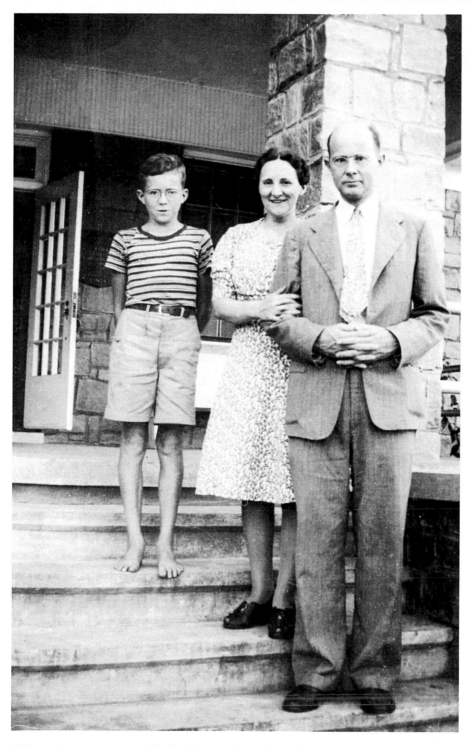

Dean C. Jones, Jr., was ten years old when he moved into the Ashe County Memorial Hospital with his parents, Dr. Jones, Sr., and Lettie. The family would make their home in the hospital until 1956. Stories abound of the youngster bouncing a basketball down the long hallways (photograph, circa 1941, courtesy Evelyn Jones).

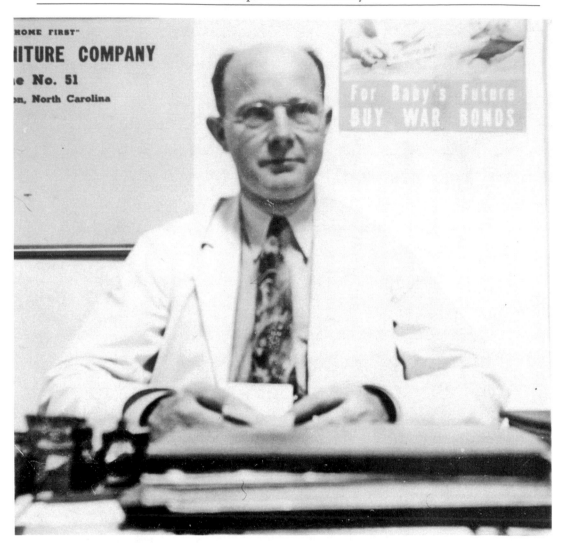

Hospital records indicate $10,000 of the hospital fund was designated by the executive committee for the purchase of War Loan Victory Bonds in 1943. A poster for war bonds is visible over the left shoulder of Dr. Dean Jones, Sr., seated at his desk in Ashe County Memorial Hospital (photograph, circa 1943, courtesy Evelyn Jones).

busy today." When he did get a day off, Dr. Dean enjoyed his two favorite pastimes—fishing and hunting, mostly for grouse. The first day of trout season was a high priority, of course, but the doctor had to move fast to get away. One Wednesday morning, a man and his wife drove up in Dr. Dean's front yard. The doctor was already dressed in his fishing gear, had on his lucky fishing hat and his bait in hand. The man rolled down the window of his car and called to the doctor, "I want you to check out my wife." Dr. Dean stepped over to the car, looked in the window, and said, "Yeah, that's your wife," turned and headed off to his fishing.[15]

When Dr. Dean left the hospital, whether for a fishing trip, dinner at a restaurant or family night at the movie theater, he left word where he could be reached if he was needed.

There were no cell phones or pagers; a network was set up to telephone where Dr. Dean was to be. Where there was no telephone, as was the case when he was fishing, people were dispatched to track him down at his favorite fishing spot. The designated posse would take a car as far as they could into the woods and then blow the horn until the doctor showed up. If that didn't work, they hiked in to fetch him. Once in the 1950s, Dr. Dean was fishing with French Young up Woodard Hollar, near Long Hope Falls. The time got away from them, and when they started hiking back to their vehicle, which was parked some distance away, they realized it was too dark to see where they were going. Rather than risk getting lost on the treacherous path, they opted to bed down and wait until first light. Meanwhile, Lettie became concerned and rounded up a search party. When the sun came up, the two fishermen appeared in front of the party, their gear in tow, and asked in surprise, "What are you guys doing out here?"[16]

Every fisherman has a story about the big one that got away, and Dr. Charles Jones tells the story of his grandfather leaving work to go fishing one Wednesday, in such a hurry he didn't stop to take his tie off. He hooked the Moby Dick of smallmouth bass and started reeling in the prize, when to his dismay, his tie caught in the reel, and the fish got off the hook in the ensuing antics to disentangle the tie. "It was the last time he forgot to take his tie off," laughs Charles.[17]

Undeterred by poor weather conditions when it came to fishing, Evelyn Jones tells how Dr. Dean listened to a fishing buddy complain repeatedly about the water temperature in the river being too cold for wading. "I'm going to catch a cold," his friend predicted. Never much for chatter while fishing or any other time, for that matter, the doctor suddenly pushed his startled friend into the river. "Why'd you do that?" exclaimed his buddy, stomping back up the river bank, dripping wet. "Well, I can't do anything for a cold, but if you get pneumonia, I can treat you for that." Having offered this logical explanation, the doctor waded out into the freezing river and commenced to fish.[18]

Tending to your family, friends, and neighbors makes practicing medicine very personal for a small town doc-

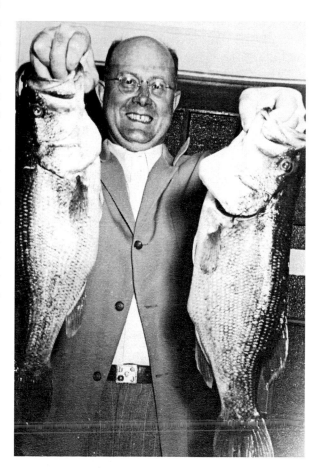

Dr. Dean Jones, Sr., maintained work was his greatest hobby, but he set aside Wednesdays for fishing, an avocation he passed along to his son (courtesy Evelyn Jones).

tor. A fishing buddy got hit by a car and was brought to Dr. Dean for treatment. "Don't think there's much you can do for me," his buddy whispered to him from the stretcher and passed away without another word. As in any era of medical practice, there are some things that cannot be fixed.[19]

A man came in for a check up and brought a decanter of Canadian Club as a gift for Dr. Dean, apparently unaware Dr. Dean and Lettie were strict teetotalers. The doctor quietly accepted the gift, and then, to the dismay of some of the staff, flushed the contents down the hopper. "But he kept the decanter," says Evelyn. "'I think Lettie might like this pretty bottle,' he said." Apparently nobody thought anything about him carrying that empty bottle under his arm on his rounds. "He didn't think much of folks having too much to drink and then showing up with some injury for him to treat as a result," Evelyn adds.[20]

Dr. Dean's intolerance for alcohol is confirmed in a story Geneva Jones Coffey tells about her father, Bernard Jones, who got his arm caught in a manure spreader. The injury was horrific, and Bernard was in tremendous pain. As Geneva prepared to drive him to the emergency room at Ashe County Memorial, her father, not normally a drinker, spoke up, "I sure could use a good, strong drink right now, but I know Doc Dean won't work on me if I do." Bernard toughed it out and walked into the emergency room on his own, held out his arm and announced, "Doc, I have a compound fracture." As it turned out, it was Dr. Dean C., Jr., who treated the injury, not the elder Doc Dean, so he might have been cut a little slack had he opted to take that medicinal drink.[21]

"Dr. Dean Jones, Sr., probably taught me more than anybody else," says long time Ashe County physician Dr. Edward J. Miller. "He did it all—ER, surgery, and delivered most of the babies, as many as forty babies a month at one point. He was a good orthopedic surgeon; he could tell if something was broken before the x-rays were ready. My mother broke both arms in a fall, carrying laundry from the upstairs. Dr. Jones put everything back, and she never had any trouble. He was good at not embarrassing you. I diagnosed a patient with appendicitis early in my career, and Dr. Dean came in and looked at the patient's throat and said, 'I believe this is the problem.' It was strep. I hadn't gotten a good history, but I learned from that experience."[22]

Doris Oliver admired Dr. Dean's calm, fatherly authority with regard to staff. "He was good to employees." It was Dr. Dean who helped orient the young nurse in her first weeks at the hospital. "He could get irritated with people who tried to impress him with what they knew, but he didn't fuss if you did something wrong, he'd just say, 'don't let this happen again.'" Dr. Dean was sewing up a patient, when one of the female staff ran back inside from the parking lot, frightened because there was a man sprawled out in the backseat of her car, obviously intoxicated. Dr. Dean didn't say a word, finished closing up his patient, took off his surgical gloves, strode out the door to the woman's car, grabbed the man by his feet, and dragged him out of the back of the car. "He was law and order," declares Oliver. Even the weather did not rattle the doctor's demeanor.[23] Evelyn Jones recalls the statewide press reported the weather conditions and rescue operation for one particular snow storm with such fanfare, that a concerned Dean C. called his father from Charlotte, where he was doing his residency, to see if everyone was okay, and staff was coping at the hospital. Dr. Dean calmly replied, in typical mountain fashion, that all was fine.[24]

Dr. Dean and Lettie were active members of the Jefferson United Methodist Church, where he served in a multitude of roles, including lay speaker, chairman of the official board, and assistant Sunday school teacher. "Dr. Jones, Sr., was a serious, quiet, and compassionate man. I think he prayed before every surgery," says Doris Oliver. "Somebody asked him once why he didn't talk much, and he said if he talked to everybody, he wouldn't get anything done."[25] The doctor was not without a sense of humor, however. Years ago, when cherry trees were prolific in Ashe County, broken arms were an everyday occurrence during cherry picking season. David VanHoy recalls falling out of a maple tree as a boy and breaking his arm. He was taken to Dr. Dean. "Were you picking cherries?" The doctor asked. "No, sir, I was climbing a maple tree," responded David. "No cherries in a maple tree," quipped the doctor as he went about the business of setting the arm.[26] Betty Avery recalls the time she was a senior in high school, and she was in the hospital for an appendectomy. She begged Dr. Dean to let her play in the upcoming basketball game after her surgery. He said no, of course. "But he did say I could go to the game if I would sit still and not do any jumping up and down and hollering. Then he added, 'I'll be there, you know, and I'll be watching.'" And he was.[27]

Accolades of many kinds were extended to Dr. Dean over his career. For his work performing physicals for pre and post–World War II draftees, he received Civil Service Citations from presidents Truman, Eisenhower, Reagan, Nixon, and Johnson. In March 1959, he was honored for his record of distinguished service, and his portrait was presented to Ashe Memorial Hospital by the Ashe County Medical Society.[28] Emory and Henry College honored him with the Distinguished Alumnus of the year award in 1972.[29] In June 1978, marking his 50 years of medical service to the people of Ashe County, Dr. Dean was honored with a scholarship bearing his name. The scholarship, which continues through the Rotary today, is made available to a student pursuing a full-time nursing or medical career. In conjunction with the announcement of the scholarship fund, the Ashe County Commissioners and the mayors of the three incorporated towns of Jefferson, West Jefferson and Lansing officially declared June 4 to be Dr. Dean C. Jones, Sr., Day in Ashe County.[30]

Dr. Dean worked as a surgeon and did obstetrics and general practice. After about 1969, he limited his practice to appointments but remained active on the hospital staff until his retirement in 1978 and continued to cover for his son, Dr. Dean C., Jr., for years after that. "I don't think he ever retired from the hospital and the interest he had in it," said Thomas Cockerham, when interviewed about Jones in the local newspaper. Cockerham worked with Dr. Dean for thirty years as the business manager for the hospital. He was right about his friend, who served on the board of directors for the hospital from his retirement until his death. Perhaps the most special tribute came from Henry Lum, Chief Medical Technologist at Ashe Memorial, who, recalling the long hours the doctor had devoted to the hospital, said, "He was the kind of fellow I'd like to think I could live up to."[31]

Although Dr. Dean, Sr., knew he had heart disease, his death was unexpected. Dean C. and Evelyn sat with him at his home the night before he died, looking at old photographs. Evelyn, who was with him at his home when he died, tried to give him CPR, but he was already gone. He died November 14, 1984, at 80 years old, and is buried at Ashelawn Cemetery, off U.S. Highway 221 in Ashe County, next to his wife Lettie, who died a year earlier.[32]

7

Ashe County Memorial Hospital: The Dream

In 1923, when Wilkes Hospital became the first permanent hospital established in Wilkes County, there were no other hospitals in the surrounding counties of Ashe, Alleghany, Watauga, Caldwell or Surry counties. Wilkes Hospital was one of the closest places for Ashe County residents to go for a major surgical procedure and remained so for many years, but North Wilkesboro, where the hospital was located, was almost thirty-five miles from Jefferson.[1] Dr. Frederick "Fred" Cecil Hubbard was the founder of Wilkes Hospital and maintained an association with that hospital that was similar to that of Dr. Dean Jones, Sr., and Ashe County Memorial Hospital in later years. Hubbard was born December 13, 1893, in Moravian Falls in Wilkes County but grew up in Wilkesboro where his maternal grandfather, Dr. James Calloway, a great-nephew of Daniel Boone, practiced medicine for forty years. Grandfather Calloway was raised and lived for a time in Ashe County.[2] Although his grandfather died long before he was born, Hubbard's affinity for Ashe County may be attributed in part to this connection, and his early interest in medicine probably was influenced by stories about his grandfather's work in northwestern North Carolina and that of his uncle Dr. C. C. Hubbard. Dr. Fred Hubbard, like Dr. Jones, would follow in the footsteps of doctors in the family and make his mark in the place where he grew up. A graduate of Jefferson Medical College in 1918, Hubbard did his postgraduate work in surgery at the University of Pennsylvania 1921–1922, only a few years before Dr. Jones completed his postgraduate study there.[3] In a letter postmarked May 2, 1939, Hubbard wrote to Jones at his office in Lansing to report on the status of a patient Jones referred to him for surgery. The correspondence is cryptic but reflects the level of cooperation and communication the colleagues maintained in such circumstances and the level of support the Wilkes facility received from its neighbors in nearby Ashe County.[4] A trip to any hospital in those days was viewed as a last resort and many, having waited too long to seek help, did not make it back home. As local historian and undertaker David VanHoy quips, it was commonly said that "everybody went to Wilkes to die."[5] Dr. Edward J. Miller remembers his mother citing the time an Ashe County relative got sick with acute appendicitis and was taken to the hospital in North Wilkesboro. By the time he got there, he didn't seem as sick, but, as it turned out, his appendix had ruptured in route, and he died. Miller's mother felt strongly that her relative would have lived had there been a hospital in Ashe County.[6]

In later years, Carpenter-Davis Hospital in Statesville and Baptist Hospital in Winston-Salem became options for surgery, but they were even farther away from Ashe County than the hospital at Wilkes. "Before the [AMH] hospital," says Dr. Miller, "you had to go to Statesville for surgery, and people came to say goodbye when they heard you were going, because you often didn't come back."[7] By the time plans were underway for Ashe County Memorial Hospital, a fundraising brochure noted that Ashe County, with a population of 22,000 to 23,000, was one of the largest counties in the state without a hospital.[8] In his address at the dedication of Ashe County Memorial Hospital, Dr. W. S. Rankin, of Duke Endowment, acknowledged the limited number of physicians in the area and proclaimed a local hospital would attract young doctors, eager to practice where the diagnostic support of a hospital was available. A local hospital also enabled a physician to increase his professional capacity at least four times, Rankin argued, because patients were coming to the physician at the hospital, rather than the physician taking the time to travel all over the county to see one patient; plus the hospital offered

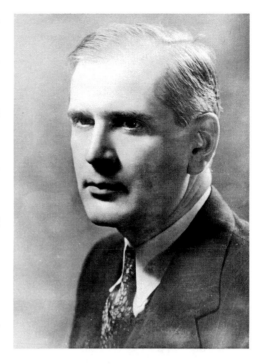

Dr. Fred C. Hubbard founded the first permanent hospital in Wilkes County and was chief surgeon and chief of staff in the early days of Ashe County Memorial Hospital, until he entered military service in 1943. He served on the N.C. Medical Care Commission, charged with assisting small, rural nonprofit and public hospitals, like AMH, with financing (courtesy Evelyn Jones).

the assistance of nurses and laboratory and x-ray facilities. A local hospital also provided a vehicle for charity care, Rankin concluded, estimating 30 to 40 percent of those who needed hospital care were unable to pay for it.[9]

With no hospital in the Ashe County area, babies most often were delivered at home, either by a midwife or by a doctor, if there was a doctor within a reasonable distance. Lack of prenatal care and poor nutrition contributed to problems with deliveries, so not having a hospital close by to address these problems could mean the difference between life and death for a newborn and the mother. And there were a multitude of other situations where a hospital was needed, including accidental injuries and acute appendicitis, when there was no time to travel a county away for help. The community recognized the need for a hospital in Ashe County long before the dream got off the ground. There were not many in the community who believed the dream could be realized, but those who did believe were a determined lot, and despite several failed attempts at establishing a hospital, those determined few continued to pursue the dream. It would take almost four years, but they would succeed.

In the January 6, 1938, issue of *The Skyland Post*, the hospital idea received a kick in the pants with the publication of a list of 15 goals for the county for 1938. The hospital was the top priority. In the same year, Iris Morphew relates her husband Paul was a high school student and wrote an essay for an American Legion sponsored competition, linking the social and economic well-being of the community to the health of its population and citing the lack of a hospital and dependence on other counties for that level of care as a handicap to the community's growth. People took notice.[10] The Jeffersons Rotary Club, whose involvement would prove critical to the success of the hospital movement, sponsored a meeting on August 2, 1938, in the office of West Jefferson physician Dr. B. Everette Reeves to discuss the idea of a hospital in Ashe County. Six committees were appointed to study the feasibility of the project and report back later that month at a meeting in the American Legion hall. The committees were chaired as follows: the Rev. R. H. Stone, the need for a county hospital committee; J. Bruce Hash, finance committee; Ed M. Anderson, public relations committee; Robert E. Lee Plummer, building and building plans committee; Dr. B. Everette Reeves, personnel committee; Roy Badger, hospitalization and insurance committee.[11]

Dr. Dean Jones, Sr., was quick to acknowledge that the Ashe County Memorial Hospital was a community effort, and without the interest and dedication of area leaders and the general population and the support of the Works Progress Administration, the hospital would not have come into being. In a brief account written by Jones and recorded in Arthur Lloyd Fletcher's *Ashe County: A History*, Dr. Dean paid special tribute to Ashe County movers and shakers Prof. Robert E. Lee Plummer, Wade E. Eller, William B. Austin, Roy R. Badger, Langdon L. Scott and the Rev. R. H. Stone, a diverse group united in the common cause of improving access to health care in their community.[12]

Roy R. Badger of Badgers' (now Badger) Funeral Home felt the need for a hospital in Ashe County every time he had to transport a patient to the hospital in Statesville, Wilkesboro, or Winston-Salem. Before there was a rescue squad or EMS or a county ambulance service, it was common practice for the local funeral home to provide ambulance service in a community, and Badgers' Funeral Home, as well as Reins-Sturdivant Funeral Home performed this function for a period of time in Ashe County. When I interviewed Badger's daughter, Gionia Badger Cook in August 2014, she recalled one time, before Ashe County Memorial was built, when Dr. Ray ran into problems with a delivery and directed the mother be taken to Wilkes Hospital immediately. Old N.C. State Highway 16 was not paved in those days, and, as anybody knows who has travelled that route, it is very curvy. By the time Badger got the mother to the bottom of the mountain, she had the baby, without the benefit of either doctor or hospital. That experience and others like it probably inspired Badger to push for a hospital and to donate the land for Ashe County Memorial. "It was a poor, poor time, and nobody had any money," but Gionia remembers her father kept a jar in the funeral home for donations for the hospital. By 1939, Roy Badger reported his firm made several ambulance trips a week, taking people from Ashe County to hospitals. He took a patient to Wilkes Hospital and made a count of the Ashe County people who were in the hospital as patients that day. There were at least fifteen, and Badger speculated there were fifteen other people who would have been in the hospital if there had been one close to home.[13]

Roy Badger became one of the first of the movers and shakers where the hospital was concerned and is representative of the diversity of people who assumed leadership roles in the project. Born near Berlin, now known as Bina, in Ashe County, May 10, 1898, he was the oldest son of John Wesley and Barbry Frances Badger. He worked for a while as a carpenter in a mining camp in West Virginia. The death of his father in 1929 brought his return to Ashe County, where he bought into the family business, Badgers' Funeral Home, working as the funeral director for 35 years. Active in community affairs, Badger was a charter member of the Jeffersons' Rotary Club, coroner for Ashe County for 14 years, and a member of the Ashe County School Board, as well as one of the original members of the Ashe County Memorial Hospital Board of Trustees.[14] It was Roy Badger and his brother Guy, partners in the funeral home business, who gave the land for the first Ashe County Memorial. According to Gionia Cook, Roy and his second wife Bessie Hartzog Badger, Gionia's mother, had planned to build a new house on the land, but "my father decided he wanted a hospital more." Badger opted to stay in his old house and renovate it. This would be the first of three donations of Badger land to the hospital. The second provided for the nurses' quarters and the third for a new sewer line for the hospital. The Badger family owned a large parcel of what is now called Mount Jefferson and built a reservoir there to furnish water for the hospital, as well as their home, at no cost to the hospital.

The Badger family had several other ties to Ashe County Memorial. Gionia's Aunt Theresa Badger was the cook at the hospital for many years, and her mother furnished eggs to the hospital. James, Gionia's brother, and his wife Erma Badger built a large home near the hospital, where some of the hospital staff rented rooms before the nurses' quarters was built. When Evelyn Price's room at the hospital was needed for patients, she moved to James and Erma's for the remainder of the summer. Dr. Dean Jones, Sr., bought the lot for his home behind the hospital from Roy Badger. "My dad just worshipped Dr. Dean," says Gionia, reflecting on their long relationship. Dr. Dean was Gionia's physician for many years and took care of her the entire nine months she was pregnant with her daughter Linda. The cost of the prenatal care, the delivery and a five-day hospital stay totaled $58.

Roy Badger suffered a stroke when he was 77 years old and lived for seven years in a rest home built by his son James. He died May 10, 1973.

Among the first and most eloquent advocates for building a hospital in Ashe County was Professor Robert E. Lee Plummer, a teacher, school builder and administrator, and active participant in all efforts to better the county.[15] David VanHoy credits Prof. Plummer with the heavy emphasis put on education in Grassy Creek. Families relocated to the area so their children could attend the schools there. Plummer was a graduate of Trinity College, now Duke University, and steered many in the region in that direction, including the three daughters of midwife and healer Mrs. Cora Reeves. According to VanHoy, Plummer's lifelong dream was to have a farm across from Healing Springs in Crumpler, his place of birth. Community leaders, including Dr. Aras B. Cox and Prof. N. C. Hurt, wanted to build a school in upper Grassy Creek. They struck a bargain with Plummer, promising he could have a school in Healing Springs, if he first would open and obtain accreditation for Grassy Creek Academy. Plummer laid the foundation for a remarkably advanced school system in Grassy Creek, and many families benefited from his efforts.[16] According to correspondence between Plummer and Congressman Robert Doughton, on file in the University of North

Carolina Southern Historical Collection, Prof. Plummer was the principal of Healing Springs High School in Crumpler at the time he advocated for the Ashe County Hospital project.

A prominent leader in civic, political, educational and religious affairs in Ashe County, Wade Edward Eller was an early and enthusiastic supporter of Ashe County Memorial Hospital.[17] He tackled fundraising with vigor, contributing to articles in *The Skyland Post*, updating readers on the hospital, urging payment of pledges, and appealing to "every man, woman, and child in the county to give as much as $1, if possible."[18]

Over the years, he served as secretary of the board of trustees and the executive committee of the hospital. An Ashe County native from Clifton, Eller was born in 1889 and graduated with honors from Trinity College in 1912. A charter member of the Rotary Club, he, like Prof. Plummer, was first an educator, serving as principal of the Helton School from 1912 to 1913 and then as co-principal, with W. L. Scott, of the new Methodist High School at Jefferson in 1913. Eller entered the banking business and became assistant cashier of the First National Bank in 1915 and continued in his employment there until he entered military service in World War I, as a member of the Marine Corps. He spent time in the mercantile business in Texas, where he met and married his wife Dempsie Smith of Lubbock, and also in Virginia and Kentucky, before returning home to Ashe County in 1931. With his roots in education, he was instrumental in the establishment of a high school at Riverview and served as its principal for twelve years. Eller also was involved in the formation of the New River Soil Conservation District and served as District Sanitation Supervisor for the District of Ashe, Alleghany and Watauga counties. In addition to his various business and community interests, Eller had a great love of Ashe County history and genealogy, devoting considerable time to collecting information on these subjects. The Wade E. Eller Genealogy Collection was donated by the Eller family to the Ashe County Library in 1977 and now is available through the North Carolina Division of Archives and History to libraries and researchers across the country.[19]

Considered one of the founding fathers of Ashe Memorial Hospital, William Bryant "Bill" Austin, Sr., served on the hospital's board of trustees and executive committee starting in December 1939, when then North Carolina Senator Austin was elected as the first president of the Ashe County Memorial Hospital Association, Inc., at a meeting of the board of trustees in the Ashe County courthouse. He would serve as president for 30 years.[20]

Born in Laurel Springs in Ashe County May 3, 1891, Bill Austin was one of two sons of George B. and Alice Woodie Austin. His father was sheriff of Ashe County in the early 1900s. W. B., or "Mr. Bill" as he was known, received his A.B. and LL.B. degrees at the University of North Carolina at Chapel Hill and was the county attorney for Ashe County for 30 years. His office was located in the little white building between the police station and the old courthouse in Jefferson. Later he and Allen Worth became law partners, and the two located their office in the downstairs of the old Northwestern Bank, where Austin served on the board of directors for many years. He practiced law in Ashe County from 1919 until 1977. Evelyn Jones recalls Austin was a good friend of her father, Dan Price. "They were both talkers," says Evelyn of the two friends. "Often they were so busy talking they didn't know what the other was saying."[21]

Active in politics, Austin served two terms in the North Carolina House of Representatives, 1926–1928 and 1940–1942, and one term in the North Carolina Senate 1938–1940. He was well acquainted with Congressman R. L. Doughton, a neighbor in Laurel Springs, where Austin was raised, and the two plotted political strategy in the Austin home on many occasions. Several letters between the Congressman and Austin are on file at the Wilson Library at the University of North Carolina, including at least one relating to the application for WPA funding for the hospital in Ashe County. Austin was a member of the North Carolina Board of Agriculture and the North Carolina Board of Conservation and Development, and president of the Ashe County Development Association, as well as active in other civic organizations.[22]

Mary Gordon Austin Tugman, Bill Austin's daughter, remembers her father as being "interested in everything that was going on and anything that would benefit Ashe County." With his impressive record of public service and active role in the Rotary, an organization committed early on to the idea of a hospital in Ashe County, Austin's support of the hospital was not unexpected, but at least two personal experiences may have contributed to his passion for the project. With no hospital in the county and few doctors, when Austin's two year-old daughter, Mary Gordon, came down with pneumonia, Dr. Fred Hubbard was hastily summoned from North Wilkesboro to tend to the young patient. A close friend of Austin's, Hubbard reportedly stayed with the family for three days, until Mary Gordon took a turn for the better. In another instance, Austin's wife, Nona Neal Austin, had one of those days mothers have all too frequently, when everything seems to go wrong at once. First one of her children and then another came in with serious injuries, and then the dog got sick. She loaded everybody in the car, including the dog, and drove down the mountain to North Wilkesboro to get help at the hospital there. All survived, but it would have been much easier for everybody concerned, including the dog, if they had not had to make the long trip to North Wilkesboro. Like the Austins, many families in the area could cite experiences, where the need for a hospital close by was brought home by some personal calamity. "When we found out we were going to have a hospital, we were thrilled," says Mary Gordon of the community's reaction to the Ashe County project.[23]

Like many children of those connected to Ashe County Memorial, Mary Gordon got her first job at the hospital. For three summers she worked answering the telephone and delivering the mail to patients. Hired by Langdon Scott, the hospital's business manager, and Lettie Jones, Mary Gordon worked under Lettie's supervision. "She was as sweet as she could be and very professional. She wanted everything to go smoothly for Dr. Jones. They were a perfect couple." The Austins and the Joneses were good friends, and Dean C. and Mary Gordon went to school together starting from sixth grade, when the Joneses moved from Lansing to Jefferson, through high school. "She was the sister he never had," laughs Evelyn Jones. "Dean C. was a part of my life forever," confirms Mary Gordon. Most often, when the two children got together after school, they came home to the Austin's house, but on those days when Dean C. had a new baby to show off at the hospital's nursery, the pair went there. Although career planning was not frequent subject matter for their conversations growing up, Mary Gordon, says there was never any doubt Dean C. would become a doctor. The early and constant exposure to the field of medicine he received from living in the

hospital and witnessing his father at work set him on a path from which he did not devi-
ate.[24]

Mary Gordon remained close to the Jones family, and Dr. Jones, Sr., was her physician
into adulthood. Over the years, she naturally formed a relationship of trust with the quiet
doctor. Sometimes it is hard to let go of that patient-doctor attachment and transfer that
trust to a younger generation, especially to someone with whom you grew up. Mary Gordon
laughingly recalls the time her young daughter needed an appendectomy, and her childhood
playmate, now Dr. Dean C. Jones, Jr., took the case at the hospital. The doctor announced
his diagnosis and the need for an immediate appendectomy and started down the hall to
the operating room, with the child on the stretcher. Mary Gordon protested—she wanted
Dr. Jones, Sr., to do the surgery. The elder doctor appeared on the scene to assure her that
Dean C. was perfectly capable of doing the surgery. When that was not sufficient to placate
the young mother, Dr. Dean stood in the operating room while his son performed the surgery, came out when it was over, and calmly assured Mary Gordon the operation was a success, and her old friend had done a good job. In April 1977, when at age 85 Bill Austin
suffered a heart attack and died a week later at the new Ashe Memorial Hospital, it was Dr.
Dean, his friend of so many years, who held Mary Gordon in his arms and told her, "Honey,
I did everything I could."[25]

A close friend of Bill Austin, the Rev. R. H. Stone was credited by Dr. Dean with
arousing the doctor's interest in the hospital. The Rev. Stone, a Presbyterian minister long
interested in assisting the sick and less fortunate, approached Jones with the idea of building
a hospital and asked him if he would run the hospital if he (Stone) got it built. With the
nod from Jones, he enthusiastically rounded up a list of pledges in a few weeks for the construction, and the dream was in the works.[26] Gionia Badger Cook recalls Preacher Stone,
who came to the area as a young man, wanted to help her father, Roy Badger, get a hospital
for Ashe County. Stone wrote to various companies, including medical suppliers, for donations of beds, kitchen equipment, linens, and anything else he thought a hospital would
need to operate.[27] David VanHoy recalls hearing about Preacher Stone's persistence in pursuing donations for the hospital. He wrote to a company that manufactured stoves and
pointed out the benefits of having one of the company's stoves in the hospital where all the
nurses would see the product in use and be so impressed they would order one for
themselves.[28] After *The Skyland Post* ran a series of columns touting the importance of having a hospital nearby, the Rev. Stone contributed an article to the paper responding to
naysayers of the project, particularly those who complained the hospital would not be self-
supporting and contending people who could pay their bills would go to a better, more
established hospital. He attacked this "spirit of defeatism" with gusto, debunking the argu-
ments against the project and likening the pessimists to those who would have been against
the first filling station for fear there would not be enough cars to buy the gas.[29] The Rev.
Stone's energy helped propel the hospital project into being and was missed when his twenty-
year pastoral relationship with his congregation in Ashe County was dissolved at his request,
so that he might assume the duties of executive secretary of the Mecklenburg Presbytery
in Charlotte, effective April 1, 1941. A month after he left Ashe County, the Rev. Stone
sent two sizable checks for the hospital from donors in Charlotte.[30]

Preacher Stone was not the only member of the local clergy to lend his support to the hospital movement. Along with him, the Rev. W. J. "Jack" Huneycutt and the Rev. W. T. Whittington were among the six county drive chairmen who helped kick off the initial fund drive launched in the local churches in early January 1939. Not only were these men key to spreading the word about the hospital within their respective congregations, they also marshaled those resources to help raise the necessary funding.[31] The June 29, 1939, issue of *The Skyland Post* included a "sermon" by the Rev. Huneycutt, pastor of the West Jefferson Methodist Church, which demonstrated the dedication of the local clergy to the hospital project. "No more significant movement has stirred the finer impulses in the hearts of Ashe County citizens since the establishment of the churches and schools. Those who follow through and see this great humanitarian institution established will write their names indelibly on the hearts of this and future generations." In a sermon delivered to the large congregation of West Jefferson Baptist Church in late October 1939, the Rev. Whittington declared, "Part of our Christian duty is to support hospitals." His forceful words were in connection with a statewide Baptist hospital campaign, part of which was directed toward support of the Baptist Hospital in Winston-Salem.[32] Meanwhile, the Rotary Club approached the Rev. Stone about the hospital idea, and the two parties decided to pool their resources.[33]

The Ashe County Woman's Club and later the West Jefferson Woman's Club played important roles in the hospital's history too, providing equipment and furnishing a room at the hospital, in addition to conducting health programs in schools and working in conjunction with the Rotary on activities related to crippled children.[34] The Ashe County Woman's Club voted to pledge $100 to the hospital for the purchase of equipment at a meeting in January 1941.[35] To help raise money to furnish a room at the new hospital, the club regularly served dinner to the Rotarians.[36] The West Jefferson Woman's Club, started in 1943 under the leadership of Stella (Mrs. Ed M.) Anderson, furnished a room in Ashe County Memorial and supported the County Health Center, the annual chest x-ray and cancer tests, and the County Welfare Department.[37]

The movers and shakers agreed the hospital should be self-supporting, and arrangements were made to seek financial assistance from the Duke Endowment and the Works Progress Administration (WPA). The Duke Endowment, established in 1924 by wealthy businessman and philanthropist James B. Duke of Durham, North Carolina, focuses on children, rural churches, health care and higher education in North and South Carolina. At the time of the Ashe County Memorial Hospital project, millions of dollars had been given to aid an estimated 166 hospitals in the two states.[38]

The Works Progress Administration, established by the federal government in 1933 under President Franklin D. Roosevelt, was a conglomeration of agencies designed to provide jobs and temporary assistance for the unemployed during the Great Depression. Initially created under the Emergency Relief Appropriations Act, the WPA went through a number of revisions and cutbacks, but throughout its existence, focused on public building projects as a means of creating construction-related jobs. Many community hospitals established in the 1930s to early 1940s were built by the WPA, and Ashe County was already on the receiving end of a number of other WPA projects. Before the demise of the federal program,

Ashe County WPA projects would include the Ashe County Clubhouse or Community Center in West Jefferson, which now houses the Ashe County Arts Council; central school buildings in Lansing, Jefferson, West Jefferson, Riverview, Fleetwood, and Virginia-Carolina; rock walls and playgrounds; sanitary service; and roads and bridges, many in need of replacement after the 1940 area flood.[39]

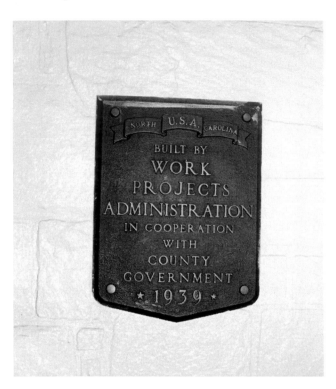

This plaque was placed at the original Ashe County Memorial Hospital to commemorate the support the project received from the WPA in helping the community realize its dream of a hospital close to home (photograph, circa 2006, courtesy N.C. Department of Cultural Resources).

Prof. Plummer, together with members of his committee, sent finished plans for the hospital, completed by architect H. N. Hains of Duke University, to the Ashe County Commissioners in December 1938, and the county commissioners voted to act as the sponsoring agency for the project. The sponsor's share of the funding was to be raised by the Ashe County Memorial Hospital Association, a nonprofit organization incorporated under state law, formed to raise money for the hospital and to operate it.[40] The final WPA applications for both the hospital and the community club house were delayed because of a misunderstanding regarding a ruling issued by the Washington, D.C., office in January 1939 and difficulties in completing requirements for the final blueprints and details on building materials. Letters from Congressman Doughton's papers in the Wilson Library at UNC at Chapel Hill indicate the Congressman was instrumental in clarifying the ruling and resolving the confusion for his constituency. The final application submitted for the hospital specified a one-story building, with stone veneer, and twenty-four beds, at an estimated cost of $44,000, with the sponsor's share set at approximately $19,000.[41] Congressman Doughton wired Finance Committee Chairman J. Bruce Hash with the official announcement of President Roosevelt's approval, March 25, 1939, of WPA funding for both the hospital project in Jefferson and the community center in West Jefferson.[42] The $25,766 in approved WPA funding for the construction of the hospital, combined with the sponsor's share of $19,000, yielded a total building cost of $45,000.

Meanwhile, the initial fund drive, launched in January 1939 with such success, lost some of its momentum because of the misunderstanding regarding the ruling and the ensuing delay, coupled with a spell of severe winter weather, making it difficult for drive chairmen and their workers to get the word out. The approval of the WPA application put the fund drive back in high gear. Construction could not begin until the sponsor's share of funding was in hand, and construction was scheduled to begin August 1939. To reach its fundraising goal, the Ashe County Memorial Hospital Association renewed its push to sell non–profit-bearing stock certificates, begun at the first of the year, and pushed for the payment of pledges already made. The cost of a share was set at ten dollars, and those who contributed amounts less than ten dollars were listed as "contributors." *The Skyland Post* printed stock subscription and contribution blanks in the paper to encourage participation in the fund drive and printed the names of shareholders and contributors as pledges were paid.[43] Within 24 hours, starting Saturday night, April 29 and ending Sunday night, April 30, 1939, a total of 44 community meetings were scheduled, with fund drive chairmen deploying 11 teams into every community in Ashe County to explain the hospital movement, answer questions and solicit memberships in the Ashe County Memorial Hospital Association.[44]

Finance Committee chairman and Ashe County Schools superintendent J. Bruce Hash appointed the following drive chairmen: the Rev. R. H. Stone, the Rev. Jack Huneycutt, the Rev. W. T. Whittington, Wade E. Eller (also general chairman of all committees), Prof. Robert E. Lee Plummer, and Ed M. Anderson. Stone and Dr. Dean Jones set about raising money through the private membership stock subscription. This initial fund drive was launched through local churches Sunday, January 1, 1939, with the help of the drive chairmen. The Certificate of Incorporation of Ashe County Memorial Hospital, Inc., authorized the issuance of 1,750 shares. Although a share had no financial yield, it did entitle the shareholder to vote on the board of trustees for the hospital, one vote for each ten dollars subscribed. People of modest means, like Dr. Edward J. Miller's 93-year-old mother, Virginia Juanita Bledsoe Miller of Nathans Creek, believed in the hospital and did what they could to support the project. Mrs. Miller raised turkeys and saved the money from their sale to buy a share of hospital stock. Her donation was touted on the front page of the May 16, 1940, issue of *The Skyland Post*. "Her interest at this age should inspire others to give, members of the board pointed out."

The largest holder of the initial stocks issued was 92-year-old Joseph Jerome Thomas (1849–1943) of Grassy Creek, who purchased 100 shares, as well as donated one thousand dollars to the hospital project. Thomas, the son of a physician who practiced in Independence, Virginia, had deep roots in western North Carolina and Virginia. He was born in Grayson County, Virginia, April 9, 1849, to Dr. Fleming S. and Emily Phipps Thomas. His grandfather on his father's side was Nathan Thomas, a North Carolinian who served with General Green in the American Revolution. A highly educated man for his time, Joseph Thomas graduated from Emory and Henry College in Emory, Virginia, in 1876. He taught school for several years in Alleghany County, North Carolina, and one of his students was the Hon. Robert L. Doughton, who would figure prominently in obtaining the federal support for Ashe County Memorial Hospital. Thomas dabbled in the mercantile business for several years, but was a farmer at heart and became one of the most noted farmers in Grayson County. He married at the age of 40, and he and his bride, Gincy Halsey, from Mouth of Wilson, Virginia, moved to Little Helton in Ashe County. In addition to his success with farming and livestock, Thomas proved an astute businessman and served for more than

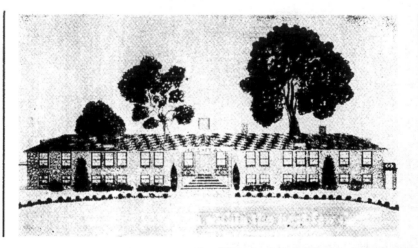
This ad by Badgers' (later Badger) Funeral Home was published by *The Skyland Post* May 25, 1939, to encourage readers to support the hospital project by joining the Ashe County Hospital Association with the purchase of a member share for ten dollars. Shareholders were entitled to vote for the board of trustees, one vote per share (courtesy N.C. Department of Cultural Resources).

thirty years as president of the First National Bank of West Jefferson, which he helped to establish. At his death he was the first vice president of the hospital board of trustees and was believed to be the oldest living citizen in Ashe County. His son, Edison M. Thomas, also served on the board of trustees for the Ashe County Memorial Hospital for many years and followed in his father's footsteps as president of First National Bank of Jefferson (later changed to West Jefferson) during World Wars I and II.[45]

The second largest subscribers were Dr. and Mrs. Dean Jones with 50 shares. Guy and Roy Badger each purchased 25 shares, and E. R. Sturdivant and Mr. and Mrs. B. Lem Hafer each purchased 20 shares. Ten dollars was a hefty sum in the late 1930s, and citizens anted up as best they could afford. The Women's Missionary Society of the Jefferson Methodist Church pooled its resources and bought five shares. Educators were targeted by fundraisers, and they responded. Local Parent-Teachers Associations (PTAs) pitched in too, with box suppers and other fundraising events. The money raised per event was modest, but it was adding up, and *The Skyland Post* regularly reported progress.[46]

A merchant in Laurel Springs offered up a quart jar of pennies he had saved to donate to the hospital fund. His total donation was $10.06.[47] John K. Reeves remembers his father, John F. Reeves, a Rotarian, as very community-minded and very aware of the need for a hospital in the county. "After work my dad would go out door-to-door to solicit pledges

STOCK-MEMBERSHIP SUBSCRIPTION BLANK

NAME _____ DATE _____

ADDRESS _____

    I hereby subscribe for _____shares, at ten dollars ($10.00), per share, of non-profit bearing stock, in the proposed ASHE COUNTY HOSPITAL ASSOCIA-TION, which proposes to raise the sponsor's share of money and materials to erect and equip a WPA Ashe county hospital, to be sponsored by the Ashe County Board of Commissioners, provided the sponsor's part is raised.

    After erection of the proposed building, it is understood that the county commissioners are to give the ASHE COUNTY HOSPITAL ASSOCIATION a long-term lease for the operation and control of said hospital. The Association will be incorporated as a non-profit organization and no one will be responsible for any more than he or she subscribes.

    It is further understood that each share of stock entitles the holder to one vote in the meetings of control of the county hospital.
    This stock is payable as follows:

Cash _____; $_____ on_____; $_____ on ____.

Material _____

Secured by _____Signed _____

    (The name of every member and contributor will be listed on the inside of the Hospital building.)

Stock-membership subscription and contributor's pledge card blanks were printed in *The Skyland Post* for the convenience of those wishing to join the Ashe County Hospital Association or make a donation (any amount under ten dollars) (image, circa 1939, courtesy AMH).

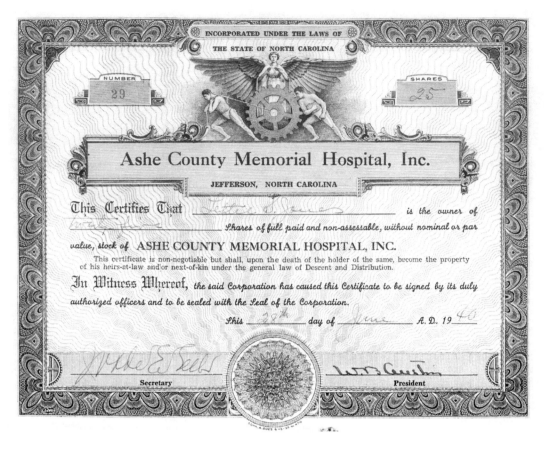

This stock certificate for Ashe County Memorial Hospital, Inc., was issued June 28, 1940, to Lettie Jones, wife of Dr. Dean Jones, Sr. Signed by Secretary W. E. Eller and President W. B. Austin, the certificate entitled the bearer to 25 shares at a cost of $250. Dr. Dean Jones, Sr., was issued a certificate for a like amount, making the couple one of the largest contributors to the hospital project (courtesy Evelyn Jones).

for the hospital."[48] The community added teas and rummage sales to a plethora of fundraising efforts, and the Jeffersons Rotary Club sponsored a series of fundraising concerts, conducted by Don Richardson.[49] Women's organizations, especially those affiliated with local churches, played a part in the fundraising too. The Women's Society of Christian Service of the Helton M.E. Church sponsored a box supper to raise money for the hospital.[50]

Support also came from individuals born in Ashe County but living elsewhere to pursue their careers. William Avery Neaves, a native of Crumpler, who was superintendent of the Chatham (Blanket) Manufacturing Company at Elkin, North Carolina, reportedly made a sizable pledge. Avery's nephew, Tom Neaves, notes his uncle still had family living in Ashe County, which, coupled with his affection for his home county, probably helped motivate his generosity. Later the Chatham company donated blankets for the hospital.[51] Several prominent doctors, native to Ashe County but not practicing in the area, supported the hospital project, as well. "I have been very much interested in this project, and I want to see my home county have a good hospital, as the people need it," stated Dr. U. G. Jones, a native of Clifton in Ashe County and owner of an eye, ear, nose and throat hospital in

Johnson City, Tennessee. Dr. Jones agreed to furnish a room in the hospital and donated several hundred dollars worth of equipment.[52] Dr. James L. Ballou, of the United States Veteran's Hospital in Portland, Oregon, also an Ashe County native, sent a check for $100 and indicated his willingness to offer consultation services to the hospital as an eye, ear, nose and throat specialist, upon his retirement from government service and subsequent return to the county.[53] Another Clifton native, Dr. J. M. Graybeal of Missoula, Montana, spoke in praise of the newly constructed hospital at the Jeffersons Rotary Club on a visit home in June 1940. "You have one of the most beautiful hospital buildings I have ever seen, and if any section of the country needs and deserves a hospital, it is certainly my home county of Ashe." Before returning to Montana, Dr. Graybeal made a donation of $50.[54] Letters of support poured in from doctors in other areas, including: Dr. James W. Davis of the Carpenter-Davis Hospital in Statesville; T. B. Goode of the Long Hospital in Statesville; Dr. C. L. Haywood, Jr., manager of the Hugh Chatham Memorial Hospital in Elkin, and Dr. A. B. Graybeal of Marion, Virginia. Dr. J. A. Smith of Lexington announced his intention to furnish a room as a memorial to Dr. S. E. Pennington, a medical pioneer in Ashe County.[55]

With funding efforts in gear, a location committee of the Ashe County Memorial Hospital Association was appointed, with original members Wade Eller, Prof. Robert E. Lee Plummer, Mrs. R. H. Stone, Dr. B. Everette Reeves, Roy Badger, and Ed Anderson.[56] By April 1939, deliberations by the committee were well underway, with the members pledging to locate the hospital within a three mile radius of Amos Graybeal's home, between Jefferson and West Jefferson.[57] In early May, the final decision was made to accept the site of the old Jefferson school dormitory, on the corner of Gentry and McConnell streets in Jefferson, convenient to the West Jefferson–to–Jefferson highway and the Warrensville-to-Jefferson highway. Two acres were donated by Roy Badger and his brother Guy; Mrs. Eula J. Neal donated an adjoining parcel; and Mr. and Mrs. V. V. (Miss Sallie) McConnell donated one acre in front of the dormitory site, on which a nurses' home could be built.[58]

With the location decided, the project gathered steam. Despite newspaper headlines warning of Hitler's continued march into Poland and England and France formally declaring war on Germany, the citizenry of Ashe County clung hard to their dream of a hospital, and thanks to donations amounting to $10,000, plus materials contributed and WPA funding of a local labor force, construction of the new 24 bed Ashe County Memorial Hospital started August 29, 1939. Of course, before a worker picks up a hammer or a trowel for a project like this, a politician has to make a speech, and Congressman Robert L. Doughton, so instrumental in obtaining the WPA funding for the project, delivered the address at the groundbreaking ceremony. J. J. Thomas took the first shovel of dirt. Other movers and shakers present included Prof. Robert E. Lee Plummer, Roy R. Badger, Jack Huneycutt, Dr. Dean Jones, Sr., and Wade Edward Eller, Sr.[59]

Arthur Frazier was selected as timekeeper and Lester Stump as foreman for the hospital project, with a crew of 40 WPA workers, including Alonzo Hicks Baldwin, better known as "O. H.," the father of current West Jefferson Mayor Dale Baldwin. Mayor Baldwin's first memory of Ashe County Memorial Hospital is as a nine or ten year old, walking the short distance from his boyhood home to the hospital construction site to take his father his

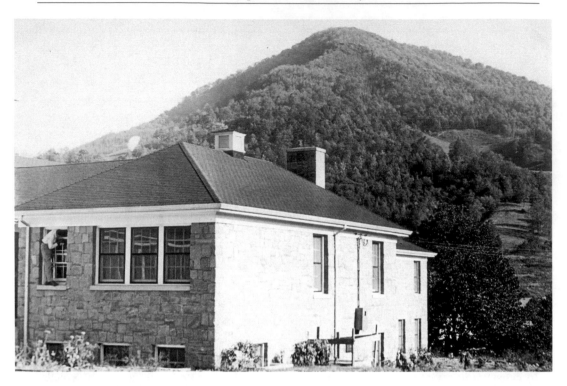

At the time the first Ashe County Memorial Hospital was built, the town of Jefferson was visible from McConnell Street, with Mount Jefferson in the background and Big Phoenix and Little Phoenix Mountains to the north and northeast, respectively (photograph, circa 1941, courtesy Evelyn Jones, published in *The Skyland Post*, October 30, 1941).

lunch. O. H. Baldwin worked on a number of projects for the WPA, including Lansing School, West Jefferson Elementary, and the community building in West Jefferson, almost completed at the time the hospital's construction began. Native stone was used in all these buildings, and O. H. was a stonemason. The columns on the front porch of Ashe County Memorial Hospital were his handiwork, more prominent in the days before the porch was enclosed. "He probably laid most of the rock on those pillars," says the Mayor proudly, "and not that stick-on rock like they use now, but real bedrock."[60]

Dr. Dean Jones was especially anxious for the hospital to be finished, and Emmett Barker remembers him coming out to see his father and some of the other men in the neighborhood to ask them if they could work a few days at the hospital construction site. "Because he asked, they came and worked for free to help the hospital get finished." In addition to their time, members of the community donated what building materials they could. The variety of brick used in the hospital's construction is visible where the plaster has broken away in the now vacant hospital building on McConnell Street, and the attic reveals a similar variety pack of wood beams holding the structure together. If it worked, they used it.[61]

As the building project neared completion in the summer of 1940, an urgent call went out to raise an additional $2,500, needed to purchase plumbing, heating and lighting fixtures and to properly equip the hospital. In response to the appeal, local churches announced Sunday, July 7, 1940, as Ashe County Memorial Hospital Day in the Sunday schools and

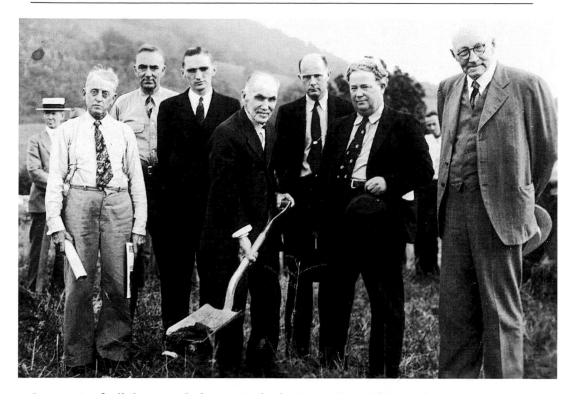

Construction finally began on the long awaited Ashe County Memorial Hospital August 29, 1939. Joe Thomas, the largest single donor to the project, took the first shovel of dirt at the groundbreaking ceremony. From left to right are Professor R. E. L. Plummer; Roy Badger; the Rev. W. J. Huneycutt; Joe Thomas; Dr. Dean Jones, Sr.; Wade Eller; and Congressman R. L. Doughton (photograph, circa 1939, courtesy Ashe County Historical Society, published in *The Skyland Post*, October 30, 1941).

churches of the county. "Every man, woman and child is being urged by the trustees of the hospital association to attend Sunday school and church this Sunday and to make a liberal contribution to the Ashe hospital," proclaimed an article in the July 4, 1940, edition of *The Skyland Post*. Sunday school superintendents, teachers, and pastors were urged to take up a special collection, and the church turning in the largest sum to hospital treasurer Roy Badger was promised "certificates of meritorious service to humanity and the county."

Joining the hospital effort in these early stages was B. L. "Lem" Hafer. His son, Gene Hafer, currently resides in Jefferson and talked with me about his father's involvement with the project in August 2014. Lem Hafer moved his family from Raleigh to Ashe County when he had the opportunity to buy the Chevrolet dealership in West Jefferson from his cousin. The dealership, renamed Parkway Chevrolet, was located where the Lifestore Bank is now, across from Boondocks Restaurant. Automobile companies, like Chevrolet, encouraged their dealers to become involved in community affairs. It was good for business, and Hafer was a businessman. Although not a charter member of the Jeffersons Rotary Club, he was one of the first members to be inducted after the club was chartered. Hafer became one of the 18 original trustees of the hospital and was soon made chairman of the finance committee with Wade Eller, Sr.[62]

Funding for the ambitious hospital project was a struggle for the community, so Hafer had his work cut out for him. Then Mother Nature threw another wrench into fundraising in August and September 1940, with two floods in less than three weeks. Bridges across creeks and the river were washed away in almost every community in the county, and many roads were closed. Sections of Obids, Idlewild, Grassy Creek, Silas Creek, Laurel Springs, Toliver and other communities were practically isolated. Many families lost everything they had. Newspaper accounts of the dire situation wrought by the flooding ran next to the latest account of Hitler's deadly blitz in London.[63]

Despite the impact of these major events, work began on the water and sewer system for the hospital in mid–December 1940, with a crew of 20 WPA workers under the supervision of Nelson Baldwin of Lansing. Thanks to the continued generosity of Roy and Guy Badger, four springs, approximately 4,000 feet from the hospital building and originating from the west side of Mount Jefferson, then known as Negro Mountain, would supply the hospital with all the water it would need. A reservoir with a 12,600 gallon capacity was built not far from the highway side of the mountain, and the water was piped from the springs to the reservoir. The sewage disposal pit was dug behind the hospital. Materials for the project were estimated to cost $800 and were the responsibility of the sponsor—the Ashe County Memorial Hospital Association, through the Ashe County Commissioners. The cost of the labor was borne by the WPA.[64]

The final fundraising drive was underway. An estimated $3,000 was needed to finish construction of the project, provide water and sewer and equip the hospital for operation. "If everyone will give a 'little,' this can be done without 'hurting' anyone," declared an editorial in *The Skyland Post*. The Rev. R. H. Stone was chairman of this final drive, and citizens who had not yet purchased a membership in the Ashe County Memorial Hospital Association were urged to do so, and those who had were urged to buy another share.[65]

Meanwhile, the homemaking department of the National Youth Administration (NYA) program in Ashe County was busy making sheets, pillow cases, towels and other linens needed for the new hospital to open. The NYA was part of the WPA and focused on providing work and education for those age 16 to 25, male and female. Mrs. Carlos Thomas, county supervisor for the program, appealed to the Women's Auxiliary of Ashe County Memorial Hospital for help getting material donated for the linen project, and the women took the donation idea to their church auxiliaries.[66]

As late as just days before the hospital was to open, *The Skyland Post* reported continuing efforts to raise the last $3,000 so that the hospital could open debt-free, with a little extra for start-up operating costs. Lem Hafer directed the last minute appeal to raise the money needed. Donors were listed in *The Skyland Post*. "Every man, woman and child is urged to co-operate. Ministers, school teachers, principals and professional men in particular are requested to assist in making this drive a success." People were making donations up through the opening ceremony, November 1, 1941, but, despite the last minute contributions, Treasurer Roy Badger reported the effort fell short of its goal by about a thousand dollars.[67] The frenzy of fund raising was reflective of the community's commitment to the hospital project. The level of support realized was remarkable for any day or time, but to have accomplished this during the hard times of the Great Depression, while contending with several catastrophic weather events and World War II in the wings, was remarkable.

While the people of Ashe County and the surrounding area worked hard for their hospital, if their leaders had not reached out to the powerful Congressman Robert Lee Doughton (1863–1954), their dream might not have been realized. His support was critical to securing the WPA funding needed for the construction of the hospital. "Doughton was a big reason we got a lot of what we have in Ashe County," says Emmett Barker of Jefferson.[68] Letters on file in Wilson Library's Special Collections Library, at the University of North Carolina at Chapel Hill, bear this out. Constituents wrote to Doughton as though he were family, and he responded in kind. Many of the letters relating to the hospital bore the signatures of familiar movers and shakers in the area. I recognized the elegant flourish of Principal Plummer's signature on his Healing Springs High School stationery, as he tracked the progress of the WPA application for the Ashe County Memorial Hospital's construction. Doughton promptly responded to Plummer's March 13, 1939, inquiry relative to "Application No. 30911" for the hospital in Jefferson, North Carolina.

My husband Louis and I visited the old Doughton homeplace, near the entrance to the Blue Ridge Parkway on N.C. Highway 18. The big Queen Anne style home was built for Congressman Doughton in 1898. Now Doughton Hall Bed and Breakfast, the home has been carefully restored and is now listed on the National Register of Historic Places. The photographs on the parlor wall reflect the political stature of the original owner, a United States Representative from North Carolina's Ninth District from 1911 to 1953. In one image, Doughton stands behind President Franklin D. Roosevelt, as he signs the bill establishing Social Security in August 1935. From the papers I read at Wilson Library, I learned Doughton was instrumental in the formulation and passage of the groundbreaking legislation and was a leader in much of the major tax legislation of the era. When his constituency urged him to run for governor in the 1930s, it was President Roosevelt who asked him to stay in Congress—his role was too critical to Roosevelt's agenda. Doughton stayed. He served a total of 42 years in Congress, chairman of the powerful House Committee on Ways and Means 1933–1947 and 1949–1953, the longest of anyone previously.[69]

The Congressman's roots went deep in the Appalachian region he represented. The son of Jonathon Horton and Rebecca Jones Doughton, his family traced back to before the American Revolution. His father pushed education, and Doughton was educated in schools in Laurel Springs and Sparta, at one time the student of J. J. Thomas, prominent citizen of West Jefferson and major contributor to the Ashe County Memorial Hospital project. Doughton, sometimes credited as one of the wisest men in Congress, never had the opportunity to attend college, although he received honorary degrees from the University of North Carolina and Catawba College later in life.[70]

West Jefferson Mayor Dale Baldwin remembers the Congressman as a tall, lanky man, known in the halls of Congress and by his constituents as "Farmer Bob," "Uncle Bob," and "Muley," perhaps a reference to his tenacity when it came to sticking to a decision and perhaps a reference to his horse trading acumen, both on the farm and in Congress. Doughton's down home, modest demeanor belied a sharp mind and a shrewd political strategist. He accomplished much in his long career, including getting the Blue Ridge Parkway moved so that it ran through Ashe County instead of Wilkes. The Parkway, which connects Shenandoah National Park in Virginia with Great Smoky Mountains National Park in Tennessee, bears a stretch named Doughton Park.[71]

When Doughton retired from Congress January 3, 1953, on his doctor's orders, he was the oldest member of Congress, at 88. He had served 21 terms, under seven U.S. presidents, and had never been defeated for public office. He died in his Laurel Springs farmhouse at the age of 90, apparently from a heart attack. His funeral was held at the Sparta Baptist Church, where he was a member and a deacon for many years.[72] Louis drove me by the cemetery after we left the old homeplace, and together we found the grave of the Congressman, his two wives, Belle Boyd Greer (died 1895) and Lillie Striker Hix (died 1946), on either side of him. It struck me that this man of humble beginnings seems never to have forgotten his roots, but rather embraced them throughout his long years of service. His name is connected to some of the most far-reaching legislation in our nation's history, yet much of what he achieved was dedicated to the specific and personal needs of those back home.

8

Ashe County Memorial Hospital, Inc.: The Reality

To commemorate the dedication of the new Ashe County Memorial Hospital, *The Skyland Post*, published and edited by Ed M. Anderson, printed a 20-page special edition October 30, 1941. "The establishment of this Hospital is a great compliment to the vision and unselfish leadership of many of our citizens and clearly demonstrates the fine cooperative spirit that prevails among our people to promote enterprises that are for the common good of all."[1] Everyone was invited to the opening, and everyone was invited to bring a gift for the hospital, "if nothing more than a jar of beans." Coal was mentioned specifically as an appropriate offering. An earlier appeal for women of the county to fill at least a dozen cans for the hospital was renewed, and it also was suggested the hospital could use "potatoes, cabbage, beans and other vegetables that could be stored."[2] During the opening week, more than 400 cans of food were donated, and *The Skyland Post* gave credit where credit was due and published a list of donors.[3]

To the sparsely populated Ashe County, the gathering of an estimated 1,500 people for the dedication of the long-awaited hospital must have seemed like a cast of thousands. The building opened for public inspection at 11 o'clock Saturday, November 1, 1941, and at two o'clock the formal dedication ceremony began in front of the hospital. Along with Congressman Doughton, other notable participants included the Hon. Frank H. Dryden of Washington, D.C., the acting commissioner of the WPA. and Dr. W. S. Rankin, of the Duke Endowment. President of the Ashe County Memorial Hospital Association, W. B. Austin presided; the Rev. R. H. Stone delivered the invocation; and Ira T. Johnston gave the welcome address. The building was officially presented by Dryden and officially accepted by the secretary of the hospital association, Wade E. Eller. Dr. Fred Hubbard introduced Dr. Rankin for the main address.[4]

In his address to the assembly, Congressman Doughton emphasized the importance of health to the community and the nation. "It has been clearly demonstrated that investments in health and security of the American people pay enormous dividends in good citizenship and increased efficiency. This hospital that we dedicate today is more than a hospital. It is a symbol of a well planned and expanding public health program, a symbol of an increasing public concern over the health of our people." The Congressman and those

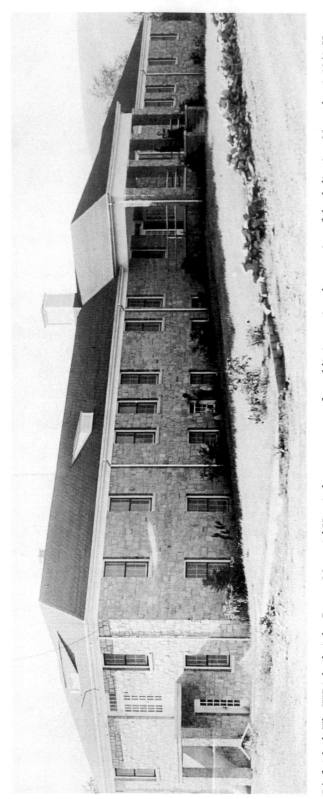

It's finished! The WPA-built Ashe County Memorial Hospital was set to open for public inspection the morning of the dedication, November 1, 1941. Here a workman puts a finishing touch on the front window while two women confer on the front porch. The woman on the right is believed to be Lettie Jones (photograph circa 1941, courtesy Evelyn Jones).

he spoke to that day were unaware the failing negotiations for peace between the United States and Japan, which shared the local headlines with the long awaited hospital, would end in the bombing of Pearl Harbor five weeks later.[5]

Having won the struggle for building a hospital, the community tackled the challenge of outfitting, staffing and operating a hospital. Once again the community anted up, with a little help from friends. Dr. Fred Hubbard donated most of the equipment in the operating room, and some furnishings and equipment came from the old Jones Memorial Infirmary in Lansing, which had closed in 1938. The estate of Dr. Lester Jones gave hospital beds, mattresses and tables as a memorial to the late doctors Thomas Jones and Lester Jones. Contributions from the community furnished rooms and wards, many as memorial gifts honoring family members. The Jefferson Odd Fellows Lodge No. 38 also furnished a ward, and the Wesleyan Guild of the West Jefferson Methodist Church furnished the office. Among the names listed as donors of rooms were the children of Dr. Arthur Lee "Bud" Jones and the children

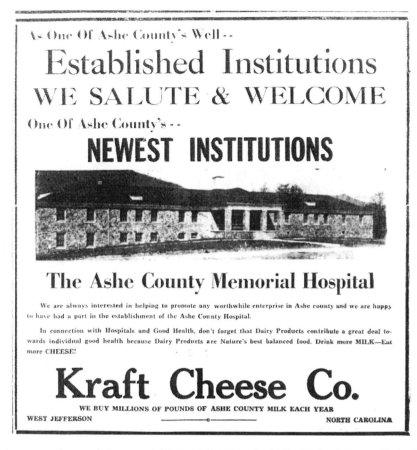

As One Of Ashe County's Well --

Established Institutions
WE SALUTE & WELCOME

One Of Ashe County's --

NEWEST INSTITUTIONS

The Ashe County Memorial Hospital

We are always interested in helping to promote any worthwhile enterprise in Ashe county and we are happy to have had a part in the establishment of the Ashe County Hospital.

In connection with Hospitals and Good Health, don't forget that Dairy Products contribute a great deal towards individual good health because Dairy Products are Nature's best balanced food. Drink more MILK—Eat more CHEESE!

Kraft Cheese Co.
WE BUY MILLIONS OF POUNDS OF ASHE COUNTY MILK EACH YEAR

WEST JEFFERSON   NORTH CAROLINA

Local businesses took out ads in a special "Hospital Edition" of *The Skyland Post*, published October 30, 1941, welcoming the new hospital and inviting everyone to come to the dedication (courtesy N.C. Department of Cultural Resources).

and grandchildren of Dr. Joseph Orrin Wilcox. A memorial for Dr. Manley Blevins, started by Ashe County farmer R. W. Hardin, was dedicated to furnishing a ward.[6] The Athens Stove Works, Inc., one of the South's major manufacturers of stoves and ranges, donated "one of their handsome all-enamel white 'Maid of Athens' ranges for the hospital," urged in their generosity by the local Rhodes Furniture Company, agent for the manufacturer in the area.[7] Despite their small percentage of Ashe County's population, African Americans did their part, contributing money for furnishing a room in the hospital. News reports specifically identified donations totaling $57.25 from African American communities in Jefferson, Crumpler, Grassy Creek, West Jefferson, and Fleetwood, and published a list of African American contributors from Cove Branch with the amount of their contributions.[8]

The Duke Endowment stepped up with an offer to match funds in the amount of $3,000, raised for the purchase of equipment and fixtures. The push was on to take advantage of this time-limited opportunity for matching funds. The heating, plumbing and lighting fixtures had to be purchased and installed at a cost of $2,000 before the Duke Endowment match could be secured. The Women's Auxiliary of the Ashe County Memorial Hospital asked local merchants to put out containers for hospital donations and came up

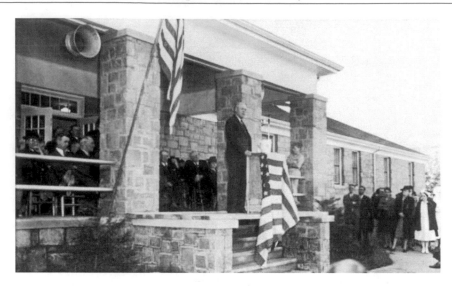

The 24-bed Ashe County Memorial Hospital was formally opened and dedicated with speeches by a host of dignitaries. The boy leaning against the stone pillar to the right of the podium is believed to be a very young Dean C. Jones, Jr. (photograph, circa 1941, courtesy Ashe County Historical Society, published in *The Skyland Post*, October 30, 1941).

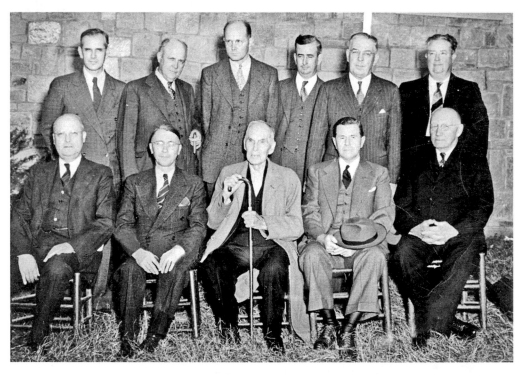

Notables participating in the opening of Ashe County Memorial Hospital November 1, 1941, included, left to right: first row—W. B. Austin; Ira T. Johnston; J. J. Thomas; WPA Acting Commissioner Frank H. Dryden; and Congressman R. L. Doughton; second row—Dr. Fred Hubbard; director of the Duke Endowment Dr. W. S. Rankin; Dr. Dean Jones, Sr.; the Rev. W. T. Whittington; State WPA Administrator C. C. McGinnis; and Wade Eller (photograph courtesy Ashe County Historical Society, published in *The Skyland Post*, November 6, 1941).

with a plan to involve school children in the fundraising with a special hospital school fund campaign. Children were asked to donate a dime to the hospital. Stella Anderson's column in *The Skyland Post* told the story of a little girl who set a goal of raising one dollar to contribute. When she fell short of her goal, she sold her treasured Easter eggs to come up with the balance. The senior class of West Jefferson High School, the largest in the history of the school with 39 graduates, presented $20 to the hospital as a memorial to the class of 1941. Other area high schools, including Elkland, Nathans Creek and Brown, made contributions too. Reid Sturdivant was tapped as acting chairman of the hospital drive with the departure of the Rev. Stone, who had served in this role December 1940 through March 1941, and the Hospital Auxiliary joined in soliciting contributions and memberships. *The Skyland Post* reported that "Mrs. B. W. Tugman and Mrs. Lem Hafer raised $106.45; in Jefferson, Mrs. W. B. Austin, Mrs. Bryan Oliver and Mrs. Glenn Little were at work fundraising; and, Mrs. Dean Jones, Miss Ruby Huddler and Miss Barker were working in Lansing."[9]

Patient rooms included a hospital bed, dresser, a table, and two chairs, with much of the new furniture purchased from the Rhodes Furniture company in West Jefferson and some beds from a firm in Bristol, Tennessee. The beds and other furnishings were touted as "the most modern that money can buy." Each regular patient room also included a sink.

The main floor of the hospital had two bathrooms, each with a toilet and bath. The new facility also boasted $1,000 worth of new surgical instruments and a modern, well-lighted operating room. A second operating room was set up next door to the general operating room and dedicated for emergency use. Each operating room had two large windows, providing "plenty of fresh air" and insuring that no odors or gases escaped to the rest of the hospital. A new $1,700 electrical sterilizer was ordered, and another smaller sterilizer was installed in the operating room.[10] When it was learned that $750 more was needed to cover the cost of the x-ray and sterilizer equipment, the Duke Endowment provided the full amount.[11] The W.M.U. of the Warrensville church held a shower for the hospital, collecting contributions of blankets, pillows and towels.[12] The Woman's Society of Christian Service of the Jefferson Methodist Church, which included a number of very active members of the Hospital

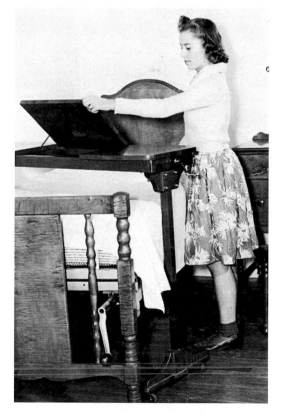

A National Youth Administration worker shows off the latest in furnishings and equipment in a patient room. Daily bed rates were set at four dollars for a two-bed room, five dollars for a one-bed room, and three dollars for a bed in a ward (photograph, circa 1941, courtesy Evelyn Jones, published in *The Skyland Post*, October 30, 1941).

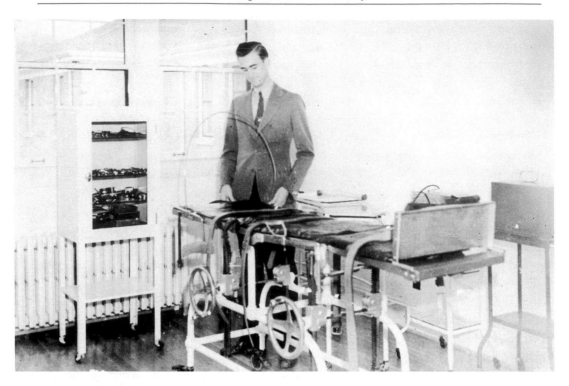

Ray Lowery looks over the new operating room before opening day of the new Ashe County Memorial Hospital. The rate set for use of the operating room for minor operations was five dollars and for major operations ten dollars. Anesthetization was five dollars (courtesy Evelyn Jones, *The Skyland Post*, October 30, 1941).

Auxiliary, contributed flatware.[13] The hospital grounds received attention as well, with donations of native trees and shrubs secured by the Auxiliary.[14]

In October 1940, with the construction of the hospital completed, Dr. W. S. Rankin of the Duke Endowment, who had offered his guidance throughout much of the organization of the hospital movement, stepped in to help with staffing the facility. The executive committee of the Ashe County Memorial Hospital Association, consisting of W. B. Austin, Wade Eller, J. Bruce Hash, Reid Sturdivant, and Ed Anderson, first pursued leasing the hospital to Dr. Fred Hubbard to run, but he declined the arrangement, citing his commitment to his hospital in North Wilkesboro. He offered, instead, to serve as head of the surgical staff and perform the major operations, charging the hospital only his regular surgical fee per patient. Dr. Rankin described Dr. Hubbard, then president of the North Carolina Medical Association, as "one of North Carolina's outstanding surgeons." Hubbard, of course, was a familiar face and well thought of in Ashe County, as he had treated and delivered many residents of the county at Wilkes Hospital. He would maintain his association with Ashe County Memorial until March 1943, when hospital records indicate Hubbard was granted a leave of absence to serve in the military for the duration of World War II. Dr. Dean Jones was designated as assistant to Dr. Hubbard, superintendent of the new hospital and resident physician. Rankin praised Jones as well, saying, "You are fortunate in having a man here in your county with his qualifications."[15]

Dr. Jones offered to take the responsibility for running the hospital, both medically and financially, receiving a salary of $3,000 for the first year of the hospital's operation, providing the hospital made that much. If not, he would take the loss in salary. If there were any profits beyond $3,000, he would share in those. This meant Jones would subsidize the hospital with a large share of his professional fees. The generous arrangement, readily agreed to by the hospital trustees, would continue for several years.[16] Former AMH business manager Mary Lou Brooks confirmed that Dr. Jones did not take any fee for his professional services until later in the life of the hospital. When he finally did get a regular salary, it was much less than the income from his fees. Lettie Jones joined her husband in this arrangement, handling the office work at the hospital without pay through the early years of the hospital's existence. Only later was she paid a small salary.[17]

The nursing staff assembled to open the hospital was impressive, not in number—there were only three—but in experience and education. From Rugby, Virginia, Miss Fannie

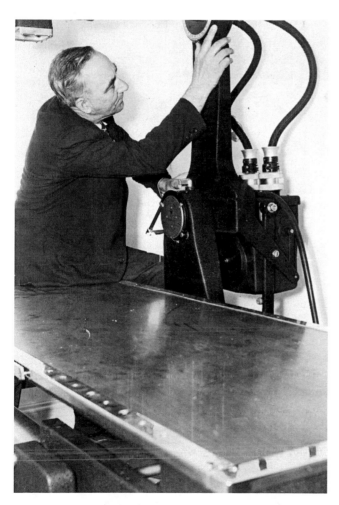

L. Perry joined the staff as operating room nurse. She was a graduate of the Maryland General Hospital of Baltimore and previously worked with a hospital in Baltimore and Grace Hospital in Richmond, Virginia. Mrs. Virginia Ashley Greene, formerly a public health nurse in Alleghany County, attended Radford State Teachers College, received her nursing degree from Pittsburgh City Hospital, did postgraduate work at Peabody College in Nashville, Tennessee, and worked there for a number of years. Mrs. Greene would donate her first month on the job. Mrs. Betha Moody of Rock Hill, South Carolina, graduated from Mt. Sinai Hospital in Philadelphia, went to graduate school, and had extensive experience with the hospital in Rock Hill. The nurses were assisted by 18 National Youth Administration girls, trained as

Roy Badger, who did so much to get the hospital off the ground, examines an x-ray machine in the new Ashe County Memorial Hospital. The cost of an x-ray was set at five dollars (photograph, circa 1941, courtesy Evelyn Jones, published in *The Skyland Post*, October 30, 1941).

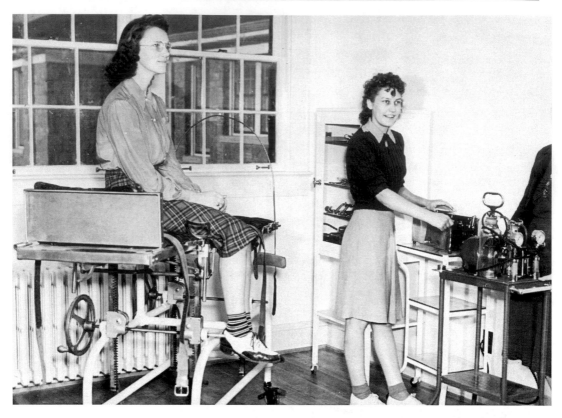

Two National Youth Administration workers help ready the new hospital for opening day—Norma Hart-zog is seated on the operating table; Myrtle Koontz is standing by the sterilizer. The NYA played a role in supplying the hospital with linens and cabinetry and later assisting with clerical duties and patient care (photograph, circa 1941, courtesy Evelyn Jones, published in *The Skyland Post*, October 30, 1941).

part of the Ashe County NYA's hospital attendant project to perform a variety of jobs, including carrying patient trays and doing some clerical work, and the janitorial work was done by several young African American men, working three to a shift.[18]

Ashe County Memorial Hospital was ready for patients, and the first patient, the morning of the dedication ceremony, was Langdon Scott, destined to become the hospital's business manager. He cut his right hand on a saw at the hospital and was treated by Dr. Jones. The first "bed" patient at Ashe County Memorial Hospital, recalls Gionia Badger Cook, was Walter Haywood Worth, cashier of Northwestern Bank, who suffered a stroke while teaching Sunday school, the day after the dedication. Before the week was out, an estimated 30 patients had received treatment at the hospital. Figures released at the end of the first month of operation reflected: 165 people treated; nine serious operations performed; 34 x-rays taken; 95 lab tests; four accident cases; nine medical cases; and three obstetrical patients. *The Skyland Post* regularly reported admissions and discharges by name.[19]

That same opening day on which Dr. Jones treated Langdon Scott's hand, Dr. Fred Hubbard performed surgery on young Mary Ann Miller (Goslen). I talked with Mary Ann in West Jefferson, August 16, 2014, and learned she grew up in Dog Creek, between Jefferson and Laurel Springs, the daughter of Thomas "Fender" Miller, a farmer, and Edna Bina

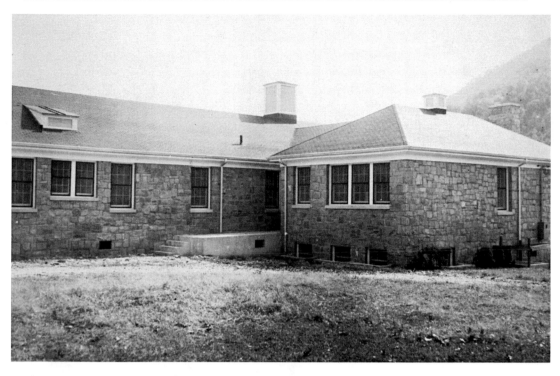

The two operating rooms were located in this outer wing of the hospital, insuring quiet and preventing the escape of any vapors or gases into the main part of the hospital (photograph, circa 1941, courtesy Evelyn Jones, published in *The Skyland Post*, October 30, 1941).

Miller. When she was nine years old Mary Ann started complaining about pain in her leg; her parents did not pay much attention, but when she developed a high fever and the pain became excruciating, her mother took her to Dr. Reid in West Jefferson. He told Mrs. Miller he thought Mary Ann had osteomyelitis, a disease of the bone, which, in children, usually affects the legs or upper arms. Treatment often entails surgery to remove parts of the bone that have died. Ashe County Memorial Hospital had not yet opened, so Dr. Reid advised that Mary Ann go to Wilkes Hospital if she was not better by morning. During the night, Mary Ann's condition got so bad she was rushed to Wilkes Hospital, where Dr. Fred Hubbard did emergency surgery that same night. She was in the hospital six weeks.

Sometime after her release, a chunk of bone was protruding from the open wound on Mary Ann's leg, and her father took her back to see Dr. Hubbard. He said the bone had to be removed, and he scheduled the procedure at the new Ashe County Memorial Hospital in Jefferson, the day of the hospital's grand opening. "Dr. Hubbard was very enthusiastic about the new hospital," Goslen recalls. "I was sitting on a chair with my leg propped up. The pain was horrible. Blood gushed out and dropped to the floor. Dr. Hubbard said to me, 'You have shed the first drop of blood in the Ashe County Hospital.' He told me I needed to remember that, because it was very important. I was considered an outpatient for the surgical procedure. I hobbled along on my crutches with my father to tour the hospital. As I remember, we saw empty beds in rooms. Patients had not yet been admitted to the hospital."

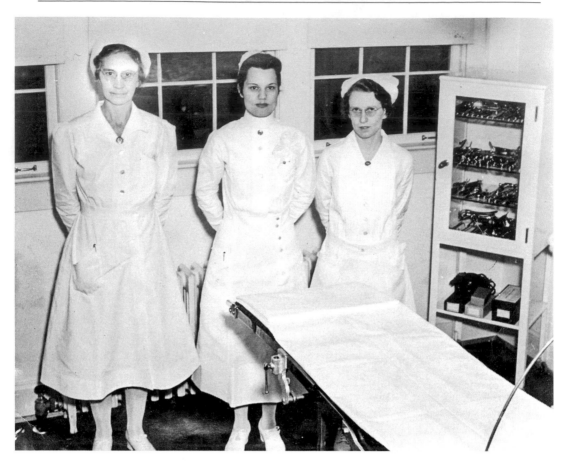

The original nursing staff of Ashe County Memorial Hospital consisted of three well educated and experienced women (left to right): Mrs. Virginia Ashley Greene, from Ashe County; Miss Fannie Perry, of Rugby, Virginia; Mrs. Betha Moody of Rock Hill, South Carolina. At the time the hospital opened, the monthly salary for a general duty nurse was $50 and for an operating room nurse $65 (courtesy Evelyn Jones).

Dr. Hubbard asked bone specialists from the hospital in Charlotte to evaluate Mary Ann's condition. "They said that I would never walk again without crutches or be confined to a wheelchair, but I was determined to walk again. When my parents were out in the field working, I would scoot over to the edge of the bed. Carefully, I would put as much weight on my right leg as I could. Then I would stand on my left, which was still bandaged, and put as much weight on it as I could. Tears rolled down my face from the pain, but I did this exercise every day. In about a year, I was able to walk again without crutches. I credit Dr. Hubbard with saving my life. He was an incredible and compassionate man."

It was not long after Ashe County Hospital had opened that December 7, 1941, came, a day that would "live in infamy," the day the Japanese bombed Pearl Harbor. The family of Amos Graybeal was sitting in the living room listening to President Roosevelt's famous speech on the radio. Lib Graybeal McRimmon's grandmother, Daisy Burkett Graybeal, got up from her chair and fell, breaking her hip. The new Ashe County Memorial Hospital was just a short distance down the road from the Graybeal home, and the family drove Daisy

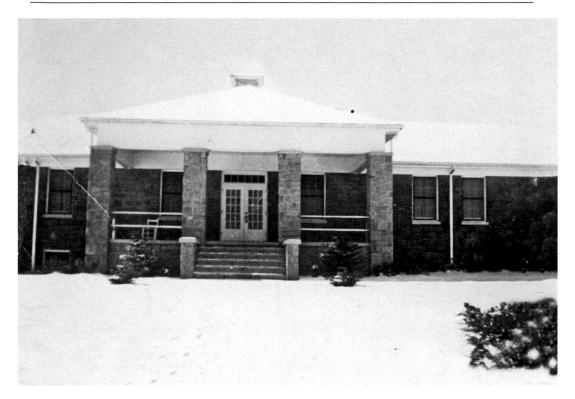

The front entrance of Ashe County Memorial Hospital was destined to undergo several renovations. The focal point of the structure were the beautiful stone pillars, the work of local stonemason O. H. Baldwin (courtesy Evelyn Jones).

there for help. Lib McRimmon filled me in on the story at the Graybeal home in September 2014. "Nobody else was in the hospital," says McRimmon, "so grandmother had the staff's full attention." One of the family stayed with her all the time, because, in those days, you didn't leave anybody alone in a hospital, but Dr. Jones and a nurse were in attendance, and Daisy was in good hands. After a couple of weeks in the hospital, she made a strong recovery, although she did rely on a cane, which she discreetly hid under her chair when people came to call.

When I started trying to identify some of the first patients in Ashe County Memorial, I thought of a story Stephen Shoemaker and I had included in our book *Stephen Shoemaker: The Paintings and Their Stories*, published in 2013. The story is about a little girl, Hopal, the daughter of James and Hattie Turner. The family lived below Stikes Hollar, near Warrensville in a house that overlooked the railroad tracks at the cut at Devil's Stairs. On June 2, 1945, the child was struck by the train on the tracks below the house, as it headed toward Devil's Stairs, coming from West Jefferson. Desperate neighbors quickly put the child on the train, and the engineer put the train in reverse and headed back toward West Jefferson—his destination, the hospital in Jefferson. The engineer maneuvered the train as close as he could to the hospital, and the child was transported from the train to the hospital, but it was too late.

Shoemaker first heard the story when he was painting the mural, *Cut at Devil's Stairs*,

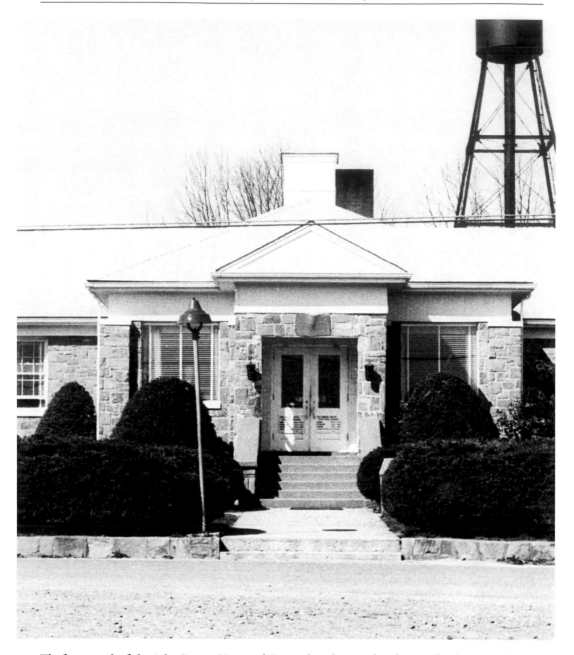

The front porch of the Ashe County Memorial Hospital was later enclosed, partially obscuring the stone pillars. Eventually, a water tower was added in back of the building (courtesy Evelyn Jones).

on the side of the Dollar Tire building, as you come into West Jefferson on Highway 16. He later completed the painting *Virginia Creeper at Devil's Stairs* that commemorates this tragic event. The hospital, of course, was the old Ashe County Memorial, and I had no way of knowing at the time I told this story behind the painting, that I would have occasion to retell it in another context, but it is part of the story of Ashe County Memorial too, as are all the happy and sad events where the hospital played a role.

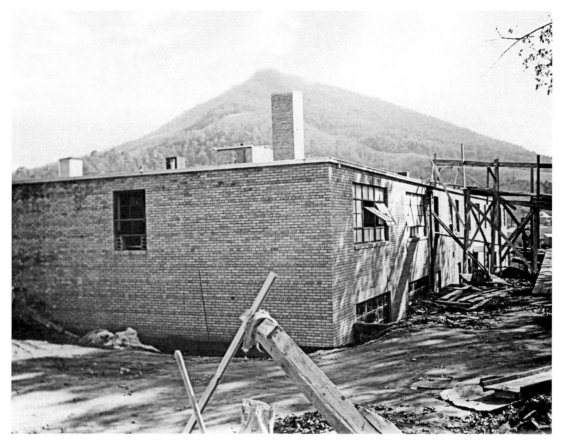

This brick addition to the hospital in 1951 added 25 more beds, an x-ray and laboratory department, and a new operating room. The brick was a departure from the stone façade of the original building (courtesy N.C. Department of Cultural Resources).

It was not long, however, before the 24 beds in the original design for Ashe County Memorial Hospital became inadequate to meet the needs of the community, and in 1951, an additional 25 beds were added, along with an x-ray and laboratory department and a new operating room. State and federal funds made up approximately 86 percent of the funding required for this project, and the hospital provided the balance. The Joint Commission of Accreditation made a surprise visit to Ashe County Memorial Hospital in 1952 and granted a provisional approval on inspection of the facility. By their next survey, full approval was granted.[20]

In the mid–1950s, a nurses' quarters finally was added behind Ashe County Memorial Hospital. Hospital records indicate plans for the project had been on file with the N.C. Medical Care Commission since 1947, with action pending fund availability. The executive committee of the board met March 23, 1953, and authorized William B. Austin, president of the board of trustees for the hospital, to file a renewal application. The financing was secured, and the nurses' quarters was built at a cost of $80,000. Hill-Burton Federal Aid was used again, as was the case with the funding for the 25 bed addition, with local funds making up a share of the cost, plus any expenses not covered by the federal funding. Doris

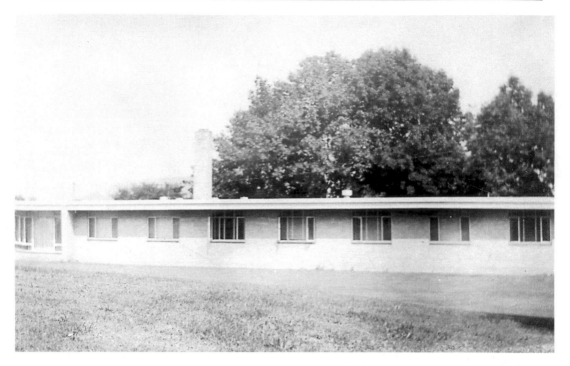

A nurses' quarters was discussed soon after the hospital opened but was not built until the mid–1950s. Lindsey Madison Gudger of Asheville, the architect for the 1951 addition to the hospital, was also the architect for the nurses' quarters. Later the building was converted to office space and now serves as a day care (courtesy N.C. Department of Cultural Resources).

Oliver remembers some staff lived in the building full-time, but it also was used as temporary lodging during severe weather events, like the 1960 snow. There was a small kitchen, but the staff who resided there took their main meals in the dining room, as they always had. The nurses' quarters served its purpose, but around the late 1960s, the building was converted to office space for the director of nursing and the business office. In more recent years, the nurses' quarters was converted to a children's day care.[21] Visible from Evelyn's kitchen window, the happy chaos of the present-day playground, which backs up to her yard, is a positive reminder of the children who came into the world in the old hospital.

By 1966, the hospital's 50-bed capacity was proving insufficient, and beds were being placed in the halls to accommodate the overflow. An additional 30 beds were needed, plus expansion of other hospital facilities, including outpatient diagnostic clinics, emergency room, and laboratory and x-ray. A promotional brochure for the Ashe County Memorial Hospital Building Fund Campaign noted, "A whole new generation of Ashe County citizens is being given the opportunity to participate in a vital community project." Statistical information covering the opening of the hospital in 1941 through September 1965 was presented in a brochure released by Ashe County Memorial Hospital, Inc. May 2, 1966: 35,129 patients treated (excluding newborns); 241,217 days of patients receiving services; 9,513 babies delivered; 3,599 major operations; 8,989 minor operations; and 12,520 emergency room visits. The average number of full-time employees at the hospital for the previous year had grown to 84. The fundraising brochure listed the total cost of the addition as an estimated

$450,000 and Ashe County was asked to come up with $250,000 to match federal Hill-Burton funds.

Despite the several additions made to the hospital, Ashe County Memorial was outgrowing its location on McConnell Street, and new accommodations were needed to meet the needs of the community. The decision was made to build a new hospital, now called Ashe Memorial Hospital, Inc., according to minutes of the November 8, 1969, shareholders meeting, which indicate the vote was taken to drop "county" from the name of the hospital at that time. D. R. Allen Construction Company, out of Fayetteville, North Carolina, got the construction contract for the new hospital. During the building process, recalls local contractor Mark Vannoy, company officials regularly flew into the county to check on progress. On one such trip their small plane crashed somewhere in the upper end of Ashe County. Fortunately and miraculously, there were no injuries.[22]

The new facility was dedicated October 31, 1971. Thousands turned out for the event, despite the rain, double parking along the nearby highway. Tom Cockerham was the hospital administrator by then and in charge of the dedication ceremony, which was moved inside. Local radio station WKSK broadcast the event and also set up loudspeakers in the hospital

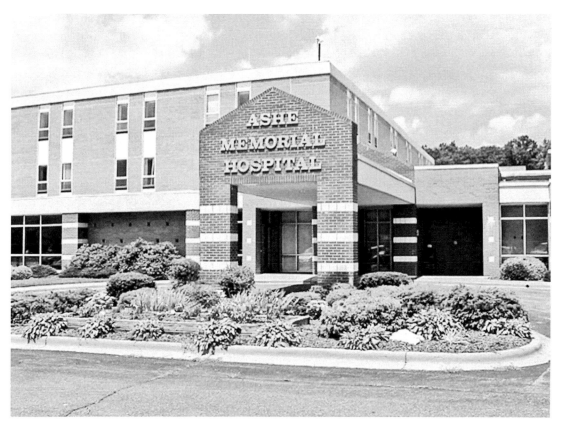

Another addition to Ashe County Memorial Hospital was made in 1966, but it was not long before a larger, more modern space was needed, and a hospital, now renamed "Ashe Memorial Hospital," was built on Hospital Drive in Jefferson. The building and its campus have undergone numerous additions and renovations since its opening in 1971 (courtesy AMH).

so everybody could hear. Dr. Dean Jones, Sr., chief of staff of Ashe Memorial Hospital, recognized the staff, and Mrs. Ed. M. (Stella) Anderson, finance chairman, recognized the fundraising committees for achieving their goal. J. Gwyn Gambill, president of the hospital executive committee and Trustee W. B. Oliver recognized the North Carolina Medical Care Commission, charged with providing part of the financing for small, rural nonprofit and public hospitals in North Carolina, through the issuance of tax-exempt revenue bonds. Also recognized were the Duke Endowment, the Appalachian Regional Commission, and other special guests.[23]

The medical staff listed in the program for the dedication included the familiar names: Robert L. Dickson, M.D.; Roy O. Freeman, M.D.; Dean C. Jones, Sr., M.D.; Dean C. Jones, Jr., M.D.; Elam S. Kurtz, M.D.; C. E. Miller, M.D.; Edward J. Miller, M.D.; and J. Lewis Sigmon, Jr., M.D. Peggy Ashley, R.N., was the director of nursing; Mary G. Brooks managed the business office; Kate Duncan, R.N., was head nurse for the operating room; Henry Lum still supervised x-ray and the laboratory; and Virginia Barker was in charge of the dietary department. Ida Marsh, C.R.N.A., headed anesthesia, and Mary Severt, R.R.L., headed up medical records. Ann Brown continued as Tom Cockerham's administrative assistant.

Ashe County native Betty Avery remembers the opening of the new hospital. "I think everybody was kind of sad to see the old hospital go but realized we needed the new facility."[24] The day for the big move came. Doris Oliver describes the task of transferring patients from the old hospital to the new. Half of the staff stayed at the old hospital to ready patients for the move, and the other half was deployed to the new hospital to receive them. "I was on the end that stayed to move patients out," she recalls, "it was sort of depressing." But there wasn't much time to dwell on the past. "We started admitting new patients the day we transferred to the new hospital."[25] "It took a little time to get used to the new hospital," Ruby Lum recalls. "When we moved to the new hospital, I thought I would never be able to figure everything out. I told Dr. Jones, Sr., I didn't know if I would ever like it there, but I got used to it. It didn't take as long as I thought it would." Among the improvements, "We had new x-ray equipment that could be moved to the patient's room, instead of the patient having to be moved to the x-ray machine."[26]

With the enlarged space at the new AMH and additional staffing to manage expanding services, the facility was bound to lose some of its former family-like atmosphere. Betty Avery, whose mother worked at both the old and new AMH, followed the changes with an insider's view. "I used to know everybody that worked in the hospital, and now I know very few people." Many staff from the old hospital continued in the new facility, but the hospital was changing and so was the population of the county and the surrounding area.[27]

9

The Ashe Memorial Hospital Board of Trustees

On December 12, 1939, Dr. W. S. Rankin, director of the Duke Endowment, addressed stock certificate members of the Ashe County Memorial Hospital Association at the courthouse in Jefferson. It was time for them to elect their board of trustees, and Dr. Rankin was there to guide them through the process. He talked about the organization of the board and stressed the importance of choosing trustees who would give the community a medical service they would use themselves. "'Don't operate a hospital you are afraid of, operate a hospital you will trust,'" he admonished his listeners.[1] His words have been heeded ever since.

The first 18 members of the new Ashe County Memorial Hosptial Board of Trustees elected that night in 1939 were W. B. "Bill" Austin; J. O. Blevins; Roy R. Badger; L. P. Colvard; C. M. Dickson; Wade E. Eller; J. Gwyn Gambill; B. Lem Hafer; J. Bruce Hash; Harris Lemly; John Littlewood; T. K. Miller; W. B. Oliver; J. E. Oliver; Prof. Robert E. Lee Plummer; E. R. Sturdivant; Joseph Jerome Thomas; and Ed M. Anderson. The following week, the trustees elected Bill Austin, president; Robert Plummer, vice-president; Joseph Jerome Thomas and T. K. Miller, vice presidents; Wade Eller, secretary; and Roy R. Badger, treasurer. An executive committee was appointed, including Bill Austin, E. R. Sturdivant, J. Bruce Hash, Wade Eller, and Ed Anderson.[2] Most of these men, so instrumental in taking Ashe County Memorial Hospital from a dream to reality, served on the hospital's board of trustees in several capacities, and some were still serving when the decision was made to build the new hospital. Over the years many of these same names continued to show up on the roster for the board, first children and then grandchildren of the original trustees. There is new blood too—even a few "not from around here."

According to veteran trustee Jim Gambill, the AMH board decided about eight years ago to place a major emphasis on insuring that every part of the county was represented on the board. "We wanted a diverse skill set—people with different world views. When we have an opening, we look for what we are missing." The strategy for diversity in the board's composition makes for better decision making. "We welcome free discussion."[3] The following represent only a few of the many who have served their community as AMH trustees.

In an article from the April 9, 1949, issue of *The State Magazine*, titled "Things of Interest in Ashe County," Ira T. Johnston penned an article, formatted as an open letter, in response to an inquiry directed to the Chamber of Commerce in Jefferson. Since there was no Chamber of Commerce in Ashe County in those days, the letter was routed to the Rotary Club, and Johnston responded on behalf of the club, describing the highlights of the community in terms of its outstanding scenery, industry and history. Among the many attractions Johnston describes are the courthouse, the old Brick Inn, the panorama of majestic mountains surrounding the town, and the following: "The new stone building over on the hill beyond the high school is the Ashe Memorial Hospital, perhaps the most successful small hospital in the state."

Johnston wrote for North Carolina newspapers, as well, supplementing his income in his early years teaching and practicing law. Described as a soft-spoken gentleman, he was born in the Pine Swamp Township in Ashe County, August 1, 1892, to John Romulus and Cisco Fletcher Johnston. He joined future Ashe County leaders Wade E. Eller, Bill Austin, Lester Segraves, Gertrude Eller Waddell, and Margaret Wilson Duncan at the Appalachian Training School at Boone, later known as Appalachian State University. He helped pay his expenses by teaching at local schools, taking his first teaching job at age 16. He entered Wake Forest College and graduated in two and a half years. Johnston continued to teach and then joined Bill Austin at the University of North Carolina at Chapel Hill to study law. After a short stint in the U.S. Army, he returned to UNC. Meantime he married Mary Adelaide Shull of Valle Crucis in Watauga County. By 1921 he was practicing law in Jefferson, where he continued his law career for more than 50 years, serving many terms as county attorney and attorney for the Ashe County Board of Education. He was elected to two terms in the North Carolina House of Representatives in 1931 and 1939 and one term in the State Senate in 1963. He authored much of the legislation forming the basis for North Carolina's public schools and was instrumental in setting up the Teachers' and State Employees' Retirement System in North Carolina.[4]

Robert G. Barr was a member of the board of trustees for more than 35 years and director emeritus at his death in late March 2000. He was one of the leaders in Ashe County who helped bring the new hospital into being in 1971. Barr was a businessman and, together with other family members, founded the Phoenix Chair Company, which later became Thomasville Furniture Company in West Jefferson. Active politically, Barr served on the North Carolina State Highway Commission and was a delegate to National Democratic Conventions. A seven and one half mile stretch of U.S. Highway 221 in Ashe County bears his name, along with at least two secondary roads in the county.[5]

Barr's Ashe County roots ran deep. He was born November 16, 1910, to Robert Clyde Barr and Sallie Gambill Barr, pioneers in the area. Barr married Charity Vannoy in 1935, daughter of another noted pioneer couple, Robert and Dora McMillan Vannoy, who moved to Ashe County from Delaware. He was educated at West Jefferson, Lees-McRae College and Oak Ridge Military Academy and devoted much of his life to civic matters, serving on the Ashe County Board of Education and as a West Jefferson fireman for a quarter century. He was a strong supporter of the Ashe County Library and the West Jefferson Municipal Park, as well as the new Ashe Memorial Hospital.[6]

In 1998, when he was chosen to serve on the Ashe Memorial Hospital Board of Trustees, Jim Gambill, of Gambill Oil in Jefferson, was following in the footsteps of his father, J. Gwyn Gambill, who gave 48 years of continuous service to Ashe Memorial Hospital. Although considered a native of Ashe County, Jim Gambill spent the majority of his growing up years in North Wilkesboro and Florida. He attended Hargrave Military Academy in Chatham, Virginia, and Wake Forest University in North Carolina, where he studied business. Next there was a three year stint in Korea with the U.S. Army in the late 1960s, followed by seven years as commander of the 1450th Transportation Company and four years as commander of the 540th Transportation Battalion of the North Carolina National Guard. During the Gulf War, he was called up again and deployed to Iraq during Desert Storm, serving with the 30th Support Group from Durham, North Carolina. He retired as a lieutenant colonel. He has served the Ashe County community through the Lions Club, the Chamber of Commerce, and the school board. Gambill continues to serve on the AMH Board of Trustees.[7]

His father, J. Gwyn Gambill, Sr. (1906–1992), was born in Crumpler in Ashe County and worked with his father Jim and his Uncle Bob Barr in the founding of a successful hardware store. The store sold so much kerosene, the two decided to open an oil distributorship, Gambill Oil Company, in Ashe, Alleghany, Watauga, and Wilkes counties in North Carolina and Grayson and Carroll counties in Virginia. Gwyn Gambill lived in Ashe County, as his family had since before the American Revolution. He was a descendant of Martin Gambill, famous in the area for his 24 hour ride to alert Colonel William Campbell that militia commanders planned to engage British Major Patrick Ferguson. His fearless ride enabled patriot forces to assemble and march to Kings Mountain, where they defeated Ferguson's forces on October 7, 1780.[8]

Gwyn Gambill had a myriad of professional and community interests, including being a charter member of the Rotary. He was particularly active in his native Crumpler community, where he donated land for the Methodist Church and Crumpler community building, started the men's Sunday school class and the Boy Scout troop. His early and passionate support of a hospital for Ashe County was a part of this community mindedness. Gambill also served on the Governor's Advisory Council of Comprehensive Health Planning, Ashe County Health Council, Blue Ridge Health Council, and Regional Health Council of Eastern Appalachia. He became a founding trustee of Ashe County Memorial Hospital in 1938, served as president 1962–1983, and as trustee emeritus 1983–1992. When his son Jim once questioned him about his reasoning for staying in the small rural community of Ashe County, he responded he preferred being a big fish in a small pond. If it were not for some very remarkable people living by this philosophy in the greater community of Appalachia, health care and education and many of the other elements contributing to a community's sound foundation would not have received the attention they did.[9]

Like many of the early supporters of the hospital, long-time AMH trustee Frank M. James was a leader in education. A product of the Ashe County public school system, James continued his education at Appalachian State University in Boone, receiving a B.S. degree in education and history. He was only 19 years old when he embarked on his first teaching job, in an elementary school. Teaching high school was next, then four years in the military, and then in 1948, Frank was named principal of Lansing High School and Elementary School, where he stayed until 1961. He finished his career as Superintendent of Ashe County Schools in 1975. Meanwhile, he pursued a master's degree in history and public school administration and received his advanced degree in 1951. James would devote 44 years to public education, play a major role in the consolidation and accreditation of the county's schools, and serve in a variety of state and regional education organizations.[10]

Nobody knows the need for communication better than a school principal trying to decide whether or not school should be closed due to inclement weather, and schools in Appalachia have more than their share of weather events. In his early years as a principal, schools in Ashe County were not connected by telephone with the central office, making consistent decisions difficult. An amendment to the Rural Electrification Act of 1936 provided federal funding to operate nonprofit telephone systems, specifically benefiting rural areas. Frank James was instrumental in getting a telephone cooperative in Ashe County—Skyline—chartered in 1951.[11]

Born in Ashe County in August 3, 1912, Frank was the son of Samuel W. and Myrtle Sturgill James. He married Lillian Sutherland, an Ashe County native and school teacher, in 1943. He gave 34 years of continuous service to Ashe Memorial Hospital, serving on the board of trustees 1961–1995 and as president 1983–1995. Calvin Miller recalls James as a very gracious man, who was a good listener and a good thinker. Frank provided sound guidance in decision-making in his long service on the AMH Board of Trustees. People trusted and believed in him, and his presence enhanced the credibility of the board and engendered the community's support. He died in 1995. His wife, Lillian James, a strong supporter of Ashe Memorial Hospital, as well, helped to honor her husband's memory through an annual Frank M. James Memorial Golf Tournament, a fundraiser for the AMH Foundation.[12]

After James R. "Jim" Vannoy retired from the general contracting business he had founded in Jefferson, he spent three to five days a week visiting at Ashe Memorial Hospital. He was not an official volunteer, he was just visiting staff and patients; they were his friends and neighbors. He spent a good part of his career working on construction projects for the hospital, and he knew a lot of people. "He knew the importance of having a hospital in the community," comments his son Mark, who now runs J. R. Vannoy and Sons Construction Company, Inc., with his brother Eddie. "He always told us we needed to support the hospital." And that is what the family has done. The company was not in existence when the old hospital on McConnell Street was built by the WPA 1940–41, but various renovation projects, such as enclosing the entrance of the hospital and updating the emergency room, were done by the J. R. Vannoy Co. Mark Vannoy was born in the old hospital, and Dr. Dean Jones, Sr., helped bring him into the world. He remembers working on a project at the hospital, when he was 16 or 17 years old, mixing mortar and carrying brick and block.[13]

J. R. Vannoy and Sons had not yet ventured into bigger commercial projects when plans were made to replace the old Ashe County Memorial with a larger, more modern structure, so another construction company got the job, but since then, Vannoy and Sons has taken on a number of renovations and additions to the "new" hospital. The company built the Professional Building, adjacent to the hospital, which houses the doctors' offices; Segraves Nursing Home, which is now used for administrative offices; and the Mountain

Hearts facility; and they remodeled the ER and the Intensive Care Unit. "We've worked on every floor of the hospital," says Vannoy. Most recently, the company built the Imaging Center and redid the parking lot in front of the hospital.[14]

Jim Vannoy was one of 12 children born to William "Will" Vannoy and Ella Mae Faw Vannoy from the Oval community in Ashe County. Jim served in the Army in World War II and returned home to marry Wilma Christine Witherspoon, daughter of J. E. and Effie Witherspoon in Jefferson. Jim was working as a carpenter with his brother-in-law, Zeb Witherspoon, and when Zeb moved to Asheville, Jim started his own contracting business, eventually bringing his sons into the business. The company started by Jim Vannoy in 1952 has come a long way since son Mark was mixing mortar and carrying brick and block at the old hospital. There are offices in Charlotte, Winston-Salem, and Asheville, North Carolina, and in Anderson, South Carolina.[15]

Jim Vannoy died in 2002, and after his wife Wilma's death in 2004, the family approached the AMH Board of Trustees about a sizable donation in memory of Wilma, who served for many years as a volunteer at the hospital. The result was the impressive birthing unit completed in 2005 and the continued adherence to Jim Vannoy's instruction to always "support the hospital."[16]

Jan R. Caddell, president and general manager of Caddell Broadcasting, Inc., WKSK, the local radio station in West Jefferson, came to Ashe County from Hartsville, South Carolina, in July 1968. He managed WKSK for ten years, including a two year stint with a sister station in Sylva, North Carolina, and in 1978, he and his wife Lucy bought the station which sits on top of Radio Hill. I interviewed Caddell at the station in August 2014, and he talked about his old friend Dean C., Jr., and the changes at AMH. Caddell joined the Rotary, and was a member for many years with the Dr. Dean Joneses, Sr. and Jr. He and Doc (Jr.) became good friends, playing basketball together on a local team, and he remembers with fondness the jokes Doc used to carry around in his breast pocket to share with people. Caddell became a member of the board of trustees for Ashe Memorial Hospital and continues to serve on the board, currently as its treasurer.

In his early days in Ashe County, Caddell says "The Hospital Report" was part of the daily morning line-up for WKSK and included the names of those admitted and discharged from the hospital. The report was well sponsored by local business, especially the pharmacies, and its 9:00 a.m. air time drew a large audience. On admission to the hospital, patients were given the chance to opt out of having their name included in the report but most agreed to keeping their friends and neighbors and everybody else in the area informed of their medical status. This never seemed to present a problem for the patients or the station, but, of course, with the institution of HIPPA and the patients' rights to privacy rules and regulations that went with this legislation, "The Hospital Report" was phased out.

The board of trustees meets once a month and represents a cross-section of the community, including business leaders, medical personnel, educators and the arts. The 18 members are elected by hospital shareholders, as they have been since the hospital was started. Caddell has seen a lot of changes with the administration of the hospital since he first came on the board, including the switch from hiring their own administrator and running the hospital themselves to contracting with a health care provider for the management of the hospital. As treasurer, Caddell already sees improvement in the financial prospects of the hospital since the implementation of the contract with the new provider, Novant Health. "The board is dedicated to seeing it work," he confirms.

AMH Trustee Jones "Bradley" McNeill is a retired educator with 40 years' service in the Ashe County school system. The former principal of the new Ashe High School has been on the AMH Board of Trustees for about seven years, and those seven years have seen a lot of changes at AMH. First and foremost there was the change in health care providers. Like many small hospitals across the country, AMH was struggling financially, explains McNeill, when we talk in early 2015. "We had to try something," He is especially proud of the hospital's investment in an innovative system that significantly enhances the effectiveness of colonoscopies. AMH is one of only two hospitals in North Carolina with the new technology and one of only twenty nationwide. This puts the small rural hospital in Ashe County "on the leading edge of technology."

10

The Hospital Medical Staff Since 1941

As the construction of the Ashe County Memorial Hospital neared completion in the summer of 1940, Wade E. Eller updated readers of *The Skyland Post*, laying out the next step for realizing the dream for a community hospital. "It has been fully agreed by the trustees and the interested physicians of our own county that the hospital shall be set up with a surgical and medical staff that will merit the confidence and patronage of all our people, and that all diligence will be given to this most vital question in order to obtain the best possible hospital service for all of us." His words would set the tone for the years to come.[1]

Hospital records indicate the average number of employees per day in the hospital was 14 in 1942. Staff at Ashe County Memorial would remain lean through the war years but gradually grew to an average of 36 employees per day in 1954. While not all of the staff at Ashe County Memorial lived on the premises like Dr. Dean, Sr., and Lettie, many did, and the atmosphere created by the couple was distinctly family-like. Most employees were native to the area, so they had much in common. When others came from the outside, they soon fell in love with the area and its people and found their niche. Dr. Jones credited several for their outstanding contributions in the early years of the hospital, including Mrs. Theresa Badger, the cook for the hospital, who managed to serve meals for staff and patients that defied the traditional unfavorable reputation of hospital food, and Mrs. Virginia Ashley Greene, a trained nurse, who donated her services for a short period at the beginning of the hospital's operation. And then there was Nurse Kate Duncan, who somehow managed, with the help of a few aides, to handle the nursing duties at the hospital for most of World War II.[2] I was privileged to interview some of those who worked at the hospital over the years and some who are employed there today. When I first started mapping out my strategy for this project, I intended to interview a cross section of AMH employees, physicians and surgeons, nurses, nurses' aides, lab technicians, administrative types, and maintenance personnel. Interviewing is like trying to eat one potato chip. Once you talk to one person, you decide you need to talk to another and another, and folks start making suggestions for additional people with whom I simply must speak, and I do more and more research and find more and more aspects of all these professions that would be wonderful to include, and finally I reluctantly admit I cannot possibly talk to everyone or write about everyone. But that doesn't mean this is not their story too.

Kate King Duncan Barker, R.N., Interview (West Jefferson, November 17, 2014)

A few special people are so much a part of the collective memory of Ashe Memorial Hospital that their names are forever linked with the early years of that institution and with Dr. Dean Jones, Sr. Nurse Kate Duncan is one of those special few. Kate, born Amanda Enola King and nicknamed Katie by her grandfather, is from Statesville, North Carolina, and received her initial nurses' training at H. F. Long Hospital, Inc., in Statesville.

I met Kate Duncan Barker at Ashe Assisted Living and Memory Care in West Jefferson, where she now resides. Her stepdaughter, Shirley Wallace, was kind enough to introduce me, and Evelyn Jones and I settled in for a chat about old times at Ashe County Memorial. Kate Duncan was a young woman when Evelyn Price Jones worked at the hospital as a nurses' aide, and Evelyn remembers how impressed she was with the attractive nurse in her crisp uniform. I listen as Kate and Evelyn commiserate on the lack of white hose and caps and crisp uniforms, standards for dress no longer in vogue for nurses. The rules were strict in nursing schools when these two women were student nurses. Kate took a friend from nursing school home with her on weekends. The friend fell in love with Kate's older brother, and the two married in secret, because nursing students were not allowed to be married while in school. Only Kate and her mother knew about the marriage. One evening Kate's father came home to find a woman in bed with his son. The father went to his wife and demanded to know what was going on in his house. His wife had to explain that the woman was his son's wife.

Kate Duncan was 96 years old when interviewed but that is nobody's business. Her business was nursing, and, by all accounts, she was very good at it. But Kate did not want to become a nurse, confides her niece, Nan Robinson of Mooresville, North Carolina. I talked with Nan by telephone shortly after my interview with Kate and learned it was Kate's mother, a midwife with a great respect for nursing, who insisted her first daughter become a nurse. Kate had such a tender heart that her work as a hall nurse was hard on her, because she became too attached to her patients and could not bear to lose them. "She loved every baby she helped deliver," adds Nan. So Kate chose the operating room, where the risk of personal involvement with her patient was minimized. Kate and her first husband had no children of their own, and, in researching some information for me, Nan heard from other family members that Kate routinely volunteered to work holidays, so nurses with children could be at home with their families. Despite her initial resistance to a nursing career, Kate found her niche, and, Nan reflects, in her own way, took on the whole of Ashe County as her family.

Evelyn always associated Kate Duncan with the operating room and remembers the high regard in which Kate was held by both Dr. Dean Sr. and Jr. Kate worked with both father and son, and although she acknowledges each had his own unique personality, they were both all business in the operating room. "They told you what they wanted, and they got it," she declares. But her career was most closely linked with that of Dr. Dean, Sr. She was his right hand, and if he was operating, Kate was standing next to him, listening to him pray before he began the surgery, as was his custom, and anticipating his next move, ready with whatever he needed.

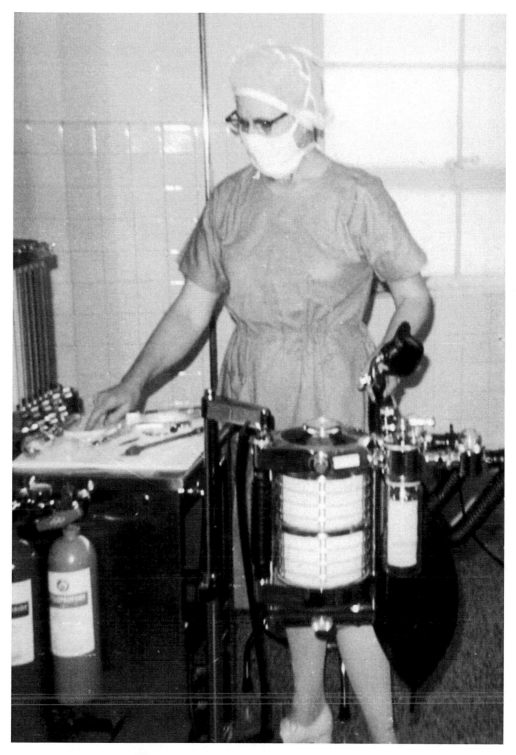

Few people are more closely linked to the early days of Ashe County Memorial Hospital than Kate Duncan, R.N., shown here at work in the old hospital (photograph, circa 1966, courtesy Evelyn Jones; published in a fundraising campaign brochure for the 1966 addition).

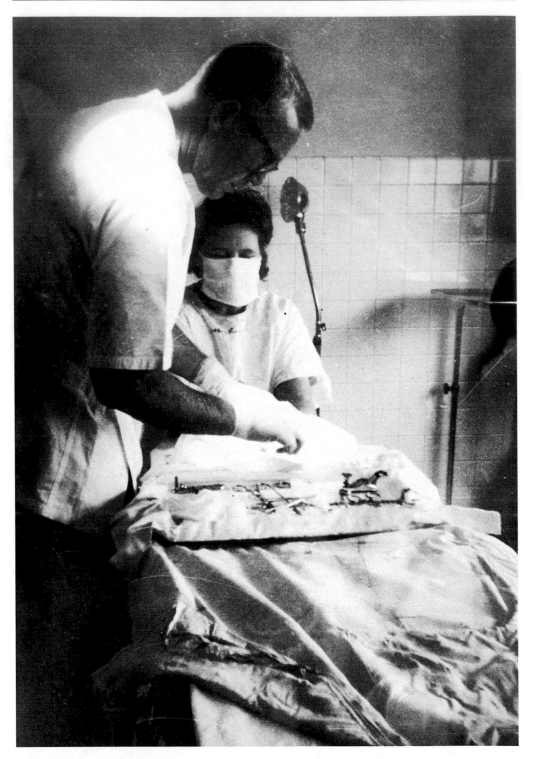

Dr. Roy Freeman, seen here at work in the operating room of the old Ashe County Memorial Hospital around 1966, was associated with the hospital in the 1960s through 1980s (courtesy Evelyn Jones; published in a fundraising campaign brochure for the 1966 addition).

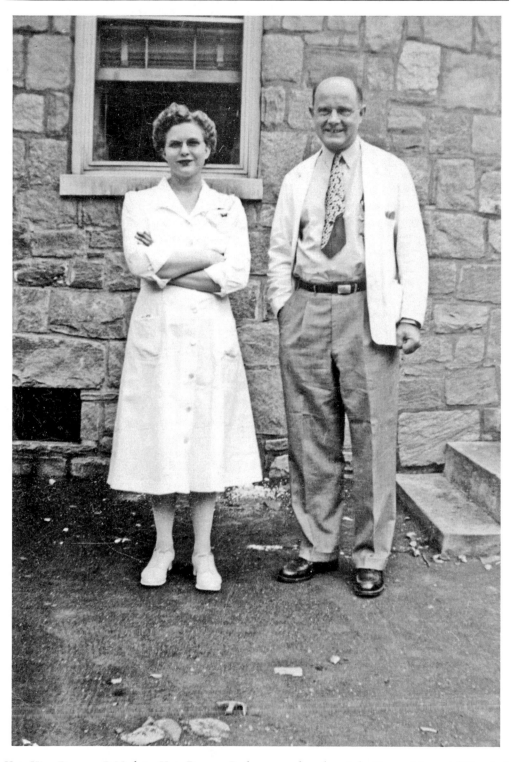

Kate King Duncan, R.N., later Kate Duncan Barker, started work at Ashe County Memorial Hospital in January 1942 and worked closely with Dr. Dean Jones, Sr. The team came to represent the beginning and end of an era in community health care (courtesy Evelyn Jones).

Duncan first started to work at the hospital in January 1942, probably right after graduation from H. F. Long Hospital. Staffing was limited at Ashe County Memorial in those early years, and she was often the only nurse on duty. This was before the days of job descriptions, and everybody did what needed to be done, and if you did not know how to do something, you learned. Dr. Jones was a good teacher, recalls Duncan. "He taught me everything I know."

Dr. Fred Hubbard, who helped with the surgeries at Ashe County Memorial initially, was in and out. He had his own hospital in North Wilkesboro, Duncan explains. Lettie Jones, Dr. Jones's wife, handled the hospital's administrative duties, and she and Dr. Jones lived in the hospital, on call 24 hours a day. "If I needed Dr. Jones, I just knocked on his door. I woke him up many a time." Duncan lived a short distance away from the hospital, off McConnell Street, and drove or walked to work, so she was on call too. Together she and Dr. Jones, Sr., set bones, delivered babies, and performed every other kind of surgery, because they were the only game in town. Duncan helped Dr. Jones when he saw his patients in the afternoons, and they worked until everybody was seen. "If he worked, I worked."

After their long history at the old Ashe County Memorial, Dr. Jones, Sr., and his nurse shared trepidations about the move to the new Ashe Memorial Hospital in 1971. "He didn't want to go," says Duncan; "he didn't like it much." Clearly, she was of the same mind, but the two left the familiar setting and stepped into the new building, with its modern equipment and fancy this and that, and they made do, like they always had. But their era was coming to an end.

After Duncan retired from nursing in 1980, she married Tom Barker, father of her stepdaughter Shirley, who sat with us for our interview. Tom fell ill, and Kate faithfully cared for him until his death—once a nurse, always a nurse.

As I look into the eyes of the woman sitting in the wheelchair in front of me, I see the familiar look of the consummate professional. I see too the remnants of a subtle sense of humor; I hear it in her response to some of my questions. That wit, says Nan, is something not everybody knows about Kate.

Langdon L. Scott

While Lettie Jones initially helped to manage the business end of the hospital's operation, the official title of business manager of Ashe County Memorial Hospital was given to Langdon L. Scott on November 2, 1941. Scott was an Ashe County native, the son of John F. Scott and Mrs. Julia Greer Scott, and a prominent local insurance man. Appointed by the hospital's executive committee, he originally agreed to serve as business manager as a service to the county. Officials of the Duke Endowment helped with setting up the hospital's capital account and uniform accounting system, and Lettie handled the day to day administration. Two NYA young women, Myrtle Jean Wyrick and Ruth Badger, received training in clerical work and were to assist in the business office, as well. Scott recruited and hired many of the hospital employees who would form the core of the Ashe County Memorial staff for years to come, including Doris Oliver and June Weaver Worth, and, together

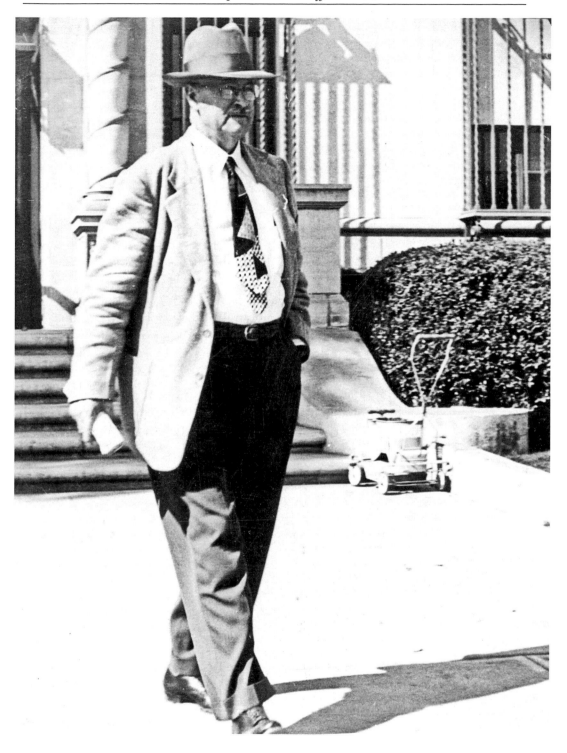

Langdon L. Scott became the first administrator/business manager of Ashe County Memorial Hospital shortly after its opening. He worked for little or no pay for the first several years (courtesy Evelyn Jones).

with them, provided a standard in dedication for those who would follow. He died Sunday, October 31, 1971, the day of the dedication of the new Ashe Memorial Hospital in Jefferson.[3]

Henry Lum; Ruby Dillard Lum, Interviews (West Jefferson, July 1, 2014, and March 27, 2015)

Ruby Dillard Lum, a native of the Obids community in Ashe County, was a nurse with the hospital in its early years. There was not too much work to be had in Ashe County then, and many young people moved away to get a job. Motivated by a friend of hers who had entered nursing training the year before, Ruby began her nurses' training at Old City Memorial Hospital in Winston-Salem. "In those days nursing had a bad name," Ruby recalls, "and our neighbors thought it was a bad thing for me to be going. They tried to talk my parents into sending me to school to learn to be a teacher or secretary instead." Ruby started work at the hospital immediately after graduating in 1947 and lived on the premises. She started out splitting her time between the operating room and working on the hall and later went full-time in the operating room, her preference. "At first, everybody did everything," Ruby recalls of the early days in the hospital, "but eventually we got a nurse for the nursery."

She met her future husband Henry Lum at the hospital. Henry was a medical technologist and came to Ashe County Memorial via Lexington, North Carolina, where he worked for a short time. But he was born in Hawaii, the son of Chinese immigrants to the islands, and grew up on the island of Oahu. Family lore has it that Henry, as a young paper boy, delivered the special evening edition of the newspaper reporting the bombing of Pearl Harbor, which occurred the morning of the same day.

Henry applied for a temporary job at Ashe County Memorial, not intending to make Ashe County his permanent home, but, like so many others, he fell in love, not just with the place but with Ruby. He liked the change in seasons he missed at his home in Hawaii, he said. Despite the long standing lack of diversity in Ashe County and the surrounding area, Lum was accepted in the community, and was a beloved and highly respected member of the Ashe County Memorial family. When I interviewed Phyllis Jones Yount, daughter of Doc Jones and Evelyn, she described working with Henry when she first got a job in the hospital in high school. "I loved Henry. I thought he was very funny. I knew he loved my family." The closeness with the Jones's would continue into the next generation. "My kids called him 'Won Ton Man,' because he made won tons for them," Phyllis laughs.

"He loved his work," relates the Lum's daughter, Dr. Tammy Thore of her father. "He was very particular and wanted everything done correctly." His daughter remembers whenever he went back to visit his parents and siblings in Hawaii, he always brought back gifts for all his friends at the hospital, and when anyone from Ashe County was lucky enough to vacation in Hawaii, Lum arranged for one of his brothers to act as tour guide during their stay. In later years, the Lums and Doc and Evelyn and their children travelled to Hawaii together, and Henry's siblings took off work and gave them the grand tour.[4]

Encouraged by Dr. Jones, Sr., to pursue a certificate as a radiation technologist, Henry Lum became head of the lab and did the x-rays too, the first to take over these tasks from Jones. The two men, both on the quiet side, became good friends and fishing buddies. With their demanding schedules at the hospital, it was hard for Ruby and Henry to share any time together, relates Ruby. When she expressed a desire to learn how to take x-rays, Henry said if she learned to take x-rays, they would never have time off together. After the two got married, Ruby moved out of the nurses' quarters on the hall, and she and Henry had a room with a bath across from the emergency room. The couple splurged and got a television before anybody else had one, and Dr. Dean and Henry often watched television together, after Ruby had gone to bed. One evening as she was wrapping up her shift on the hall, Ruby, anticipating the two men would be watching television, called out to Dr. Dean, "I'm going to

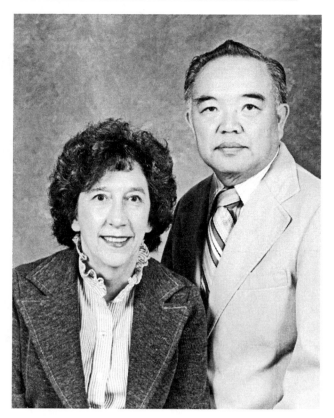

Henry Lum, who initially took a temporary job as a medical technologist at Ashe County Memorial Hospital, fell in love with Ashe County and nurse Ruby Dillard. The two married and lived in the hospital together until they moved to their own home to start their family (courtesy Dr. Tammy Lum Thore).

change into my nightgown and get in bed, so you can come on ahead." Ruby chuckles at the memory of her coworkers' reaction, "I heard a lot about that!" The Lums used the dining room for their meals. "The staff ate together, like a big family," Ruby recalls, "and if we wanted a snack, we could steal a little ice cream from the freezer." Hospital Administrator Langdon Scott, who kept a close eye on supplies, chose to overlook the petty larceny. "One time we got a watermelon, and the girl carrying it dropped it on the stairs bringing it up, and we had to clean up that big mess." Mr. Scott came out to investigate the commotion and apparently chose to ignore that too. "We had rabbit every Sunday. Laura McConnell, who lived down the road from the hospital, raised them and sold them to the hospital." The staff spent much of their time together, roller skating in the basement or playing ping-pong. Ruby remembers the hospital's matriarch, Lettie Jones as a wonderful person. "I never heard her say a bad word about anybody. She was special." Henry and Ruby were instrumental in getting Dean C. and Evelyn together. Like Henry and Ruby's courtship, theirs was hampered by conflicting work schedules at the hospital, and the more established couple helped them find the time to see each other and encouraged their romance. "We would go

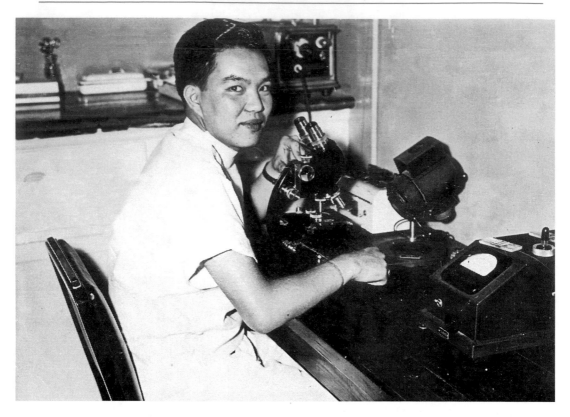

Encouraged by Dr. Dean Jones, Sr., to pursue a certificate as a radiation technologist, Henry Lum became the head of the lab and did x-rays too, the first to relieve Dr. Jones of these responsibilities (courtesy Dr. Tammy Lum Thore).

places together, like ball games. We just sort of talked them into it," Ruby confides with a smile.

When they started their family, Ruby and Henry moved from their room at the hospital to their own house, but they were close enough to walk to the hospital. "Dr. Dean delivered all my children," says Ruby proudly. The Lums had three children: Butch, Phillip and Tammy. When Ruby and Henry were both on call, they would take the children to the hospital with them, and everyone would help take care of them while they worked.

Ruby was admired and respected by doctors and staff, and patients appreciated her kindness and professionalism. Fourteen-year-old John Reeves was hospitalized at Ashe County Memorial with double pneumonia. When I interviewed John in September 2014, he described the experience. He found the hospital a scary place and wanted his mother to come back and stay with him. The food was not like his mother's cooking, so he awarded no stars on that front either. But one thing about his brief hospital stay did favorably impress the young man—nurse Ruby Lum. "I thought she was the prettiest thing I had ever seen."[5]

Among her lifetime of memories of the Jones family and the hospital, is Ruby's recollection of the night Dr. Dean and French Young fished at Long Hope Falls until it was so dark they could not find their way back safely and had to stay the night. It was Ruby who accompanied a worried Lettie on the drive out to wait in the car for their return. "She was not normally anxious, but she was worried that night. He did always come home with fish," Ruby adds.

Dean C., Jr., was only in high school when Ruby started work in the hospital, and she remembers when he worked as an orderly. She also remembers Dr. Dean doing the physicals for the draft board and the community getting together a petition to keep Dr. Dean C., Jr., from being drafted for the Korean Conflict, because they needed him in the county. She worked in the operating room with both Dr. Jones, Sr. and Jr., and Dr. Charles Jones joined Ashe Memorial before she left. "Dr. Jones Jr. and Sr. worked together so well. I never remember hearing a harsh word between them. They had a good working relationship." Doc and Ruby were working in the ER when Dr. Dean died. "They didn't bring him to the hospital; he was already gone; he died in his house. He had a picture of my oldest in his wallet when he died."

Ruby was on the scene with Doc and nurse Edith Blevins when the bridge at Silas Creek collapsed in 1966. When the call came in at the old hospital, Doc, Lum, and Blevins jumped in Doc's car and sped to the site. Doc was the coroner at the time, and he didn't know if he would be acting in that capacity when he arrived at the scene or dealing with a live victim. A front page article in the local paper shows a photo of Doc and the two nurses wading out of the river, after assessing the driver's condition and administering a shot of morphine, before rescue workers extracted the victim from the wreckage. While it was not unusual for the doctor to be called out to the scene of an accident, Ruby says, it was unusual for the nurses to go, and the situation reflects the commitment of AMH staff to providing help when and where it was thought to be required, even when it meant wading through a river.

Many admired Ruby's dedication to her work, including Dr. Thore, who worked with her mother for 14 years as a surgeon at Ashe Memorial. Ruby retired from the hospital with 50 years of service and worked for a couple of years as a nurse in Thore's practice before hanging up her nurse's cap for good. She continues to live in Ashe County at Forest Ridge Assisted Living. Her husband Henry worked with the hospital for 39 years before he retired in 1989. He died in 2009. Ruby and Henry Lum are remembered by all as a vital part of Ashe Memorial's history and growth and the legacy of caring which has come to characterize the Ashe County community. It was welcome news when AMH announced Dr. Thore was returning to Ashe Memorial, effective June 1, 2015, bringing the Lum family legacy of care in Ashe County full circle.

Betty Ball, R.N., Interview (West Jefferson, August 15, 2014)

One of the things I miss about nursing, says Betty Ball, "is when people would come up to me and tell me, "You were there when I was sick, or you took care of me when I had my baby, or you took such good care of my father or my mother when he or she was in the hospital. It's so nice to hear that." Betty lives in West Jefferson. Her father was from Ashe County, and her mother was from Whitetop, Virginia. The family lived in West Virginia for a time, while Betty's father worked in a sawmill, sawing timber for the mines. That is where Betty was born. The family moved to Sparta, North Carolina, and Betty worked as an inspector for Atwood, Inc., in Sparta, a textile mill that made men's pants. She saved her money for nursing school, received her nursing training 1953–1956 at Mercy Hospital in Charlotte, and returned to Ashe County at age 21 to work for Ashe County Memorial. "I sure liked nursing better than making pants."

By the time Betty started at Ashe County Memorial, there was a separate building for the nurses' quarters, and she moved in. Seven months later she was married to Joe Ball, and moved out of the nurses' quarters. Eventually the couple moved to a brick ranch house on East Buck Mountain Road, where they continue to live today. Betty's commute to work was relatively short, compared to some of her coworkers, who had to rely on Tom Cockerham or Jack McClure to fetch them to work in the snow. At the hospital, Betty worked on the hall and in the ER, when the need arose. In those days, there was no staff specifically dedicated to the ER; whoever was on duty reported to the ER when a patient came in.

I ask Betty to tell me about a story I heard where she was recruited to accompany Dr. Carson Keys on a helicopter to pick up a patient, during one of the area's big snow events. "That was the only time I ever rode a helicopter," she laughs. "The helicopter landed in West Jefferson Park, where the library is now, and took us up toward Lansing. We landed in an apple orchard." The patient had an infection in his leg, and there was danger of gangrene if he did not receive attention. There was no time to prepare for the trip; Betty got the call to go; Doris Oliver was called in to relieve her; and Betty was transported immediately from the hospital to the park. "It was so loud, I had to scream to be heard," she recalls. The mission was accomplished, however, and the patient recovered, with no loss of limb.

"It was great having Dr. Dean and Lettie so close," says Betty. With the doctor and his wife right down the hall at the hospital, staff didn't have to run far to get help in an emergency. Betty recalls one of the many times she was involved with bringing a baby into the world. The patient's obstetrician was not there, and the baby started to come. Betty delivered the baby and shouted to another nurse, "Get the doctor!" Doc appeared shortly. "Get some gloves," she called to him, "there's another one in here." "Looks like you're doing fine," he calmly replied. He held the mother's hand while Betty delivered the second of the twins. "It was so much fun!"

If Henry Lum was not in the hospital, Dr. Dean instructed the nurse to drip the anesthesia in a surgery, under his close supervision. "Now, just a few drops. Now let up. Now a few drops. Now let up." Nowadays, there is an anesthesiologist or nurse anesthetist to handle this task. Other things have changed too. In the old hospital, male orderlies provided all the personal care to male patients. Nurses still administered medications, but they did not bathe or assist with the toileting of male patients. During the days of segregation, there also were designated rooms for nonwhite patients, and those patients were admitted separately, as well. The African American population in Ashe County was less than 1 percent during that time, so there were few patients and fewer staff who were African American.

Betty was in the old Ashe County Memorial when the transfer was made to the new hospital. "We had more long term patients, then, because there was a lack of nursing homes in the area, but they (the patients) were excited about the move too." Betty was stationed at the new hospital to receive the patients coming in by ambulance or private car from the old hospital—a busy day, but the job got done.

From 1960 to 1964, Betty left Ashe County Memorial to work for Dr. Keys and again from 1981 to 1991, when he returned to the area and set up his office in the Professional Building, behind the new AMH. Later she worked at Watauga Hospital in Boone, retiring in 1999. But caregiving is not completely out of her system. For the last fifteen years, she has volunteered for Meals on Wheels in Ashe County, covering the familiar back roads of her home, helping, like she always has.

Toby Younce Hartzog Interview (West Jefferson, October 23, 2014)

"I got in on the very beginning," says Toby Hartzog about Ashe County Memorial Hospital. Toby was in about the sixth grade at Fleetwood School, when the children were given the opportunity to help raise money for the hospital. The student in each class who collected the most money got a bus ride to the dedication ceremony for the Ashe County Memorial Hospital in Jefferson. Toby had two uncles who made sure she had enough money to make the trip. The day of the dedication was a cold one, especially standing on the hill where the new hospital was situated, and muddy. "There was a big crowd, and I was afraid to get away from my group. I was so short, I couldn't see anything. It was too far from home, and Grandpa wasn't there." A stop for ice cream on the way home saved the outing from being a total letdown.

A few weeks before Toby graduated from high school, Business Manager Langdon Scott offered her a job at the hospital as a nurses' aide. She worked at the hospital from about 1947 to December of 1950 and lived in the hospital during that time. This was before the separate nurses' quarters was built, and five women shared a large room, with a common bathroom at the end of the hall. Toby had never seen the need for a bathrobe until faced with that long walk to the bath and shower. Dean C., Jr., was in school then, and Toby did not see him much, except during the summers, when he worked at the hospital, relieving the orderlies when they went on vacation. Nurses' aides worked everywhere in the hospital, but Toby loved the nursery. It reminded her of the baby brothers and sisters she had left at home. "One February we had nineteen babies in the nursery. The mothers made it to the hospital to deliver, but the weather was so bad, they couldn't get back home." Meals were taken in the hospital's dining room, and the doctors and nurses ate separately. "We were a pretty calm bunch," declares Toby. "We were all raised in homes where you had to walk the straight and narrow." Toby spent her off hours knitting. There was no television at the hospital then. "The first TV I ever saw was when Miss Lettie took some of us to watch a ball game on a TV somewhere." Toby was so fascinated with Lettie's tatting, she doesn't remember watching much of the game on the tiny screen. Lettie later gave her a pair of pillowcases for a wedding present, with her beautiful tatting on the hems.

Toby married Willard Hartzog in December 1950, leaving the hospital to raise a family and help her husband with his furniture building business. She returned to Ashe Memorial for the birth of her children, delivered by Dr. Dean. On the occasion of her first baby's delivery, she remembers Lettie bringing her baby clothes, a baby blanket, and other baby paraphernalia—enough to completely outfit her newborn. Toby and her husband stayed in touch with Dr. Dean, her husband hunting with the doctor on occasion. She did not go to the dedication of the new hospital in 1971, because the rainy weather made travel difficult from her house, so close to the river. Her daughter drove her around to see the old hospital awhile back, and she was saddened to see its state of disrepair. She is a patient of Dr. Charles Jones now and lives in her home near the Idlewild community in Ashe County.

Doris Oliver, R.N., Interview (West Jefferson, July 28, 2014)

By the time Ashe County native Doris Oliver made her decision to enter nurses' training at Charlotte Memorial Hospital, now Carolinas Medical Center, the profession had evolved into an accepted career choice for women. Langdon Scott was a patient of Oliver's at Charlotte Memorial and talked her into going to work at Ashe County Memorial. She started her job there in January 1952.

There was no separate building for nurses' quarters yet, and Oliver lived in the hospital, rooming with Ruby Lum. Their room was between the delivery room and the labor room. When visiting hours were over, recalls Doris, "We put on our pajamas and sat up front visiting with Lettie, until Dr. Jones finished his rounds, and then we all turned in." She managed to stay about six weeks before the continual racket of stretchers being wheeled down the hall outside her door became too much, and she opted to board with the James Badger family a short distance from the hospital.

Later that first year, Oliver left Ashe County Memorial for a brief stay in Pennsylvania, returning in 1957 to stay with the hospital for the remainder of her career. She assisted Dr. Dean with the first organ donation performed at Ashe County Memorial in September 1962. Laura Faw Shatley of Jefferson stipulated that her eyes were to be donated, and, at her passing, the hospital arranged for the transfer to a recipient in Winston-Salem. The Highway Patrol, assisted by the Lions Club, set up a relay at the county lines to assist with the rapid transport needed to accomplish this groundbreaking task. The recipient reportedly fared well with the transplant. As an interesting sidelight to this story, the son of the first donor later received cornea transplants for both eyes.

I ask Doris if she ever had trouble getting to work in bad weather. "I've never been so scared in my life," she exclaims, as she describes trying to get to the hospital during one particularly bad snowstorm in the 1960s. After experiencing two white-outs, she stopped at a house and asked the man there if he could drive her to work. He obliged, as one would expect in this part of the world, and she made it, albeit shaken.

Oliver retired in 1983, after 25 years with Ashe Memorial, and lives in West Jefferson. She is the daughter of J. E. and Vista Oliver, both of Ashe County. J. E. Oliver was one of the original 18 members of the Ashe County Memorial Hospital Board of Trustees.

Christie "Chris" Phillips; Betty Avery Interview (Jefferson, January 5, 2015)

Betty Avery's mother Christie "Chris" Phillips worked with both Dr. Dean and Doc at the hospital and when the two shared an office in the Professional Building. An Ashe County native from the Silas Creek community, Chris had no formal nurses' training but learned on the job at the old hospital. She started out working on the hall, progressed to the nursery, and then the ER. Although she loved the ER, her time in the nursery happily coincided with the birth of her granddaughter Charlene, delivered by Dr. C. E. "Johnny" Miller, and Chris spent every spare minute rocking her new granddaughter. Kate Duncan, Doris Oliver, and Betty Ball were working at the hospital, and doctors Keys, Freeman and Kurtz as well as Johnny Miller were on the medical staff. The staff was small, and Chris was called in wherever she was needed, including the operating room. Her work and her opinion were respected by the medical staff. Accustomed to having the run of things at AMH, the petite Chris raised a big fuss when her granddaughter Marlene was taken to the

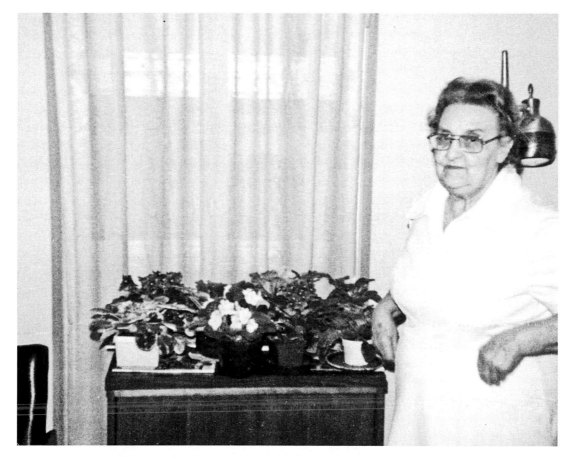

Christie "Chris" Phillips worked for both Drs. Dean Jones, Sr. and Jr., at the hospital and in the office the two doctors shared, until she finally retired at age 74. Although she had no formal nurses' training, she worked everywhere she was needed, including the operating room (courtesy Betty Avery).

hospital in Winston-Salem with a broken elbow, and the staff there would not allow Chris in the operating room. "I don't see why I can't go back there—I work in a hospital, and that's my granddaughter!"

Chris loved working with Dr. Dean and Doc and stayed on the job until age 74, when she fell and broke her shoulder and pelvis at her daughter's home, across the street from Doc and Evelyn's house on Northwest Drive. "She wasn't going to go to the hospital," relates her daughter, "so Doc came down to the house to check her out. She wasn't going to let anybody else touch her." In later years, when Chris was persuaded to go to an adult day care program, she referred to her time there as "going to work," occupying herself with diagnosing and looking after other participants. Some habits are hard to break.

Edith Brooks Blevins Interview (Lansing, January 7, 2015)

"She was one of a kind. She was the best," says Edith Blevins, when I ask her about coworker Chris Phillips. Blevins was a nurses' aide too and worked alongside Phillips for many years at the old and the new hospital. Both women later went to work for both Dr. Jones, Sr. and Jr., in the Professional Building. When people asked Edith when she was going to retire, she always answered, "When Doc Jones retires." She meant what she said, and her long career came to an end when Doc left his practice. In the meantime, Blevins worked with three generations of doctors Jones, starting with Dr. Dean at the old hospital and ending with Dr. Charles Jones. While working for Doc, Blevins was diagnosed with cancer, and Doc performed the surgery. "She took her chemotherapy treatments during her lunch break," recalls Dr. Charles Jones, when I interview him a week or so after talking to Edith. Much later, there was a recurrence with more chemotherapy, but Blevins was too tough for cancer again. She continues to live on her own, with a little help from an old friend and coworker, Rob Black, who runs errands for her and helps to maintain her property.

Born and raised in Ashe County in Griffith Holler, Edith worked first in hospitals in Pennsylvania and then Knoxville, Tennessee, before coming home to Ashe County. Her training, like that of Chris Phillips, was on-the-job. "Work was hard to come by," she recalls. "You took what you could get." She liked the second shift at AMH, which started at 3:00 p.m. and ended at 11:00 p.m. and left her time for her other obligations. "I lived on a farm, and I had cows to milk." But she worked all three shifts at one time or another and did anything that needed doing. She was called on to accompany Doc Jones and Ruby Lum to the scene of the bridge collapse at Silas Creek in July 1966. "Ruby and I were just hanging onto our seats," Edith says of the car ride to the scene. "Doc was driving his Pontiac. I thought he was going to kill us getting down there."

By the time the new AMH opened, Blevins was working in the ER. She also worked for Dr. Freeman at his office in Lansing and then with Dr. Keys, when he joined Dr. Freeman in his practice, and the office was moved to a location between the towns of Jefferson and West Jefferson. "I worked until I was dead old."

Ella Pennington Baldwin Interview (West Jefferson, November 24, 2014)

For Ella Pennington, like many young women growing up in the area, there were few jobs close by and suitable for a young lady, other than waitressing or clerking in a store, and those opportunities were limited in a small town. Thomasville Furniture, located where Jefferson Station is now in West Jefferson, was the only other large employer, besides Ashe County Memorial Hospital. The hospital offered a safe place for women to earn a decent wage, plus housing away from home, but sometimes applicants had to wait for a position to become available. In late 1948-1949, Ella, who hailed from around Little Laurel in Ashe County, was working in Pennsylvania when her parents telephoned to tell her she had received a letter from Langdon Scott at the hospital, offering her a job as a nurses' assistant. She was on the next bus home. Her parents dropped her off at the hospital, and she started to work the next morning. She moved into a ward in the old hospital dedicated to female staff. "I lived right across from the new mamas and babies," says Ella. There were six single beds, and if somebody new arrived and there was no bed available, the women doubled up. The bathroom, shared with patients, was a long walk down the hall.

Ella soon made friends with Doris Oliver and Ruby Lum and settled into the routine, which was pretty much anything that needed to be done, including cleaning and rolling cotton tips and folding bandages. There was no such thing as Q Tips or the prepackaged bandages and dressings that run up hospital bills now. Ella worked in the nursery too, bathing the infants and mixing formula. "I made fifty dollars a month, and I bought my own uniform, although the hospital laundered it." Later her salary was raised to $65 a month. "It was hard work, but I enjoyed it."

Ella met her future husband, Dale Baldwin, when the young women living at the hospital used to go to the old Parkway Movie Theatre, where Dale was the manager. He started calling on Ella, picking her up on the porch at the hospital. "Dr. and Mrs. Jones were just like parents," she recalls. Lettie kept a close eye on men calling on the young women under her wing. "Lettie felt it was her responsibility to the parents to look after us." Accordingly, Lettie questioned Ella about her new beau, just to be sure he was a suitable companion. He must have passed muster, because the two got married, and Ella left her job at the hospital to start a family.

June Weaver Worth, R.N., Interview (West Jefferson, November 25, 2014)

When Langdon Scott talked to June Weaver of Smethport in Ashe County about working at Ashe County Memorial Hospital as a nurses' aide, she assured him she would be 15 years old in a few days. He decided that was all right and put the 14-year-old girl to work immediately. Training was on-the-job, and June was instructed to see that everybody got water. She didn't know that some of the nurses were living in the hospital, so she delivered water to their rooms too, catching some of the night shift asleep. "I was giving everybody water." Despite this initial faux pas, she continued work at the hospital through high school, working weekends and summers. The hospital never had enough help in those days, and June remembers Langdon Scott coming to her house to see if she could come in to work. "We didn't have a telephone until after I graduated," she explained.

After high school, June attended nursing school at Presbyterian Hospital in Charlotte. Transportation was always an issue, and June's father had to drive her to North Wilkesboro to catch the bus back to school in Charlotte. On one such trip, a young man pulled up behind them at the gas station, struck up a conversation with them and offered to drive June to the bus station. He ended up driving her all the way to Charlotte. Long story short, they got married. The couple lived in Asheboro about three years, and June worked at the hospital there. Then it was time to come home to Ashe County, where she worked as an R.N. for a while at Ashe County Memorial. "I always worked the night shift." Normally, there was only one nurse and two aides on duty, so if the nurse was in the operating room, there was no nurse on the floor. One evening a man came in the door carrying his wife. "Get the baby," he called out. The woman had delivered her baby between the car and the hospital front door. The newborn had dropped onto the sidewalk. Thankfully, the baby survived the rough arrival.

There was no hospital security in those days, unless you count Dr. Dean, and maybe you should. But it was a small community, and people didn't worry about things like that. For a brief period, a homeless man was allowed to sleep on a sofa downstairs at night. "He would be gone by daylight." But the hospitality was abruptly rescinded after the man's impaired speech was interpreted, and June realized he was asking her, "Care if I kiss you?"

Worth eventually left the hospital and began teaching nursing at the local high school. Her student nurses were qualified at a level she describes as somewhere between a nurses' aide and an L.P.N. When the new Ashe Memorial opened in 1971, Worth took her students to the hospital before the patients were due to arrive, and they cleaned every patient room and made up all the beds—a lesson in mitering corners they probably never will forget. Worth still runs into some of her former students at Ashe Memorial today, and she is proud to see them doing their jobs the way she taught them. Reflecting on her career at Ashe Memorial and the evolution in services she has witnessed over the years, June adds, "And I am proud of our new hospital too."

Tom Cockerham; Clairene Cockerham Interview (Jefferson, September 29, 2014)

In April 1952, Thomas "Tom" Franklin Cockerham replaced Langdon Scott as business manager of Ashe County Memorial Hospital and served in that capacity and as a member of the board of trustees for 40 years. Cockerham's father-in-law, William "Bryan" Oliver, of Ashe County, suggested the job opportunity at the hospital in a tactful and low-key effort to persuade his daughter and her husband to move back to Ashe County. Born in Elkin, North Carolina, June 8, 1923, Cockerham served as a medic in General George Patton's Third Army, Sixth Armored Division in World War II. He graduated from Appalachian

State University and got a job coaching and teaching math and physical education in Surry County, North Carolina, where he met Clairene Oliver, a graduate of Women's College at Greensboro, who was teaching English at the same school. Clairene, daughter of Maude Phipps and Bryan Oliver, did office work at the hospital in the summers before and during college, filling in for Lettie Jones, when she took a summer break from her duties at the hospital and visited her parents in Pennsylvania. Clairene worked with Langdon Scott, who eventually left Ashe County to move out West for health reasons. When Cockerham took over the administrator's job at the hospital, he worked with Lettie in the office. Later Ann Brown would join him as his private secretary.

Mountain winters are not for sissies and getting to work can be a challenge, but staying home by the fire when there is a major snow event outside is not an option for medical professionals, and Tom Cockerham was aggressive in his approach to getting hospital staff to work.

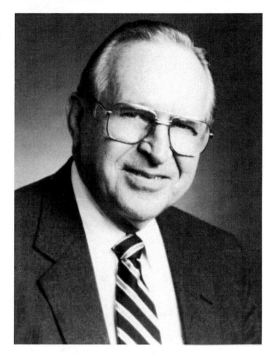

Tom Cockerham replaced Langdon Scott as administrator of Ashe County Memorial Hospital in 1952 and served in that capacity for forty years (courtesy Clairene Cockerham).

If somebody could not get to work, he sent one of the maintenance staff to pick them up. One time, Doris Oliver remembers Cockerham came to pick her up himself. "He was right behind the road grader!"[6] Apparently, Cockerham had a good rapport with the county's snow removal crew, as he routinely directed them to plow the roads between Doc's house on Northwest Drive and the hospital, even riding on the road grader himself to be sure the way was clear for the surgeon to get to work. "I didn't even see him when it snowed," says Clairene, the exception being once during a big snow in the 1960s, when she was in the hospital for the birth of her second daughter.

Not everybody had their own car, like nowadays, so living in the nurses' quarters at the hospital, where you didn't have to worry about getting to work in the bad weather, was a real advantage. Mary Lou Brooks tells me after she got married and moved from the nurses' quarters to her own house, Cockerham, her immediate boss, saw that she got to work in the snow, frequently picking her up himself.[7] During the famous snow event in 1960, Dale Baldwin remembers it snowed about 14 inches every Wednesday for four or five consecutive weeks, starting in February. Snow drifts were as high as 20 feet, so high there was no place left on the sides of the roads to put the snow. There was no phone service and trees were down, blocking many of the roads. The Red Cross and National Guard were called in, although for what reason some hardy mountain folks could not fathom; natives to the area had managed to cope with whatever nature threw at them for generations, without assistance from the outside. People were supposed to leave a message in the snow, visible from the air, if they needed help. According to Dale Baldwin, one desperate fellow wrote in red paint in the snow next to his house "DROP HOOCH"—to be used for medicinal purposes, no doubt.[8]

Jack McClure Interview (West Jefferson, August 12, 2014)

Ashe County native Jack McClure was 18 when he started work as an orderly at the old Ashe County Memorial Hospital. His training was on-the-job. "Orderlies then did everything for the men patients. There were two orderlies on each shift, taking care of as many as twenty-five patients. By that time, Dr. Dean and Lettie had moved out of the hospital and into their house behind the hospital." When Jack was working the third shift, he remembers regularly seeing the tall figure of the doctor walking across his backyard toward the hospital, flashlight in hand. "If Dr. Dean had a patient who was not doing well, he'd get out of bed, walk over to the hospital, pick up the patient's chart, and head down the hall. He didn't say much to anybody, just nodded and went about his rounds."

"At the hospital, he was strictly business, but when he went fishing or squirrel hunting, he was in a different world," says Jack, recalling some of those precious Wednesday afternoons with the doctor, fishing trout streams all over the county. "Dr. Dean loved fried squirrel and gravy." When he got too old to hunt squirrel, Jack would kill the squirrels and get his mother, Mae McClure, to fix them for the doctor. Toward the end of his life, Dr. Dean went through a spell when he had no appetite. "Do you think he'd eat some fried squirrel, Ms. Lettie?" Jack asked. She thought it was worth a try, so Jack killed three squirrels, and his mother and wife, Joy, fixed them up. Lettie told Jack her husband ate so much of the delicacy, she was afraid he was going to be sick.

Jack's parents, Walter and Mae McClure, worked at the hospital in their younger years, and while Jack was employed with the hospital, his Aunt Hazel Barker McClure worked in the dietary department at the hospital. In the old hospital, before there was a cafeteria, staff walked into the kitchen and told the ladies there what they wanted, and they would get it right out of the pot on the stove. "You couldn't have found a better meal anywhere," says Jack—a claim still made by many about the current AMH cafeteria. In true Mayberry fashion, when the new hospital was built, the county jail contracted with the hospital kitchen to provide the three meals a day for the prisoners, a practice that continued until the new jail was built.

Jack left his orderly job and moved into maintenance at the hospital, taking over his Uncle Scott McClure's job when his uncle's health failed. Maintenance entailed a little bit of everything, and one of Jack's main responsibilities in bad weather was to transport clinical staff and other necessary personnel to and from the hospital. "We used to have snow here," quips Jack, with the typical perspective of a High Country native. Transporting staff was an around the clock task, as he had to take home one shift and pick up the next at the same time. "The kids and I hardly saw him in the winter," remarks Joy. The hospital owned a pickup truck, and Jack put a snow blade on the truck to clean the parking lot and areas around the hospital. By the time Rob Black came on board to provide some back up in the maintenance department, the hospital had two trucks with chains on all four wheels, one a Chevy and one a Jeep. Black drove the second vehicle, and the two men worked all three shifts. "We went all directions in the county—Lansing, Fleetwood, everywhere." In later years, the hospital put people up in the hospital or at the Best Western Motel in Jefferson. Meantime, the maintenance crew of two kept the boilers going and the road scraped. "I pulled many a vehicle out of a ditch," says Jack. "I had to keep Dr. Freeman's long, steep driveway scraped when he was on call."

When Doc joined his father at Ashe County Memorial, Jack fished some with him, like he had with his dad. "He was like his father as far as his patients were concerned." Once, when a patient went to Winston-Salem for surgery, the staff at the prominent Bowman Gray Hospital asked, "Why did you come down here? You've got one of the best surgeons in the country in Ashe County." They were referring to Doc. Dr. Dean Jones, Sr., had a reputation as an excellent diagnostician, adds Jack. "Dr. C. E. Miller used to say if Dr. Dean says somebody has appendicitis, you may as well take him to surgery."

Jack McClure left the hospital after 23 years and did contract work. He and Joy live in Jefferson, where he was born and raised.

Joy McClure Interview (West Jefferson, August 12, 2014)

Jack McClure's wife, Joy, grew up in Little Horse Creek. She started with Ashe Memorial Hospital in 1970, answering the telephone. "Mary Lou Brooks, the business office manager, hired me, and Tom Cockerham was the administrator of the hospital at the time." When Joy worked the 1:00 p.m. to 9:30 p.m. shift, she too would see Dr. Dean, Sr., coming through the side door of the hospital at night to check on his patients. By April 1970, Joy moved to the business office at the hospital and worked in bookkeeping. "By the time the new hospital building was underway, Jack was working in maintenance, and we were so excited to have a new facility, we would go to the site to see the progress of the building. When the facility opened, most of the ladies from the business office acted as tour guides, showing people around."

Around 1979 or 1980, Joy recalls Tom Cockerham announcing to her, "We will have to computerize, and we need your assistance with the computer system." Joy, Mary Lou Brooks, and Ann Brown were among those sent to Atlanta for computer training, and later Joy became the data processing manager. She continued her education in the late 1980s to early 1990s, going to school while working. She received her degree in accounting from Wilkes Community College and continued on to Appalachian State University, graduating in 1994 with a bachelor of technology degree. From 2001 until her retirement in April 2015, Joy was the CFO (chief financial officer) for Ashe Memorial, overseeing patient financial services, information systems, accounting, and materials management, and a couple of the physician office practices, and reporting to the hospital's CEO (chief executive officer) Laura Lambeth and the board of trustees.

When I first talked with Joy, she had been with AMH for 44 years and had seen the impact of the changing population of the county. "Ashe has always been a poor county, but people were so proud that they tried to pay their bills. Not everybody could, however, and minutes from board meetings in the early 1950s show that Wade Eller, secretary of the board, was "authorized and empowered to receive and to collect all the past due accounts of the hospital...." "When Tom Cockerham was the administrator," recalls Joy, "the hospital didn't use a collection agency. Mary Lou Brooks and Mr. Cockerham would work up a list of those who owed money, and the collection agent, Mr. Hartsog, would drive around the county in a little red car with 'Ashe Memorial Hospital Collector' on the side, drive up in people's driveways, and talk to them about the importance of paying something on their bill. It was considered a great embarrassment to have the red collection car in your driveway." Apparently, Mr. Hartsog was persuasive, as he reportedly would come back from his calls with cash in hand to pay on the accounts. Today there are more indigent persons than in the years when Joy first learned her bookkeeping skills under the tutelage of Mary Lou Brooks. "We define charity care as those who can't pay their bills, and we define bad debt as those who won't pay their bills."

    "When I started at the hospital, it was like one big family," says Joy. "Ruby and Henry Lum, Dr. and Mrs. Jones, Tom and Clairene Cockerham, and Kate Duncan were all family. When I had our boys, Ruby Lum, Kate Duncan, Doris Oliver, Helen Barker, Ida Marsh and Susanne Stoltzfus all took care of me. Kate Duncan and Dr. Dean, Sr., delivered Jack, and Dr. C. E. Miller delivered our sons. There still are members of the same family employed at the hospital, but we do make an effort to keep them under separate supervisors." With the growth and expansion of the hospital, the employees have maintained a team spirit and attitude. "There still is a sense of caring and concern, and we still treat patients like we would treat our own family."

Robert "Rob" H. Black Interview (Lansing, January 7, 2015)

    I met Rob Black when Evelyn and I were visiting Edith Blevins. Rob is a handyman and does odd chores for a living now. "I got about twenty-eight widow women I do for," he says, as he hauls in a big bag of kitty litter for Edith and sets it in the kitchen. He went to work at the old Ashe County Memorial sometime after Jack McClure and worked in the maintenance department with Jack. He worked on the boilers and the emergency generator, stoked the old coal furnace mornings and evenings, repaired the appliances in the kitchen, painted, plumbed, mowed grass, plowed snow and fetched nurses and other hospital staff in the big three-quarter-ton hospital pickup truck when it snowed. "There was one nurse up Mount Jefferson Road I picked up all winter." He answered to the head nurse for his transportation duties, but it was Mr. Cockerham who hired him. In the summer, people sometimes donated vegetables, when they had extra in their gardens. Other times, Rob picked up produce for the hospital kitchen at Bare and Little Wholesale and drove to North Wilkesboro to get beef. He ate his meals at the hospital and vows the food was good, although he never seemed to get enough salt.

    Rob ate lunch in the hospital's cafeteria with Dr. Dean the day the doctor died. Faye Green, who acted as a caregiver for Dr. Jones in his last years, brought him to the hospital to eat, and the three sat together. Faye took the doctor home, and he passed away soon after, Rob remembers sadly. Black left the hospital after 40 years of service, but he is still helping people.

Nancy P. Edwards, R.N., Interview (West Jefferson, September 17, 2014)

Nancy Parker Edwards, Sue McMillan Hampton, Evelyn Jones, and I sat at the Edwards' kitchen table one morning, talking about the old days at Ashe Memorial and the new days and everything in between. Nancy and Sue, both Ashe County natives, from well-known Ashe County families, worked together at the hospital for many years.

Nancy did her nurses' training at Charlotte Memorial, got married in 1961, moved to Columbus, Georgia, for a time, and then came home to Ashe County and started to work for Dr. Elam Kurtz in his Lansing office. She was the only R.N. he had working in his office, which operated almost like a satellite hospital to Ashe Memorial, offering a closer alternative for folks who could not easily travel to the hospital in Jefferson. Nancy worked four years for Dr. Kurtz before moving to the hospital. Dr. Kurtz had his own drug room or pharmacy, says Nancy. As he dictated his notes on each patient, his staff would listen for the prescription and have it filled before he finished his notes.

Dr. Dean was still there during the days Nancy and Sue spent working at the hospital, but most of their job experience was with his son, Doc. "You never caught them on a mistake," remarks Nancy, a veteran of 27 years with AMH. "They were on top of everything." "Both Senior and Junior had a good relationship with the nurses." Once when a nurse wanted to take off work and go to a dance, Dr. Dean, Sr., said, "You go ahead, and I'll take over for you." And he covered the rest of her shift himself.

People grow attached to their doctors in a small community. Dr. C. E. Miller, noted for his excellent bedside manner, delivered so many babies, people looked on him like he was divine. Dr. Dean Jones, Sr., had so many babies named after him, it became confusing. Sue says the worst accident victim she ever saw in her career was a man hurt when his tractor fell over on him. He insisted he wanted Dr. Dean to take care of him; he did not want to be sent to Winston. He survived, his trust in his doctor intact.

Nancy and Sue reflect on their years in Ashe Memorial, agreeing "it was a privilege to do the job, but it was hard." "It's been eighteen years since I retired," says Nancy, "and I still have dreams where I can't get through—it's 12:00, and I haven't done the 8:00 pills yet."

Sue Hampton, R.N., Interview (West Jefferson, September 17, 2014)

Sue McMillan Hampton graduated from nursing school at Cabarrus Memorial Hospital, near Concord, North Carolina, in 1969. The Director of Nursing at Ashe County Memorial and Administrator Tom Cockerham together hired her. Nursing was different in

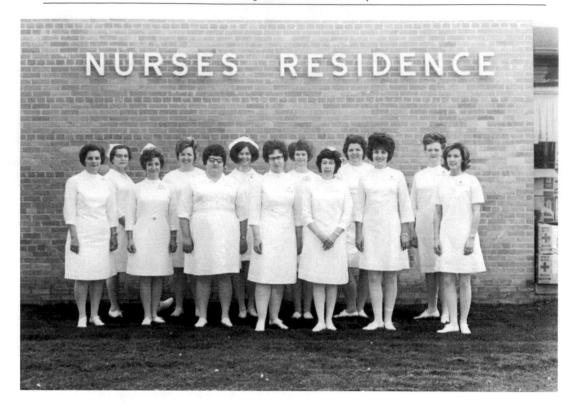

Nursing staff standing in front of the nurses' quarters at Ashe County Memorial Hospital left to right: front row—Mary Wilcox Iles; Nancy Edwards; Peggy Ollis; Doris Oliver; Ruby Lum; Juanita Greene; Sue McMillan (Hampton); back row—Kate Duncan; Sylvia Allen; Doris Stoltzfus; Nancy Testerman (Lewis); Betty Ball; and Peggy Ashley, the director of nurses (photograph, circa 1970, courtesy Doris Oliver, published in *The Skyland Post,* **June 4, 1970).**

those days, Sue relates. "Nurses not only did patient care, but anything else that needed doing, we did it." Nurses filled prescriptions, organizing daily doses for patients from big stock bottles, like those seen in a pharmacy. "We didn't have a registered respiratory therapist, so we trained a nurse assistant to administer breathing treatments." Scheduling was different too. Dr. Dean, Sr., told his patients who needed a post-op visit to come in at 1:00 p.m. so they all showed up at the same time, and staff just worked on into the evening until everybody was seen. Oxygen tanks were rolled around from room to room as needed, instead of fixed in place in each room, as they are now. There was little in the way of disposable equipment and supplies then, and considerable time was devoted to sterilizing everything from needles and surgical instruments to gloves. Despite this, there was little incidence of post-op infection in the hospital. The consensus at the kitchen table was that smaller hospitals give better care and have fewer infections. The incidence of infection in Ashe Memorial today continues to be relatively low. Infection control and employee health at AMH eventually came under the direction of Sue Hampton and Dr. Don McNeill.

In the old hospital, there were separate wards for men and for women, in addition to private rooms for those who could afford them. When the hospital was full, beds were put in the halls, as necessary. A dressing cart was moved from room to room. Dr. Dean missed the cart when it was taken out of use, finding it more efficient for his purposes than the new way of doing things. Sue remembers Dr. Dean regularly studying the clipboard with all the patients' vitals recorded for the day. "He had his finger on the pulse of every patient in the hospital." In those days before there were computers, nurses had to spend more time sitting with a patient to monitor his condition. And then there were times when Mother Nature did not wait on the doctor to handle a delivery, and both Sue and Nancy found themselves in the right place at the right time to "catch a baby."

Staff at the hospital were not afraid to try something new if it could help a patient. Sue's father, Warner McMillan, had a heart attack. It was around 1970, and he was in the old hospital on McConnell Street, experiencing "a lot of arrhythmia." Dr. E. J. Miller was his doctor and consulted with Sue. He had been reading about the use of the drug lidacain to treat arrhythmia after a heart attack. "Let's try it," he suggested, and Sue agreed, volunteering to monitor the patient, using an EKG machine and running strips over and over again, because there was no monitor for this specific purpose and no IV controller at the nurses' station. "We mixed our own fluid," says Sue, using the kind of lidacain that was on hand for numbing for stitches, a primitive version of the lidacain drip that now comes prepackaged for cardiac use. Sue stayed with her father all night, monitoring the homemade drip, using her watch and counting the drips per minute. "My father survived," she relates. Their ingenuity had saved him.

Sometimes people came out of the hills to bring their loved ones to the hospital and were caked with dirt from tending their crops or livestock. The hospital was probably the cleanest place they had ever stepped foot in. This presented a problem for the maintenance of a sanitary environment, and Dr. Dean and Doc addressed the delicate issue with a direct order on the patient's chart to "bathe the family," leaving it to the nursing staff to carry out the order in such a manner as to cause no offense. The challenge was met by an enthusiastic staff, ready with soap, hot water, and fresh towels. "You just needed to make people feel at ease," says Nancy with a smile.

"Doc never forgot a face," remembers Sue. "One time I was making rounds with him; we passed this one patient; and Doc said, 'Don't I know you?' The patient nodded, 'Yes, you operated on me. I am sorry I could never pay you, Doctor.'" Doc did not hesitate. "That's okay," he said and moved on. It would not be the first or last case where a patient did not have the means to pay his or her bill at the hospital.

The day came when history sheets were required for every patient, but Sue recalls a simpler time when Dr. Dean had only two questions for his patients: "How's your appetite?" and "How are your bowels moving?" Sue worked forty years for Ashe Memorial and had plenty of time to observe both Dr. Jones, Sr. and Jr. The thing that impressed her the most was the calm demeanor the two shared, no matter what crisis was at hand.

Judy Davis Interview (West Jefferson, August 7, 2014)

Judy Davis made the move from Waynesville, in Haywood County, North Carolina, to West Jefferson in 1971, with her husband, who was one of two Highway Patrolmen assigned to Ashe County. Temporarily without a job, she spent some time at the old Ashe County Memorial Hospital on McConnell Street, visiting with her next door neighbor, who worked in the emergency room and in the lab, where the other Highway Patrolman's wife worked as a lab technician. Her friends encouraged her to seek employment with the hospital, and after waiting a year for a job to open, Judy started to work as a ward secretary in the new Ashe Memorial, making rounds with the doctors, taking notes and transcribing the orders the nurses would need for the patients. "Reading the handwriting was a challenge." She worked the third shift, from 11:00 p.m. to 7:00 a.m. The new hospital had 76 beds when it first opened, and with the less restrictive Medicare rules in place at the time, the beds were full.

When Davis moved to a position in the lab, there was only one shift, and then staff was on call to come in if something was needed. This kind of schedule meant employees often had to bring their children to work with them. "But somebody was always there to take care of them for you. It was very family oriented." In the lab, Judy worked with Henry Lum. "I consider him my mentor. He put a lot of faith in me, and I tried to live up to his expectations." Henry was strong on education, and Judy took advantage of opportunities to broaden her knowledge through conferences and going back to school to expand on her biology major. Her hard work paid off, and she became the lab manager at Henry's retirement.

During her time at the hospital, Judy saw dramatic changes in the lab work required. There were five in the lab in the first years she was working there, and they would get through the tests they needed to run by noon, take an afternoon break, and come back in the evening to run the next batch required. "When I started, we used Bunsen burners and Erlemeyer flasks to check blood sugar and heart enzymes, etc., one test at a time. Now large, robotic chemistry analyzers are capable of running hundreds of tests at one time. "And you still can't do it fast enough," she laughs. "It sometimes seems like improved technology just increases expectations for productivity, and you never catch up." X-rays were done in the lab too and stress tests, EKG's—all in one department. "If the lab got a new piece of equipment, like when the first ultrasound machine arrived, lab employees always were the guinea pigs for the new equipment, but Doc could detect the minutest abnormalities using his finger tips and a physical examination of the patient. He could estimate the size of a lump and be within a centimeter of what the ultrasound would show."

Dr. Dean and Doc were working at the hospital when Davis started, but she worked the longest with Doc. "I was always amazed at his recall; he never forgot a patient. He knew who he (the patient) was and who his daddy was and everything that had ever been wrong with him. That is something all those tests required now can't provide." Staff wondered if Doc ever slept, but Davis says she saw him do it more than once. "He would come in my office and ask if I had heard any good jokes; I would have to take a telephone call; and when I finished, I would look over, and he would have fallen asleep. I would just leave him sitting there and quietly leave."

Davis worked in the lab for 15 years, and then, continuing her education, studied her way out of the lab and into the position of compliance officer, navigating patients through the red tape of Medicare and Medicaid rules and regulations to insure they got the benefits they were supposed to get. She retired in April 2014, after 42 years with the hospital. At the time of our interview, she continued to work two days a month.

Elam S. Kurtz, M.D.; Kevin, Orpah and Michael Kurtz Interviews (West Jefferson, July 13 and 16, 2014, and January 16, 2015)

Of the relatively few doctors practicing in the Appalachian region, a significant number, like Dr. Bud and the two Dean Jones, were home grown, but every now and then a doctor "not from around here" ventured into the mountain communities to offer his or her services. In 1955, Dr. Elam Kurtz was just beginning his internship at St. Luke's Hospital in Shaker Heights, Ohio, when Aquilla Stoltzfus, a Mennonite pastor in Ashe County and originally from the same area of Pennsylvania as the Kurtz family, put the young doctor in touch with Dr. Dean, who was in need of backup at the growing Ashe County Memorial Hospital. Kurtz was the son of a Mennonite pastor, a faith which renounces violence and refuses to take up arms. The rural Ashe County location, with its scarcity of physicians, offered Kurtz, a possible opportunity to obtain his CO (conscientious objector) status. Dr. Dean, impressed with the young doctor's credentials, was willing to take a chance on him, despite some opposition from the hospital's board of trustees. Kurtz and his wife Orpah moved to Ashe County in 1956, thinking they would stay about two years and then begin a mission in Ethiopia, in the planning stages before Ashe County was an option. At the time they had a four-year-old daughter, Karen Joyce, and a one-year old son, Michael David. Orpah remembers they got a call from Ashe County Memorial asking them what color paint they wanted for their house. The Kurtz family started out in the small house two blocks from the hospital, custom built for the new doctor and his family by Roland and Faw Builders, as a gesture of gratitude to Dr. Jones, Sr., for saving the life of a friend.[9]

Kurtz was born in Pennsylvania, April 1, 1924, the eldest of five sons, and raised on a dairy farm. His father anticipated Elam would stay on the farm, but young Elam had an interest in learning, which his mother Elsie supported, and his father grew to accept. At an early age, he was impressed by a letter his grandmother received from a cousin, a missionary physician in India. In 1947, Elam left farming for good and entered Eastern Mennonite College in Harrisonburg, Virginia, where he devoted a year to premedical education with an emphasis on biology. In 1948 he moved to Lebanon Valley College, passing the farm to his brother John. At the College, Elam married Orpah Horst, his sweetheart from home, who was born and raised between Lancaster and Reading, Pennsylvania, near the Kurtz family. After his graduation from Lebanon Valley in 1951, Elam and Orpah moved to Cleveland, Ohio, where Elam graduated from medical school at Western Reserve University (now Case Western University) in 1955. A one year internship at St. Luke's Hospital in Shaker Heights, Ohio, followed. It was during that year of internship that Kurtz was put in touch with Dr. Jones, Sr., at Ashe County Memorial.[10]

Kurtz and Jones made a good team, and Elam often remarked that his time with Dr. Jones was as good as an internship. He and Jones rotated shifts, working 24 hours on and

24 hours off. Kurtz's presence afforded Jones some much needed time off and Elam a chance to perform surgical procedures he had not been allowed in his internship with St. Luke's. Soon he was treating fractures, breech deliveries, and acute appendicitis. His first solo appendectomy was performed when he was on call for Jones, who had "gone fishing." After two years with the hospital, Kurtz started his private practice. The death of Dr. Joseph Robinson a year before Elam's arrival in Ashe County left a critical need for health care in the community of Creston, where Robinson had maintained a clinic. Kurtz started working on his day off and every Monday evening in Creston, taking care of Robinson's patients. Many of those patients from Robinson's practice remained with Kurtz until he retired in 2003. Bartering was still in practice as a payment option during this time, and Kurtz took payment in firewood and hams and an assortment of services. In 1958, Dr. Roy O. Freeman decided to join practices with Dr. Keys in West Jefferson and left his office in Lansing. Kurtz acquired Freeman's Lansing office and continued hours there from 1958 to 1995, dispensing medicines from his own pharmacy, located on the premises. He also had his own x-ray equipment. From the Lansing office he served people from the northwestern portion of Ashe County and patients from southwest Virginia. Orpah helped with the office work, and gradually a staff of as many as ten was assembled to run the Lansing office.[11]

Transportation to a doctor's office in those days continued to be a challenge for patients. One patient from Horse Creek rode on horseback to see Dr. Kurtz at the Lansing office. He parked his ride on a convenient patch of grass next to the office. Kurtz had patients who could not get to his office, even on horseback, so he went to them. During his early days in Ashe County, he made house calls in his Volkswagen Beetle, an uncommon vehicle in the mountains at the time. He would take his leather doctor's bag, some morphine and penicillin, and somebody would meet him at the road and show him up to the patient's house. Dr. Kurtz gained somewhat of a reputation for being a fearless traveler over the rough terrain of the area. Once he was making a call accessible only by pole boat. Before there were roads in some parts of the county, the only way to get across the river was for someone, in this case the patient's husband, to "pole" you across in a small boat. For some reason, when Kurtz arrived at the river, the pole boat was on the opposite side. Undeterred, the doctor drove his Volkswagen into the river and crossed to the other side to get to his patient. This feat quickly made the rounds in the storehouse of mountain doctor tales.

Paying forward the learning experience afforded him during his time with Dr. Dean Jones, Sr., Kurtz became involved in mentoring medical students and did this from the late 1960s until the early 1990s. In their book, *Crossings,* which served as background for these interviews, Kurtz and his son and coauthor Michael D. Kurtz, record a total of 56 students in 25 years. Dr. Kurtz's last student was his son Kevin. Reading that Michael Kurtz had gone with his father on many of his house calls, I was interested in getting his personal observations of his father's relationship with his patients and his philosophical approach to practicing medicine. I got the opportunity to talk with Michael in January 2015. As is often the case with the eldest son, Michael begins, there were differences between him and his father that sometimes made communication a challenge. Dr. Kurtz, like his colleague Dr. Jones, Sr., was not a big talker, while Michael is very much the extrovert, choosing a career as a pastor, licensed marriage counselor and family therapist. But despite his father's

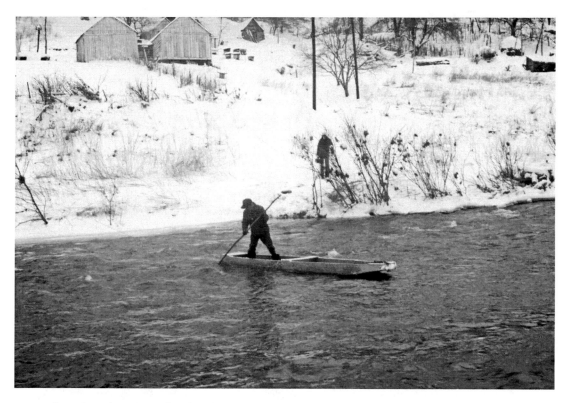

Dr. Elam Kurtz (1924–2010) had a reputation for overcoming obstacles to reach his patients. In this image, he stands on the bank of the river with his doctor bag, waiting for his patient's husband to come pole him across to get to his patient on the other side of the river (courtesy Dr. Kevin Kurtz).

taciturn and somewhat eccentric nature, Michael witnessed firsthand "the connection and trust" the doctor achieved with his patients, an ability Michael probably inherited and applied in his own way in his career. "His approach to medicine was holistic—he cared about his patient as a whole person, body, mind and soul." He developed a great passion for mental health education and advocacy and was involved in volunteer work for the New River Mental Health, a multicounty network. Daymark and Smoky Mountain Mental Health now provide mental health services for the region, but funding in the area of mental health has suffered in recent years.[12]

Even though he might not have talked as much as Michael would have liked, his father instilled in him lessons by example. "He gave me the confidence to try new things—to step out of the box. Pop was not a box person." One has only to look at his break from his strict Mennonite upbringing and his own father's traditional expectations for his eldest son to see that Elam Kurtz was not afraid to take an unchartered course. A story Michael tells me provides an interesting window into his father's adaptation from the strictures of his youth to a man accepting and often passionate about new ideas. Michael played high school basketball, and in his first year of play, his father dutifully came to the games but brought a book to read, so as to make productive use of his time. In the second year, he left his book at home and watched the game. By the third year, he was cheering on his son's team. By year four, he was getting on the referees, fiercely defending plays. "I call it the evolution of a fan," laughs Michael.

Unlike the Drs. Jones, "Pop didn't fish, but we all had time with him, despite his demanding schedule." The father and son particularly enjoyed climbing Mount Jefferson together, making the climb at least a dozen times. Michael credits his mother with managing the family's time in such a way that outings and vacations and sitting down to dinner together were viable parts of their lives. "Mother is a stickler for scheduling."

January 1, 1995, when Dr. Elam Kurtz was 71 years old, he joined his son Dr. Kevin Kurtz and Dr. Leigh Bradley at High Country Family Medicine and practiced there until his retirement in June 2003. Over his career, he delivered hundreds of babies, worked ER shifts, and remained on active staff at Ashe Memorial. And he and Orpah made friends, many friends. Dr. Elam Kurtz died April 26, 2010, at the age of 86. He practiced medicine in Ashe County for more than 47 years. Ashe County was his home for almost 54 years.[13] Orpah Kurtz still lives in West Jefferson.

Ann Day Brown Interview (West Jefferson, October 21, 2014)

Ann Day Brown started to work at the old Ashe County Memorial Hospital in 1954, right out of Jefferson High School. Dean C. Jones, Jr., had not finished medical school yet, and Mary Lou Brooks had not started to work in the business office. The hospital had about fifty employees. Ann would remain with AMH for 51 years. "It was my job from beginning to end," she smiled, as Evelyn Jones and I took our seats in her living room to talk about her career and her recollections of the hospital and its staff.

The daughter of Claude and Minnie Day, Ann was born and raised in Jefferson and has lived in the area her entire life. Tom Cockerham was the hospital administrator then and hired the petite Ann to work in the business office at the hospital. Her brother, Oscar Day, fresh from a stint in the Army medical corps, worked in the hospital too, for forty-plus years, as an orderly or nurses' assistant and then in maintenance. Ann's sister, Evelyn Woodie, worked briefly as a nurses' aide at AMH and then moved on to the hospital in Wilkes, where she became a respiratory therapist. Ann's daughter, Diane, worked part-time at the hospital during her high school years, filling in on the switchboard and doing some office work after school, on weekends and during the summer.

Ann's training was on-the-job, and Lettie Jones and Tom Cockerham both worked with her to hone her business skills. "Mr. Cockerham taught me bookkeeping, and Lettie helped me learn the general office work." The hospital, especially the administrative end, was a simple affair in those days, without the range of specialized personnel and various divisions and sections which even a small hospital supports today. "It was just Lettie, Mr. Cockerham, and me," Ann recalls. Among the responsibilities were admissions, discharges, birth certificates, insurance billing, billing for patients, cashier, payroll and statements, reception desk, and telephone. The business office was the front line for the hospital, situated at the main entrance where patients and visitors checked in. "We were the first ones they saw." Ann wore a white uniform in those early days. For patients entering by way of the ER, in the basement of the hospital, admission forms were filled out with the help of family, while the patient was treated and placed in a room. If the patient came in alone, the admission paperwork was done after the patient was treated. "Of course, at that time, it didn't take as long to admit a patient." All checks were signed by hand for years. Ann's was one of the authorizing signatures recognized by the bank, and she cosigned with the hospital administrator. There was a board in the reception area, where the names of patients were listed. Visitors would peruse the board when they came to see family or friends and determine if there was anyone else staying at the hospital they should stop in and visit while they were there. It was the neighborly thing to do, and if a patient did not want their name on the board for all to see, staff did not put it there. Of course, in a small community, everybody knows everybody's business anyway, so it is doubtful a patient could remain anonymous, despite this precaution.

The main level of the hospital, where the business office and reception area were, had the nursery, operating rooms, separate wards for men and women, and private and semiprivate patient rooms. The lower level or basement had the ER, the doctors' offices, Henry Lum's lab and x-ray, the kitchen and dining area, and central supply. When Ann first started to work, the nurses' quarters building was almost complete. She lived at home for a few weeks until the building was ready for occupancy. Probably the first to live in the quarters who was not a nurse, Ann made the modest room her home for several years, sometimes sharing accommodations with a roommate. "You brought anything personal that you wanted, and your clothes, of course," but space was limited. And although the young women were not so much under the watchful eye of Dr. Jones and Lettie as they had been when everybody lived under one roof at the hospital, the feeling of being looked after was still there, and it was a safe environment in which to work.

While the hospital was responsible for laundering her uniform, when she had to wear one, personal laundry was done in a laundry room in the nurses' quarters. Ann took all her meals in the dining room on the lower level of the hospital building, and a modest fee was deducted from her paycheck for meals. "We'd just go in the kitchen, and they'd fix us a plate." Theresa Badger, Ella Lambert and Virginia Barker made sure there was a good meal available. "It was like a family," recalls Ann. "Everybody knew everybody."

Ann left the nurses' quarters in 1957, when she married Ray Brown from Alleghany County. Getting to work in the Ashe County winters was not a problem for Ann, as her husband drove her. Her brother, Oscar Day, was often called on by nurse supervisors to pick up nurses for the next shift on his way to the hospital, especially at night. Oscar continued this accommodation after the new hospital was open. This service was part of the looking-after-your-own atmosphere of the hospital and the community.

Ann's long career at AMH included the move from the old hospital to the new in 1971. Moving day was busy for everybody, including the administrative staff, charged with getting patients to the right rooms and then making sure families and other visitors knew where to find them. At the spacious new hospital, staff was so spread out, the hospital lost a little of its close family atmosphere. Progress brought more departments and more specialized staff.

Manual typewriters were replaced with electric and then with computers. Ann went from administrative assistant, to interim administrator, to payroll supervisor. She retired from full-time work in 2000 and continued to work a flex schedule until 2006.

Mary Lou Brooks Interview (West Jefferson, August 1, 2014)

In 1959, Mary Lou Griffin Brooks had just finished business school in Winston-Salem, returned home to Ashe County, and was working in the five and dime in downtown West Jefferson, where the Ashe County Chamber of Commerce is now. Tom Cockerham and Scott McClure came into the store and asked Mary Lou if she would be interested in working at the hospital. Their bold recruitment strategy was successful, and Mary Lou started a career in business management at Ashe County Memorial that would last 51 years and three months. She started out doing anything she was given to do, working mostly with Mr. Cockerham on the business side. Mary Lou moved into the new nurses' quarters building behind the hospital and continued to live there until she married. "It took him [James Brooks] a long time to make up his mind," quipped Mary Lou, regarding the length of her courtship and subsequent time she lived on the hospital campus.

Everybody ate in the dining room. "People brought fresh vegetables and donated them to the hospital. The food was good. We had good cooks—Theresa Badger and Virginia Barker worked in the kitchen." The camaraderie extended past mealtime, and the hospital even had a women's basketball team. "We played against the Winston-Salem All Stars," says Brooks proudly. There was a convenience to living in the hospital which was missed when she moved out and had to face the challenges of getting to work in bad weather. But Mr. Cockerham made sure she got there—he picked her up. "He had chains. There was no four-wheel drive in those days. On snow days, you often had to put in extra hours to cover for the ones who couldn't make it to work."

One of Brooks's responsibilities was to admit patients. She asked them all the necessary questions like name and address, etc., and then collected the medical history, which she passed on to the medical staff. If a patient came in during the night, staff on duty would put the patient in a room, and Mary Lou gathered the admission information the next morning. "Sooner or later everybody has to come to the hospital for something," so Mary Lou knew everybody in the county; all the last names were familiar. By the end of her career, however, she could not say as much. One of the questions asked at admission was whether or not the patient wanted their name announced on the local radio station's daily "hospital report," sponsored by a local pharmacy. Admissions and discharges were duly noted for the benefit of the small community's thirst for information about their friends and neighbors. Patient names were also listed on a board in the hospital lobby, so if folks had an afternoon with nothing much to do, they could stop in at the hospital and check the board to see if there was anybody in the hospital they should call on. If the visitor didn't know any of the patients, they might just pick out somebody and drop by their room, introduce themselves, sit down, inquire as to the patient's state of health, and have a nice chat.

Mary Lou also received the payments from patients. "Most people had to pay in installments. I would be in the grocery store shopping, and people would come up to me and give me ten or twenty dollars to put on their account. I would send them a receipt when I got back to the hospital." Of course, with the move to the new hospital building in 1971, some of that relaxed atmosphere was lost to rules and regulations, but the hospital remained a family affair. Mary Lou's first two children, Cindy and Jim, were delivered by Dr. C. E. Miller at the old hospital, and she was expecting her third, Chris, when the new hospital opened. It was exciting to move to the new building. On the day staff transitioned to the new space, Mary Lou's task was assigning patient rooms, a process she remembers as running smoothly. There were many changes in the years to come. "If they had a new program, they wanted me to start it. I was sent twice a month to help with the urology clinic in the Professional Building. I interviewed patients and got their history." By the time Brooks retired in 2010, everything was done on the computer. She concluded her career in accounts payable. The days of folks handing her money in the grocery store to put on their account were over, as were the days when she recognized every name of a patient. Looking back, she says, "I miss the people but not the work." Her ties to the hospital, the new and the old, like her ties to the hospital family, are strong. Mary Lou's sister, Peggy, worked at the hospital for a while, her mother, Alice Griffin, worked in the hospital cafeteria, and Dr. Jones, Sr., delivered her son Chris at the new hospital.

Cindy Brooks Baucom Interview (West Jefferson, August 1, 2014)

The children of hospital employees typically got their first summer jobs at the hospital. Cindy Brooks Baucom, daughter of Mary Lou Brooks, remembers her older brother Jim working in the lab when he was in high school and college, while Cindy's first job, at age 15, was as receptionist and switchboard operator at the front desk. "It was pretty intimidating if a nurse called and wanted a doctor paged 'stat.' It was a big responsibility, but it helped lay the groundwork for handling stressful situations later in life, by putting me in situations where I had to deal with people who were not at their best," as is usually the case when you are in the hospital. Cindy also delivered flowers to the patients' rooms, sometimes reading the cards to the patient, fluffing a pillow, or getting a glass of water—whatever the patient might need. "There was no such thing as 'that's not in my job description.' Everybody pitched in and did what was needed to help a patient be more comfortable."

"Probably the biggest percentage of the housekeeping staff was made up of children of employees, especially the boys. The girls usually worked at the front desk, like I did. I always found it a very welcoming environment. Everyone became a part of a family, and we banded together for meals. Some of my best memories are of the Christmas parties, where employees got to bring their whole family."

Pat Bare Cooper Interview (Glendale Springs, October 22, 2014)

Like so many other Ashe County natives who were employed by Ashe Memorial Hospital, Pat Cooper worked almost her entire career at AMH. The daughter of Effie and Ernest Bare, the principal at Glendale Springs School, she was delivered by Dr. Dean Jones, Sr. Cooper grew up on a farm behind the Trading Post on the Blue Ridge Parkway at Glendale Springs. After graduation from Ashe Central High School in 1965, she worked briefly in the office of Jefferson attorney Ira T. Johnston and then went to work at the old hospital in 1968. Although she spent most of her years at the new hospital in the business office, working with Ann Brown, Mary Lou Brooks and Tom Cockerham, she first interviewed for her job with Director of Nursing Peggy Ashley and was put to work handling admissions in the ER. When she moved to the business office, she got her training on-the-job, working under the supervision of Mary Lou Brooks. She enjoyed working for Tom Cockerham and served as his secretary for many years, while Ann Brown was his administrative assistant. Her job expanded along with the hospital, and she worked as executive assistant to the hospital CEO, including 17 years with R. D. Williams II, the job she liked best. She also was medical librarian, director of volunteers, personnel coordinator, and worked with Joe Thore with the AMH Foundation. There were 68 volunteers under her supervision, and Cooper went to great lengths to make them feel appreciated for the work they were doing for the hospital. Before the days of a digital library for medical reference, the medical library consisted of a carefully maintained collection of medical reference books, magazines, and periodicals, which doctors could access through the librarian. Cooper's various responsibilities were reassigned to several different departments at her retirement.

Pat Cooper has fond memories of Dr. Dean Jones, Sr., and Doc. "Dr. Dean was a quiet man," she reflects, "but when he spoke, everybody listened." She remembers how hard it was for him to make the move from the old AMH to the new, leaving the hospital he had worked so hard to see built and that had been his home for so many years. Doc nicknamed her "Cat Pooper" and shared jokes with her. Once her family physician instructed her to make an appointment with Doc about a knot he discovered in her neck. When she saw Doc in the hall at the hospital, she mentioned it to him. He stopped right then and there in the hall and examined the knot, "This has got to go," he declared. Surgery soon followed, and when Pat showed Evelyn Jones, sitting in on our interview, the wisp of a scar on her neck, Evelyn smiled proudly at her husband's fine handiwork. "He was always known for his excellent suturing."

Pat and Larry Cooper's daughter April grew up in the hospital, like many children of the AMH staff, dropping by after school, and later working as a Candy Striper and in the hospital pharmacy. The exposure influenced her chosen field of study, and now Dr. April Laney is a clinical pharmacist at Ashe Memorial.

Cooper retired in December 2011, after 43 years with AMH. She retains a place on the board of directors of the AMH Foundation, which is charged with raising money to support various hospital needs.

Polly Osowitt, R.N., and Elliott Osowitt Interviews (West Jefferson, October 17, 2014)

Polly and Elliott Osowitt represent another love match made at Ashe Memorial Hospital. Polly Parsons was born in Ashe County, delivered by Dr. Dean Jones, Sr., and grew up in the Baldwin community, the daughter of Ruth and Wintford Parsons. She started to work at the old Ashe County Memorial Hospital in 1969 as a nurses' aide, combining a job and the pursuit of higher education for many years. She got her L.P.N. at nearby Wilkes Community College and was in the first class to graduate from the Ashe Memorial Nursing program. She received her R.N. at Caldwell Community College, and in May 1991, she received her bachelor's degree in nursing from Gardner Webb College in Boiling Springs.

Polly met her future husband, Elliott Osowitt, while both were working at Ashe Memorial. Elliott was the first surgeon's assistant in the county and came to work for Doc, who was willing to take on someone "not from around here," as his father had done with Henry Lum and Dr. Elam Kurtz. Elliott was from Los Angeles, California. He first made it to North Carolina via the U.S. Army and Fort Bragg. While stationed at Fort Bragg, he had the opportunity to vacation in the western part of the state and fell in love with the mountains. He entered a surgeon's assistant program at the University of North Carolina at Chapel Hill, graduating in 1975, and started looking for a job in the mountains of North Carolina. The concept of a surgeon's assistant was new at the time, but Elliott had an ace up his sleeve—his mentor at Chapel Hill was a former roommate of Doc's. Doc and his new surgeon's assistant worked well together, complementing one another's skills. Doc would make his diagnosis and announce the need for surgery, with his usual as-few-words-as-possible-style, and Osowitt, a big talker, would follow up with the patient, offering a more extensive, reassuring and chatty explanation of the procedure to be performed, drawing pictures where appropriate. Meanwhile, Doc was on his way to his next patient. This method of operation resulted in Osowitt's spending a lot of time looking for Doc, but he learned to track him down. "He was an awesome teacher. He taught commitment and dedication with a sense of humor."

While Evelyn and I sat in the living room of the Osowitts' home on one of those beautiful, Ashe County autumn days, Elliott reflected on his years with Doc and Dr. Dean, describing the similarities in the two men, both devoting so many hours to their patients— "working like bumblebees, never stopping until their wings wore out. I feel like I came in (at Ashe Memorial) at the end of an era, when there was more time to spend with patients and their families." Osowitt made house calls when patients could not get to the hospital for post-op visits. Care extended beyond the office. "I am privileged to have experienced that era."

The atmosphere at the hospital reflected the emphasis on family, as well. "Every Sunday, the whole Jones family, children and grandchildren, came to the hospital for lunch. It was like a huge Walton Mountain thing. It was the only time I ever saw Dr. Dean C., Jr., in a suit and not scrubs." Coming from Los Angeles, of Polish descent, and raised in the Jewish faith, Osowitt might have had trouble fitting in, but he was welcomed by the Jones family immediately. "I don't think I would have been accepted (in the community) if not for Dr.

Dean C., Jr.," says Elliott, recalling Doc's introductions at the Rotary and to his fishing buddies. He was included in Jones family outings, taking leaf looking drives on the windy roads of Ashe County until he was car sick and playing with the children, hanging a young Charles Jones upside down. The partnership with Doc turned into a friendship, and when Elliott and Polly married in 1978, their witnesses were Doc and Evelyn.

In 1982, working out of the basement of their home, Elliott and Polly Osowitt started Mountain Air Home Oxygen, bringing the latest in home respiratory assistive devices and advanced home health care equipment to Ashe County. The electric machine, called an oxygen concentrator, generated oxygen on site, was not combustible, and was lighter and more portable than the old oxygen tanks it replaced in the homes of patients needing oxygen. The old 150 pound tanks, delivered by a local drugstore, had to be manhandled into position, often by an elderly caregiver in the home. Dr. Roy Freeman and Dr. Edward J. Miller were early supporters of the couple's business endeavor. The Osowitts coordinated their efforts with the Ashe County Health Department and Hospice. Recognizing the need for a comprehensive line of health and sickroom supplies, Elliott and Polly started Ashe Home HealthCare Consultants in 1986, operating out of Ashe Memorial Hospital. Their service included rental of wheelchairs and beds, but never medications. It was not long before the company, now with three full-time employees, moved from the hospital to the shopping center below the hospital. As Ashe Home HealthCare Consultants continued to grow, another move was made in 1991, to Dr. Roy Freeman's former office, between the towns of Jefferson and West Jefferson, and a second location was opened in Sparta to serve Alleghany County. The company relocated again to North Main Street in Jefferson in 1994, and eventually was bought by Lincare. Elliott was president of the North Carolina Association of Medical Equipment Services for three years and successfully pushed a bill through the North Carolina General Assembly in 1994, enforcing the protection of patients receiving home medical services from unethical suppliers.[14]

Polly worked in the ER for 28 years. With the growth of Ashe Memorial Hospital, came new responsibilities, and she held a number of positions, including staff nurse, acute care nurse manager, and hospital education coordinator. Polly retired from Ashe Memorial in October 2013 and now works for Appalachian Student Health Service on the campus of Appalachian State University in Boone. Elliott exchanged his devotion to the physical care of people to the spiritual, becoming pastor of Faith Fellowship Church in Jefferson in 2003. He misses the hands-on part of his first career and the joy of seeing patients repaired, but seems at home with his life as a Christian and pastor.

Tammy Lum Thore, M.D., and Joe F. Thore Interviews (Jefferson, September 19 and 16, 2014)

The contribution to health care in the region made by Henry and Ruby Lum lives on through the practice of their daughter Dr. Tammy Lum Thore, a general surgeon at AMH. Her first job was as a phlebotomist (somebody who draws blood) at Ashe Memorial Hospital, under the supervision of her father, Henry Lum. Eventually she was cleared to run some of the tests in the lab. The Lum children grew up in the old hospital, brought to the hospital when both Ruby and Henry had to be there, which was often. Staff kept an eye on the children while the couple worked. "Sometimes," recalls Dr. Thore, "Dad would put the patient to sleep, and Mom would be the nurse."

Dr. Thore's interest in medicine came naturally, then. "It is all I knew." Henry Lum encouraged his daughter to become a surgeon, declaring if you were going to do something, like have a career in medicine, you needed to do it at the highest level you could achieve. Tammy liked the idea of being able to see immediate results from her work, as is the case with surgery, more so than treating chronic illnesses. She graduated from East Carolina University Medical School, Brody School of Medicine, in 1986 and did her residency with Spartanburg Regional Medical Center in South Carolina, where she met her future husband, Joe F. Thore, on a blind date. Joe, a native of Alleghany County, had graduated from the University of North Carolina at Charlotte and was working as an account manager for Kraft in Greenville, South Carolina. The two married in Tammy's last year of residency. They looked around for a place to settle, and Jefferson looked like a good fit. In 1992, Tammy began a 14 year career with Ashe Memorial, working closely with Dr. Dean C. Jones, Jr., with whom she enjoyed an excellent and mutually beneficial working relationship. "I taught him laparoscopic cholecystectomies, and he taught me how to do hysterectomies."

Phyllis Jones Yount, oldest daughter of Doc and Evelyn Jones, witnessed Dr. Thore's surgical skill firsthand one day when she was on call at the hospital, and Thore was on duty. An elderly man came in with a leaking aortic aneurism, a desperate situation, and there was no time to transfer the man to another, bigger hospital with specialized heart care. Thore repaired the aneurism, and the patient lived.[15]

The same year Dr. Thore started to work at Ashe Memorial, Joe went to work with the hospital as the first director of the AMH Foundation. He wrote the by-laws for the foundation, handled public relations, and created his own job description. His father-in-law, Henry Lum, had retired from the hospital by the time he came on board, but Ruby Lum was there for a few years after he started with the hospital. "She loved her job," says Dr. Thore of her mother. Locals, familiar with Ruby and her caregiving for so many years, sometimes lent more credence to her recommendations than those of her daughter, the one with the M.D., but then there is something to be said for fifty plus years of experience in a small community, says Tammy. Ruby was known to recruit patients for her daughter in the post office and other places of business, where she met and greeted people anxious to describe their state of health to the friendly nurse.

In 2006, Dr. Thore left AMH for Sparta and Alleghany Memorial Hospital. She and Joe continued to live in Jefferson, and Tammy covered surgical calls in Ashe County every other weekend. Effective June 1, 2015, Dr. Thore gave up the winding commute to Sparta and returned to full-time work at AMH. Joe is in his 23rd year with the hospital and is AMH's Chief Operating Officer (COO). The couple have two daughters.

I asked the Thores how they felt about their decision to forego city life and bigger paychecks to return to western North Carolina. Joe reflected on the question and responded, "We've been able to live in a small community and make a difference." I was not surprised by his answer—it is consistent with the perspective I often find in talking with people in this community, and it is one of the things I admire most about this place.

Charlotte Caddell Thompson, R.N., Interview (Telephone, January 19, 2015)

Charlotte Caddell Thompson is part of the future in nursing. I talk to her right before her weekly 6:00 p.m. to 9:00 p.m. shift, which she works from her home. Charlotte is employed with a health management company, based in the Triad. Her patient load or membership assigned is approximately 400. She has never met any of them face to face and never will; she tracks their status via telephone. Some of her patients are on the other side of the country, and those are the ones she is contacting on this once-a-week 6:00 to 9:00 p.m. shift, to accommodate the West Coast time difference. The rest of her work week, Tuesday through Friday, is 9:00 a.m. to 6:00 p.m. With two sons, 10 and 15, this is a happy marriage of work and family, and, Charlotte assures, "They know to be quiet when I am on the phone." She communicates with her coworkers via email, and they share their individual expertise on cases that require some brainstorming. They just don't do it sitting at a conference table, passing around a box of doughnuts and wearing scrubs.

But it wasn't always like this, and Charlotte probably would not be as good at her job now if she had not worked her way up in a more traditional medical environment. In 2002, while she was still an L.P.N. and working on becoming an R.N., she joined the staff at Ashe Memorial Hospital, starting off as a hall nurse on the second floor, the medical surgical floor. When she graduated as an R.N., she went to Watauga Medical in Boone for about two years, in the intermediate care unit and pediatric unit. Then it was back to Ashe Memorial, now as an operating room nurse, cross-trained in Mountain Hearts and x-ray. During her six years as an operating room nurse, AMH, in a collaborative effort with Appalachian State University, offered some of the nursing staff the opportunity to bump up their credentials to a bachelor of science degree in nursing. Eight or ten signed up for the program and were in the first class to graduate from the program at ASU. It was a good way for a working mother to continue her education, because class started right after the shift ended, and it was conducted at the hospital, so the students did not have to move their cars.

During her second tour of duty with AMH, when Charlotte was an R.N. and working in the OR, she had the opportunity to work with both Doc Jones and his son, Dr. Charles Jones. Having been born and raised in Ashe County, she was well aware of the Jones family legacy. She remembers Doc as quiet and soft-spoken and very serious about his job. "He was a very wise man. Sometimes during a surgery he would step away from the operating table and think through the mechanics of what he needed to do, working out his next move." In many ways she sees Dr. Charles as a younger version of his father. "He is very interested in educating the people around him—the nurses and technicians with him in the OR. He'll say, 'Glove up and feel this. This is what cancer feels like.'" As a result, his team is extremely knowledgeable about the various surgical procedures in which they assist and can anticipate the surgeon's movements and what he will need. "I have learned things from him I could not learn in a textbook, and I am thankful for that. He has respect for his OR team; he listens to what they have to say, and he has complete control of the OR." The team Charlotte worked with was like a family. "That is the closest knit group I have ever worked with, and my time with AMH is one of the best job experiences I have ever had. I was blessed to be a part of it."

But Charlotte acknowledges the stress of working long shifts. The job in health management, which she started in 2011, offered her a break from that stress, the opportunity to expand on what she had learned and combine it with the skill set from her initial degree from ASU in communications. She attended a four month orientation for the job, which she describes as "like going to nursing school all over again," except with a focus on diseases, her specialty. Charlotte misses the face-to-face contact with the patients, but she has adapted to this new way of nursing and is comfortable talking to her patients or members by phone, educating them on the risks of their disease, answering their questions, and following up on their concerns.

11

Dr. Dean C. "Doc" Jones, Jr.: Third Generation of a Family Legacy

"For an only child, Dean C. ended up with a lot of brothers and sisters," begins Evelyn Jones, when I first interview her about her husband's life. The son of Dr. Dean Jones, Sr., and Lettie, Dean C. Jones, Jr., was born February 12, 1931, in Charlotte, where his parents were living and working at the time. Doctors later advised his mother not to have any more children, but, every time a baby was delivered at Ashe County Memorial, Dean C. would go down the hall to the viewing window of the nursery to see his new "brother" or "sister." He would announce the arrival of the new baby with as much pride and enthusiasm as if the new addition was blood kin. Always optimistic the baby was a permanent addition to his family, he regularly rebounded from the disappointment of not getting to keep the new baby, but, in his own way, reflects Evelyn, he was brother to everyone born in the hospital.

His father did not have much time to spend on entertainment, but he did enjoy taking his wife and son out to the movie on "family night" at the local theater. On more than one occasion, Dean C. voiced his despair over the lack of siblings in their little group, since none of the hospital babies were keepers, and declared when he got grown, he was going to have a real family, with lots of children to sit with on family night at the movie show. With Evelyn's cooperation, he followed up on this life goal with five children of their own— a respectable showing for family night. And he got to keep them all, although, as he acknowledged later in life, "Evelyn raised my family for me. If it had been up to me, they'd just have been 'jerked up.'"

Nell Jones Taylor, first cousin to Dean C., grew up in Charlotte, but her parents, Hunter and Mattie Jones, maintained a cabin in Helton and visited often, especially in the summer. Nell, who was my primary source for Dr. Bud Jones, also supplied me with information about Dean C. Close in age to her cousin, Nell remembers visiting the family in the old Ashe County Memorial Hospital. "Dean C. and I were buddies. Going into a hospital to visit my cousin was exciting." Dr. Dean and Lettie had two rooms and a bath in one wing of the hospital, across the hall from the nurses' ward. "They were always saying 'Don't run in the hall!'" There are stories about Dean C. dribbling a basketball down the halls of the hospital and riding his bicycle, but Nell claims she was not involved in these rowdy antics. She does remember Dean C. loved to take her on hospital tours, showing her the sites and

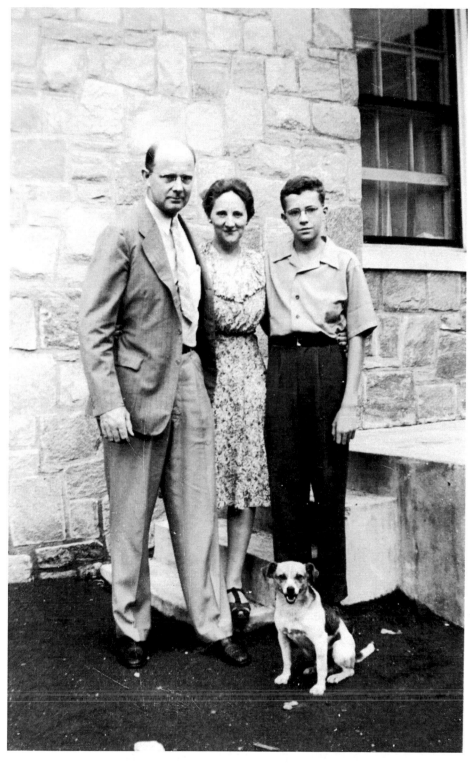

Dean C. Jones, Jr., lived with his parents, Dr. Dean Jones, Sr., and Lettie, in Ashe County Memorial Hospital until he left for college. The dog's name was Jasper (courtesy Evelyn Jones).

the secret places he liked to hide. Her playmate did not talk about becoming a surgeon, but it seemed obvious to Nell and others that he would. Friends already called him "Doc," because he lived in the hospital.[1]

Dean C. and his father were similar in height and build, and, like his father, Dean C. excelled at basketball and played at the intramural level in college. He played point guard and was an excellent shooter, relates Dr. Charles Jones, when we talk about his recollections of Doc in early spring 2014. Dean C. was captain of the team for two years at Jefferson High School, where he graduated in 1948. As was the case in Dean Sr.'s days on the court, the game was pretty rough, says Charles, and the rivalries with area teams were fierce, especially between Jefferson and West Jefferson. After one particularly close game, where Jef-

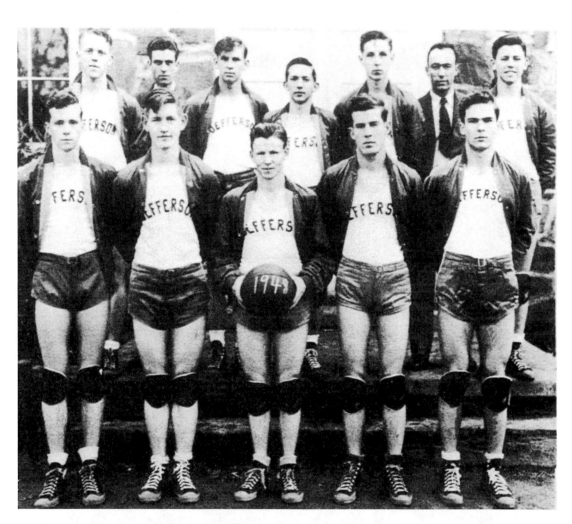

Dean C. Jones, Jr., excelled at basketball, was captain of the Jefferson High School team for two years, and played at the intramural level in college. He was inducted into the Ashe County Sports Hall of Fame in 2008. Those identified in this photograph of the Jefferson High School team include, left to right: first row—Dean C. Jones, Jr.; Howard Jones; Ford Rash, center; and Edgar Burkett, far right; second row—Ralph Colvard; Principal Orvil Jackson; Bill Calloway, fifth from the left; teacher and coach Colonel Francis, sixth from the left; and Clayborn Sheets, far right. (courtesy Evelyn Jones).

ferson lost to West Jefferson, one of Dean C.'s teammates picked a bit of flesh out from under his fingernail and commented, "Well, we may have lost the game, but we got us some Barr meat," referring to Duke Barr, a player on the opposing team. During one hotly contested basketball game between rivals Jefferson and West Jefferson, which no doubt will live forever in the annals of local sports lore, Dean C. made a last second shot from past half court and sank it to win the game. Charles says he still has people come up to him claiming to remember when his father made that winning shot. Although Doc reportedly never got in a hurry and was more than fashionably late for all kinds of engagements, including fishing dates, his deliberate approach clearly did not extend to basketball, even into adulthood. He attended at least 36 ACC basketball tournaments over the years and watched all the UNC games on television. Doc's dedication to sports was recognized when he was inducted into the Ashe County Sports Hall of Fame April 26, 2008, for his contributions to basketball on the Jefferson High School team 1945–1948 and for his 40-plus years as sports physician for Ashe Central High School and Ashe County High School. His presence on the sidelines was a reassurance to parents of athletes. The Ashe County Sports Hall of Fame is an exhibit in the Museum of Ashe County History in Jefferson.

Dean C. was still living at the hospital with his parents and home from medical school when a pretty young nurses' aide caught his eye, and he asked his mother to introduce him to Evelyn Price. The two had a hard time getting the romance off the ground. "We didn't get to go out on a date at first, because I was always working when he was off," remembers Evelyn. "Henry and Ruby Lum were trying to fix us up. They had met at the hospital, got married, and were living in the hospital, across from the emergency room." Evelyn admits she was dating another boy steady at the time, but Dean C. soon had the advantage, aided, to some extent, by living across the hall from the nurses' quarters and a prophesy in Evelyn's high school newspaper that she would be a nurse, marry a doctor, and run a free clinic.

"When we had a date, he would say goodnight at my door and walk across to his," Evelyn laughs. She thought it would be a summer romance, but a long distance courtship developed when Evelyn started to school at Emory and Henry College in Emory, Virginia, and Dean C. continued his studies at UNC at Chapel Hill. The couple regularly made the commute between the two schools to see each other. Between Dean C.'s third and fourth year of medical school at UNC and during Evelyn's last year of nurses' training at Johnston Memorial Hospital in Abingdon, Virginia, the two married, in August of 1955. The wedding came two weeks after Dean C.'s cousin

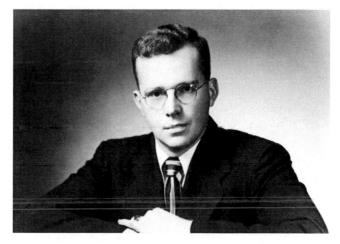

Dean C. Jones, Jr., was home from college and working in the hospital when he first met Evelyn Price, who was working there as a nurses' aide (photograph, circa 1955, courtesy Evelyn Jones).

Nell and her husband Tom Taylor married. Nell and Tom went to the Jones-Price wedding while still on their honeymoon at the family's cabin in Helton, says Nell.[2]

Dean C. and Evelyn would have to continue their long distance relationship for a little longer, commuting between Chapel Hill and Abingdon. There were rules then which prohibited married student nurses from living in the student nurses' quarters, so Evelyn moved to an apartment. Before that last year of school was over, Evelyn was pregnant with their first child, Phyllis. After Dean C.'s graduation from UNC Medical School in 1956, the two moved to Charlotte for a one year internship and three and a half year surgical residency at Charlotte Memorial Hospital, now known as Carolinas Medical Center. Their first three children were born during their stay there, Phyllis in 1956, David in 1959, and Tommy in 1960. His fellow surgeons at Carolinas Medical were eager to have Dean C. stay, especially the plastic surgeons, who were impressed with his suturing. "When he closed up a thyroidectomy, his sutures were so fine they left an almost indiscernible scar in the natural wrinkle of the neck," declares Evelyn proudly.

"Between the internship and residency, we lived with Dean C.'s parents for about six months, because we thought he (Dean C.) was going to be drafted into the service to go to Korea." But locals got up a petition saying his medical services were needed in the rural communities, and Doc was deferred from service. At the end of the surgical residency, with the three children in tow, the couple moved from Charlotte to Louisburg, where Doc had a one and one half year surgical fellowship with Dr. John T. "Jack" Lloyd at Franklin Memorial Hospital. He honed his surgical skills and was encouraged to continue at the hospital in Louisburg, but there was never any question that Doc would move back to Ashe County and join the Ashe County Memorial staff with his father. "It was always agreed we would go home," says Evelyn.

When the young family moved back to Ashe County around 1963, Doc went straight to the hospital, and father and son worked together until Dr. Dean retired. They made a good team too, and in one case pooled their talent with Dr. Elam Kurtz to prepare a noteworthy report on penicillin allergy, which was printed in the *North Carolina Medical Journal* (volume 19, number 3, pages 112–115, March 1958). The report was based on an unusual case in Ashe County where a patient was so sensitive to penicillin that she experienced a severe reaction just from physical contact with another person who had taken penicillin. There was concern about her eating dairy products from cattle receiving penicillin. The doctors conducted a controlled experiment, which confirmed the patient's extreme sensitivity to penicillin, and their report warned of the risks involved in incorporating antibiotics in various cold remedies. More recent medical research has supported the concerns expressed in this report by Drs. Dean Jones, Sr. and Jr., and Elam Kurtz. Not only did the three Ashe County doctors probably save a patient's life by recognizing and treating this extraordinary medical condition in a timely manner, but they conducted valuable clinical research, shedding light on problems associated with the overuse of antibiotics—impressive accomplishments for doctors in a small, rural community.

Charles recalls his father and grandfather collaborated on another remarkable case involving the son of Rufus Stuart of Ashe County, the patient for whom a rare form of hemophilia is named. Rufus Stuart experienced severe bleeding from infancy. Eventually he was treated by Dr. Dean, Sr., who noticed that when he gave Stuart a donor's blood, his bleeding would stop. Dr. Dean, Sr., recognized the case as very unusual and referred Stuart to Winston-Salem and then to UNC at Chapel Hill for further testing and study. In 1955, Drs. John B. Graham, E. M. Barrow, and Cecil Hoagie were credited with discovering the true nature of the Stuart factor, also known as the Stuart-Prower factor, after another patient, and as factor X deficiency. Factor X is a protein in the body that helps the blood to coagulate or clot. People with factor X deficiency, estimated to be as rare as one per million, experience bruising, nose or mouth bleeds, and excessive bleeding after an injury or surgery, Charles explains. Severe deficiencies may result in joint and gastrointestinal bleeding. Factor X can be passed down in families where both parents carry the gene. If only one parent has the gene, the child may be a carrier, while having no symptoms. During the lengthy evaluation process at UNC, the whole Stuart family in Ashe County was tested. Meanwhile, the son of Rufus Stuart came into Ashe Memorial with a bleeding ulcer, requiring immediate surgery. Drs. Dean, Sr. and Jr., recognized the name and the extreme risk involved. They asked the son if he had the Stuart factor. He replied he had been tested but had yet to receive the results. The two doctors made a judgment call and went forward, performing the critical surgery together. The call was right, and the surgery was a success—the son of Rufus Stuart did not have the factor X deficiency; he was a carrier.

This case involving the Stuart factor may have inspired Doc to start the blood bank in Ashe County. Previously, when blood was needed for a patient, Evelyn would call a donor

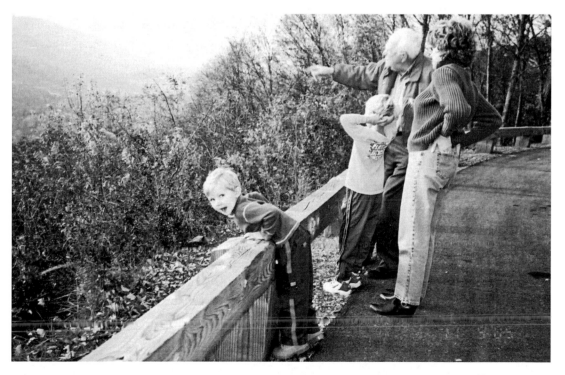

Dr. Dean C. "Doc" Jones, Jr., delighted in showing off the sites of his beloved Ashe County. Grandchildren Cameron and Lane Patterson with their mother Linda Patterson enjoy a day with "Grandoc" on Mount Jefferson (photograph, circa 1999, courtesy Evelyn Jones).

from a list maintained for this purpose, and the donor would come to the hospital and make the donation. Evelyn became very active in the Ashe County Hemophilia Foundation and served as president.

Doc and Evelyn bought a house on Northwest Drive in Jefferson, and Doc immersed himself in the job at the hospital and his community, Evelyn relates. He was a member of the North Carolina Medical Society, the American Medical Association, and the American Board of Surgery. He helped get numerous worthwhile projects off the ground in Ashe County, including the Red Cross Blood Mobile and Meals on Wheels. His contributions were not confined to community health care; he also helped start Ashe County Park. The church was and still is an important part of the lives of the Jones family, and Doc was an active member of the Jefferson United Methodist Church, served as chairman of the administrative board, and played many other roles during his lifelong membership. "The Rotary was near and dear to his heart, and he personified the Rotarian philosophy of 'service above self'," Charles adds. Doc served as president of the Rotary Club, and, in the 1970s, his community honored him as Ashe County Man of Year for Civic Service.

Doc and Evelyn and Nell Taylor and her husband, Tom, maintained their close friendship over the years, playing bridge, watching ball games on television, and sharing outings. According to Nell, Doc's Aunt Frances taught him to play bridge when he was about nine years old, and he became an avid player. "Dean C. loved taking his family, including us, all over the mountains in his Jeep," she recalls. "He loved to get out and roam these mountains," confirms Evelyn, "he knew every peak and ridge and stream and was quick to point them out." Nell laughs, "And we never argued with him, because he was always right."[3]

Those who had the opportunity to work with both Doc and his father cite their similar work ethic and devotion to patients. Senior was certainly the more serious of the two. Doc, like his father, was not a big talker, but, as his son Charles relates, "he was never at a loss for words when it came to telling a joke," and he delighted in bestowing nicknames on his acquaintances and the hospital staff.[4] Some staff I interviewed commented they knew they were accepted into the hospital family when they got their nickname. Pat Cooper, who worked with both father and son, as secretary to the hospital business manager, recalls Doc periodically coming up to her desk, looking around to assure they were alone, and then pulling a slip of paper from his front pocket as he said, "I got a joke for you."[5] He set such great store by his collection of jokes that once, after falling into the river on a fishing excursion, his friend Dr. Don McNeill recalls finding him painstakingly spreading his pocketed jokes out on the hood of his car to dry.[6]

Like his father, Doc never aspired to be a wealthy man, says son Charles. His profession was a passion; it was not about money; it was about the patient. Doc was operating one day when a car pulled up to the hospital and dumped out a man who had been shot. Staff got the man inside, and Doc set to work on him. A telephone call was patched through to the emergency room. The call was from a friend of Doc's—turns out this friend was the man who shot the fellow Doc had on the operating table. The friend had been arrested and taken to jail, and he wanted Doc to come post bail for him. Doc informed his friend he was too busy trying to save the man's life, so he (the friend) would not get charged with murder.

Doc maintained an office in the basement of the old hospital, across from that of his father. Later, he and his father would have an office in the Professional Building behind the new hospital, where Dr. Charles has his office now. Doc's fees were billed out of his office rather the hospital's business office, and sometimes, recalls business office staffer Ann Brown, when he would peruse the list of accounts owed, he would point to a name and say simply, "mark that off; he can't pay."[7] Dr. Charles says when he first joined his father at Ashe Memorial, staff advised him he needed to help with the "Doc specials." "When I inquired as to what that might be, I was told it referred to people who traveled some distance to see Doc and had no means to pay him but came anyway, knowing they would be cared for."

As one fellow doctor quipped at Doc's retirement party roast, Doc was famous for not disseminating a lot of information. But although Doc was a quiet man by reputation, especially to those who did not know him well, when he spoke, people listened. His daughter-in-law, Dr. Leigh Bradley, recalls his taciturn nature with patients. Like other staff, she quickly learned to follow-up with his patients, explaining that the doctor had made his diagnosis and was scheduling surgery, as Doc would already be on his way to the next patient or to scrub for surgery, leaving his patient uninformed. The same was true for post-op. His patients might have no idea what their surgery involved or what their prognosis was, if not for Doc's surgical assistant, Elliott Osowitt and other staff who knew to do the necessary hand-holding.[8]

Doc and Evelyn lived in the house on Northwest Drive almost 24 years until it was destroyed by an electrical fire in December 1986. No one was there at the time, says Evelyn. By then only their youngest, Linda Noel, was still living at home. When the couple's oldest son, David, asked his father what he managed to salvage from the fire in the way of clothing, Doc pointed out he was at work at the time of the fire, so the only clothing he had left was the underwear he was wearing under his scrubs.[9] The family moved into a friend's house for about a year and then into the brick ranch above the hospital, where Dr. Dean and Lettie had lived. They were both gone by then, Lettie first in 1983 and then Dr. Dean in 1984. Evelyn continues to live there now with her son David.

Doc did not want to retire, says Evelyn. He said he needed to stay on awhile longer and work with Dr. Tammy Thore, Henry and Ruby Lum's daughter, and then he said he needed to stay on awhile longer to work with Charles. Finally, in May 2007, after a career in surgery spanning 44 years, serving as chief of staff and as a member of the board of trustees for Ashe Memorial Hospital, he grudgingly took down his shingle. He quit, he maintained; he did not retire. He always insisted he did not want a going away party or retirement party, so, of course, his family rented the Blue Ridge Dinner Theater and put on a big surprise bash for him.

Unfortunately, Doc did not get the chance to enjoy his leisure for long. He fell ill and was in and out of the hospital and Margate Health and Rehabilitation Center the last two years of his life. He did not like being sick any more than anybody else does, but being accustomed to such an active lifestyle made his confinement especially frustrating. Dr. Leigh Bradley recalls Doc disappeared once while he was a patient at AMH. The staff went into panic mode, searching for him everywhere. They called Evelyn and then Charles to see if Doc had gone home or someplace else off the hospital campus. Dr. Bradley was working in the ER at the time and discovered him sitting in the call room in the ER, watching the

Carolina game on the TV. "People have been looking everywhere for you," she scolded. Unrepentant, Doc explained he couldn't pick up the game on the TV in his room.[10]

Doc died Tuesday, December 29, 2009, at Ashe Memorial Hospital. He is survived by his wife Evelyn Price Jones; three sons, David Jones, Thomas Jones and his wife Dr. Leigh Bradley, and Dr. Charles Jones and his wife, Debbie; two daughters, Phyllis and husband, Dr. Keith Yount, and Linda Noel and husband Dale Patterson; ten grandchildren; two step-grandchildren, and one step-great-grandchild, and a legacy of health care passed down from his father and grandfather.

Donald D. McNeill, M.D., Interview (Jefferson, October 29, 2014)

Although he did not share his father's interest in hunting, Doc was an avid fly fisherman. When he was working, Doc regularly set aside Tuesdays for fishing. Since fishing was such a big part of his life, I wanted to gather recollections from the perspective of his longtime fishing buddy, Dr. Don McNeill. McNeill is a physician and hospital pathologist, originally from Charlotte. He moved to Lenoir after his service with the U.S. Army and became affiliated with Ashe Memorial Hospital in April 1974, when Dr. Dean, Sr., was still practicing, and Henry Lum was manager of radiology and the clinical lab. "Dr. Don McNeill brought modern pathology to Ashe Memorial," says Dr. Charles Jones, "and he and his wife Ann, a physical therapist, started the first physical therapy program at Ashe Memorial in 1975."[11] McNeill was serving as consultant for six hospitals when he retired in 2008, giving up all but Ashe Memorial, his "home away from home." He continued to be involved in committee management with the hospital until he retired for good in July 2015.

McNeill went fishing with Dean, Sr., and Henry Lum a few times in his early days with Ashe Memorial, but he soon became a good friend of Dean C., who introduced him to a group of his fishing buddies. The group, as described by McNeill, included: Dale Shepherd, a pharmacist and original owner of the New River Christmas Tree Farm; Earl Hightower, veterinarian, Mayor of Jefferson, and long-time secretary for the Ashe Memorial Hospital Board of Trustees; Tom Weaver, native of Ashe County and retired Navy chief petty officer; and Duke Barr, who competed against Dean C. in high school basketball, earned a degree in forestry at North Carolina State University, and became director of the Cherokee National Forest. For forty-some years, the friends made a fishing trip every May and October, usually setting up camp at Gentry's Creek in the Cherokee National Forest in Tennessee, a prime site no doubt assured by Duke Barr's position as director. Others joined the group over the years, including Frank Gentry from Erwin, Tennessee; Edgar Burkett, who also played basketball with Dean C. and Duke; and John D. Weaver, of Weaver Tree Farm. McNeill joined the party in May 1975, at Dean C.'s invitation.

Dean C. and Earl Hightower both had phenomenal memories and could go for hours without repeating a joke, says McNeill. "Dale Shepherd, Tom Weaver, Duke Barr, and Frank Gentry each had their own unique sense of humor, storytelling style and voice. One May in the early 1990s, we all went to Frank Gentry's campsite on the Hiwassee River below the

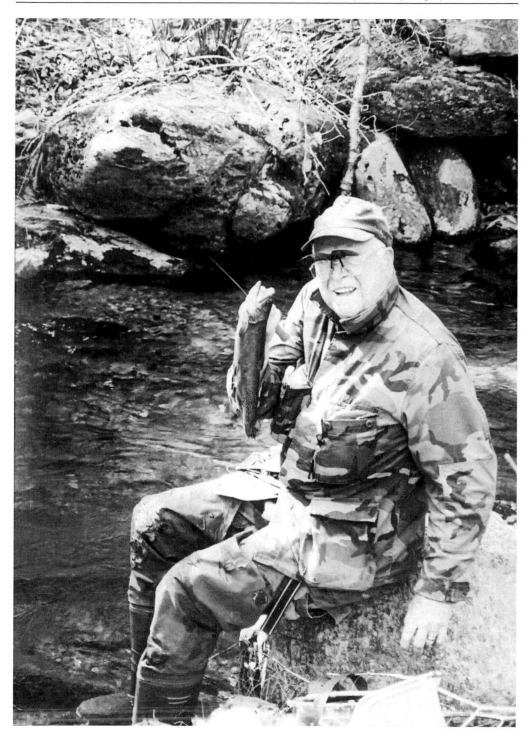

Dr. Dean C. Jones, Jr., caught this 15 inch rainbow trout on the Gayle Price section of Helton Creek in Virginia. He is cleaning his fish on upper Cabin Creek (photograph, circa April 18, 2008, courtesy Dr. Don McNeill).

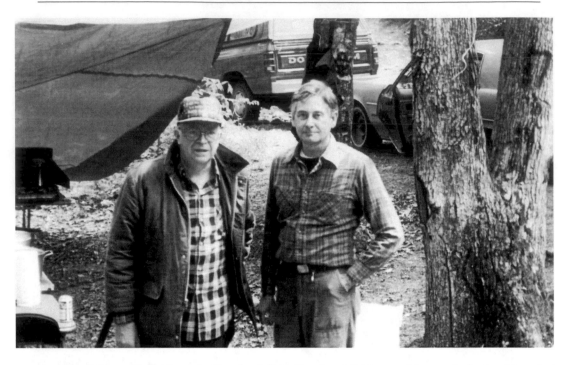

Dr. Dean C. Jones, Jr. (left), worked hard and played hard, and fishing was his way of relaxing. He and his fishing buddy, Dr. Don McNeill (right), are at their campsite at Gentry's Creek, Tennessee (photograph, circa 1978-1979, courtesy Dr. Don McNeill).

dam, fished the area extensively and returned exhausted. I had picked up Dean, Earl and Dale for the trip. The jokes started immediately, and in the first two hours, I had to pull off the road to readjust my contact lenses. I laughed so hard, my tears floated my contacts."

McNeill saved a notebook full of Dean C.'s jokes, numbering over three hundred. Here is an example of one that is fit to print:

A woman accompanied her husband to the doctor's office. After his checkup, the doctor called the wife into his office to speak to her alone and advised, "If you don't do the following, your husband surely will die: (1) Fix him three nutritious and delicious meals a day; (2) Be pleasant at all times; (3) Don't burden him with chores; (4) Don't upset him by discussing your problems; (5) Have sex with him several times a week." On the way home, the husband asked his wife what the doctor had told her. She replied, "He said you are going to die."

The trips weren't all fishing and jokes; there was card playing too, affording Doc the opportunity to exercise his powers of concentration outside of work. One evening, after dark, relates McNeill, Dean C. was sitting in a folding chair, with his back to the stream, about five feet away. Four or five others were around the table, when they noticed Dean C.'s chair sinking, little by little, into the soft mud on the stream's bank. He had to stretch further and further to reach the table to play his cards. Gradually the rear legs of the chair sunk so deep into the mud, he tipped over backwards, as if in slow motion, still in a sitting position, and still holding his cards. His friends jumped to his rescue, but Doc, completely focused on his hand, simply rolled over and out of his chair, got to his knees, still holding his cards, and muttered, "I'm going to win this hand." And he did.

Evelyn Price Jones Interview (Jefferson, June 26, 2014)

The high school newspaper prophesy that Evelyn Price would become a nurse, marry a doctor and open a free clinic was not without foundation. During her high school years at Konnarock Lutheran School in Konnarock, Virginia, she served as the school nurse. She had no formal training for this job, but apparently the only qualification was an interest in nursing.

Evelyn was born January 12, 1936, in Whitetop, Grayson County, Virginia, just over the North Carolina line from Ashe County. She was delivered at home by Dr. Dean Jones, Sr., her future father-in-law, but that was not the first time the two families crossed paths. Dr. Bud Jones, father of Dr. Dean was acquainted with Evelyn's grandfather, Hugh C. Price, and presented him with a mortar and pestle he no longer needed for making medicines, figuring Price might be able to put it to use in tending his cattle. Evelyn's parents were Dan and Zola Kilby Price, and their families' roots go back generations in Whitetop. Like many during the Depression, Evelyn's father moved his young family to the city to find work. Evelyn was the only child when her parents moved near Baltimore, Maryland. One day while her mother was busy with her chores, 18-month-old Evelyn climbed out of her crib and pulled a laundry washtub of boiling water over on herself. She was burned over 80 percent of her body and stayed in isolation in the hospital in Baltimore for a month. The treatment of burns was not far advanced then; there were no antibiotics, and recovery was slow and painful. Her arms and hands were strapped down to prevent her from scratching her damaged skin, and she was painted regularly with gentian (or gensen) violet, a dye used as a bactericide and applied topically in the treatment of skin infections at the time. Back home, after her time in the hospital, a neighborhood doctor came to their house to dress and check her burns, as she continued to heal. Thanks to the care she received, she made a full recovery, and her scars are not noticeable, but until her death in the early 1990s, Zola Price continued to caution Evelyn when she was around anything that could burn her. The family returned to Whitetop, and Dan Price opened a sawmill and lumber business.

Prior to entering nursing school in 1953 at Emory and Henry College in Emory, Virginia, Evelyn traveled the short distance from her home in Whitetop to Jefferson, where she worked as a nurses' aide at Ashe County Memorial Hospital and lived in the nurses' ward in the main hospital

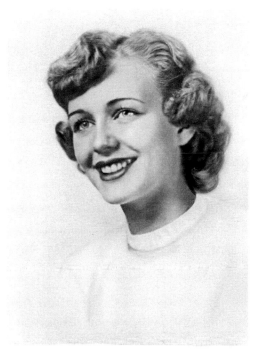

"She was the prettiest girl I ever saw," said Dr. Dean C. Jones, Jr., of his wife, Evelyn Price Jones. The two met while Evelyn was working as a nurses' aide at Ashe County Memorial Hospital (photograph, circa 1955, courtesy Evelyn Jones).

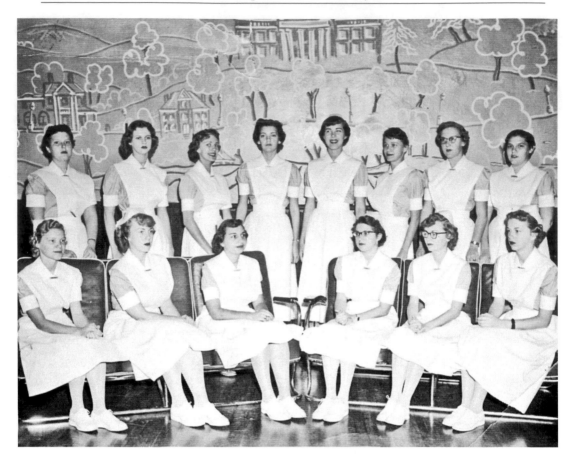

Evelyn Price Jones, third from the left on the second row, with her class at Johnston Memorial School of Nursing in Abingdon, Virginia (photograph, circa 1954-1955, courtesy Evelyn Jones).

building. She graduated from the four year program, with two years at Emory and Henry and the last two at Johnston Memorial in Abingdon, Virginia. The March 8, 1954, issue of *The Roanoke Times* hailed Evelyn's class as the largest class in the history of Johnston Memorial Hospital School of Nursing. Caps were awarded to 46 student nurses of the first-year preclinical classes. But Evelyn was not destined to pursue a career in nursing. She did some private duty nursing when she and Dean C. moved back to Ashe County, but most of her time was devoted to raising their growing family. She is active in the Jefferson United Methodist Church, as her husband was, and continues to be involved in the administrative board. Over the years, she tackled a variety of projects, including the Heart Fund and Ashe County Hemophilia Foundation, and devoted much of her energy to the Girl Scouts. Much later she ran a health food store for awhile in West Jefferson and then in May 1992, she acquired full ownership of Ashe High Country Realty, a real estate business she founded with friends Jim Reese and Cleta Colvard. Evelyn sold the company, and it is still in operation.

Evelyn's role as a stay-at-home mom was very different from that of her mother-in-law Lettie, who played such a vital role in managing the day-to-day affairs of the hospital, but being a doctor's spouse still gave them much in common. "She warned me before we were married, that I wouldn't see Dean C. as often as I would like," recalls Evelyn. The situation was helped to some extent in that Dean C. was a surgeon, rather than a family physician, so he did not make house calls as a general rule, but his responsibilities at the hospital still took time away from his family and his fishing. And, of course, practicing medicine in western North Carolina has the additional challenge of coping with extreme weather conditions, even in modern times. When the phones were out, Doc and Evelyn set up regular times for him to check on things at home, using the children's walkie talkies to communicate.

One would think that having two doctors in the family, both working at the hospital nearby, meant one would not have to worry about medical attention in the event of an emergency, but when things were hopping at the hospital, family took their place

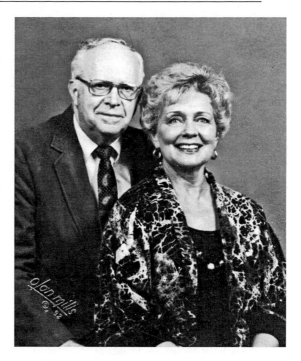

Evelyn and Doc were married 54 years, raised five children, and enjoyed a yard full of grandchildren, despite Doc's demanding schedule as a surgeon (courtesy Evelyn Jones).

in line, like everybody else. Evelyn recalls the time her son Tommy fell and hit his head at school. She had taken him with her to meet with his teacher about a school party. He was sitting on the desk, waiting for her, and it tipped over. She took him to the hospital, but both the Sr. and Jr. Jones were in surgery, so she put Tommy on a stretcher in the hallway of the hospital. Evelyn could tell his injury was not life-threatening, but his skull was shining through the wound, and it looked terrible. "People were passing by and saying "Why don't they do something for this poor young'n?" Evelyn was too embarrassed to tell them the boy's kinship with the two doctors.

12

The Role of Ashe County Practicing Physicians

Headlines in the June 6, 1940, issue of *The Skyland Post* announced "Hitler Claims Victory Is Near." The Allies had abandoned Dunkerque, and battle lines were shifting to defend Paris. Sharing this front page story was another, declaring doctors pledged cooperation with the newly constructed Ashe County Memorial Hospital. The community was determined to focus on bringing their dream of a hospital to reality. The success of the hospital depended on the cooperation of local doctors, and Dr. Fred Hubbard of Wilkes Hospital and Dr. Haywood of the Elkin hospital added their pledge of support to that of doctors Dean Jones, Sr., B. Everette Reeves, W. Joseph Robinson, Lester Lee Long, Carlton Reeves Eller and Burgess Cox Waddell.[1]

In looking back on the start-up of the hospital, Dr. Jones, Sr., agreed that, in addition to the support of the community and the dedicated service of his staff, much of the credit for the success of the hospital lay with the cooperation received from Ashe County's practicing physicians. Among those he singled out were: Doctors C. E. "Johnny" Miller; Ritz C. Ray, Sr.; Ritz C. Ray, Jr.; Roy O. Freeman; Dean C. Jones, Jr.; Carson M. Keys; and Elam S. Kurtz. Other physicians offering service or consultation to the hospital in the early years included Doctors James L. Ballou, Robert L. Dickson and Carlton Reeves Eller.[2]

In Appalachia, as in many regions in North Carolina, the survival of many in sparsely populated communities could be attributed to the medical treatment they received. That was the case in the days of the horseback doctors, and it continued to be the case in more modern times. Doctors might not be riding a horse to reach their patients, but many continued to make house calls in hard-to-reach areas, walking in or fording rivers in their cars or being poled across the river to get to patients on the other side. Some of their feats, like those of their predecessors, became legendary. There were those who may have had limitations in their ability, but for the most part, they operated within their limitations.[3] More importantly, these doctors were people who cared. They could have lived anywhere, but they chose this place in the far flung mountains of Appalachia, some because they were born here, and this was where they belonged, and some because they came here, fell in love with the region and its people, and this became where they belonged.

At the time Ashe County Memorial Hospital was opened, Dr. W. S. Rankin of the

Confucius Say:

"You May Need Doctor First. Don't Make Him LAST To Pay."

How true that is. So many people make the doctor the last to pay regardless of how quickly they wanted him when they needed his services.

When there's serious illness in your home you expect your physician to give you the very best he has. You know that he is prepared to serve you, and you know that he is your friend.

You know the physician had to spend lots of money and many years of hard work to become the professional man he is. You feel at ease when he is bending over the bed of your loved one administering the best he has that a life might be spared.

You, too, know that physicians are necessary, sometimes when nothing else will do. And you know that when you need a physician you generally need him in a hurry—and he comes in a hurry.

Now why not get yourself in a hurry and go to your physician with a payment on your account. You've just neglected it, but remember:

Confucius Say:

"You May Need Doctor First. Don't Make Him LAST To Pay."

Physicians practicing in Appalachia often treated patients who were unable to pay for the services rendered. In support of local physicians, *The Skyland Post* ran a series of ads like this in the summer of 1940, encouraging people to pay their doctor bills. This one appeared in the July 18, 1940, edition (courtesy N.C. Department of Cultural Resources).

Duke Endowment noted that in Ashe County there was one physician for 3,250 people, compared to the state average of one physician for every 1,356 people and the national average of one physician for every 751 people. The Ashe County statistics reflected a total of seven doctors to serve the area, half the number in 1925. "Furthermore, of your seven physicians, three are over seventy years of age. Only one is under fifty. Alongside this limited and dwindling supply of physicians, we have to consider the fact that your sick are scattered over a large area of 427 square miles, and that some sections of this large mountainous area, especially in the winter, are not easily accessible."[4] It is not possible to tell all their stories or even to accurately report all their names, but what follows is a cross-section of the physicians who played a role in the health care of Ashe County and the surrounding region over the years.

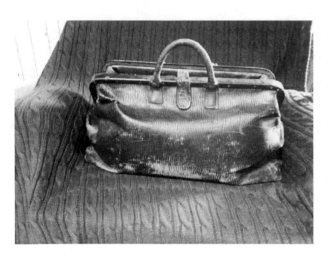

Starting in 1941, with the opening of Ashe County Memorial Hospital, local physicians were elected annually by the board of trustees or its executive committee to serve on the hospital's medical staff. This doctor's bag was used by Dr. Bud Jones, who was elected to the medical staff in January 31, 1942, as recorded in the minutes of the board (photograph, circa 2015, courtesy Louis Pittard).

Dr. James L. Ballou and his wife Iona Mae Shugard of Pennsylvania, left a legacy of philanthropy in Ashe County, particularly with regard to Ashe County Memorial Hospital and to the West Jefferson United Methodist Church, where they were members. Dr. Ballou was born in the Crumpler community of Ashe County August 11, 1873, just a decade after the Civil War, one of the 14 children of Uriah and Mary Jane Witherspoon Ballou. Uriah was known to be astute in matters of politics and religion and was well versed in geology and mineralogy, an interest he inherited from his father, Napoleon Bonaparte Ballou and grandfather, Owen Meredith Ballou, a founder and operator of iron manufacturing plants in the area. Uriah and Mary Jane apparently had a high regard for education and passed this interest in learning on to their children. Uriah and his father and father-in-law built a one-room school for the Ballou children, next to his house on the North Fork of the New River in Grassy Creek. James Larkin received much of his early education there.[5]

Determined to pursue their education, James Ballou and two of his brothers reportedly built a rowboat and traveled on the New River from Ashe County to Hinton, West Virginia, where the enterprising young men sold the boat and proceeded to their respective schools. James graduated from the University of Nashville, later the University of Tennessee at Nashville, receiving his degree in 1901, and from Jefferson Medical College in Philadelphia, receiving his M.D. in 1907. He served his internship at St. Mary's Hospital in Philadelphia. He did postgraduate work at Johns Hopkins Institute and specialized in eye, ear, nose and throat. He practiced in Ashe and Alleghany counties in North Carolina and Grayson County in Virginia. After serving in the U.S. Navy, aboard the U.S.S. *Harrisburg* during World War I, he signed on with the U.S. Public Health Service in Washington, D.C., and was transferred to the Veteran's Medical Service and stationed at the Veteran's Hospital in Portland, Oregon. He became head of the Ear, Nose and Throat (ENT) section at the Veterans Hospital in Portland and served in that post for 18 years. In 1942, he returned to Grassy Creek with his wife and acquired a 320 acre parcel of land from his relatives, including the family home where he grew up. Major renovations followed, and a cottage, office, barns and outbuildings were added. Completed by 1940, the old home became a showplace.[6]

Besides his medical practice, which he maintained for 20 years, Ballou was an inventor of agricultural systems and held hundreds of patents, which added considerably to his wealth. He employed his inventions on property in Grassy Creek, installing underground drainage pipes and building a 26,000 gallon reservoir to provide running water to his house and all the outbuildings on his property. The Ballous devoted much of their wealth to helping young people further their educations and established the Ballou Memorial Scholarship Fund at the University of North Carolina at Chapel Hill in 1953.[7] Lonnie Jones, who grew up in Grassy Creek, commented on the generous nature of Dr. Ballou, who made him his first pair of glasses in 1964—at no cost. Dr. Ballou died of a heart attack January 6, 1966, in his home in Grassy Creek, at the age of 92. His widow, Iona, died in 1968.[8] Their home is now known as the River House Inn and Restaurant, owned and operated by Gayle Winston, who purchased the property in 1989. Among Winston's treasured possessions are Dr. Ballou's stethoscope and eye charts; his old office is room number one of the inn.[9]

Cornetta Price remembers her great-uncle, Dr. Robert Lee Dickson as a big, blustery man with a kind heart, who brought his significant talent back home and made a difference. When Dr. Dickson came home to Ashe County, he bought a house in Jefferson Heights and set up an office in Ashe County Memorial Hospital. Although initially in family practice, by the time he joined the staff at Ashe County Memorial, he was a specialist in otolaryngology (ear, nose and throat) and served the community in that capacity for about 13 or more years, before retiring in June 1978.[10] According to Evelyn Jones and Ruby Lum, Dickson claimed he started working on noses because somebody botched a job on his nose, and he wanted to learn to fix noses without messing them up. He practiced medicine for a total of 53 years.[11]

Robert Lee Dickson, or "Bob," as he was called, was born to David Allen and Malinda Koontz Dickson June 17, 1894, on a farm at the headwaters of Old Field Creek in Ashe County. He enrolled in the Appalachian Training School, where he received his teaching certificate. He taught in Ashe and Alleghany schools and served as principal of West Jefferson High School, before attending Duke University and the two-year medical school at the University of North Carolina at Chapel Hill. He earned the money to enter the Jefferson Medical School in Philadelphia by selling Dr. LeGears Stock Powder, a medicine for livestock. Thanks to his good salesmanship, he was able to enroll by around 1920 and continued to pay his own way, working a variety of jobs, including washing dishes, waiting tables and, according to some accounts, doing a little boxing for money. He received his medical degree from Jefferson around 1925 and while in Philadelphia, was on staff at Frankfort, St. Joseph, and Jefferson hospitals. When Dickson returned to Ashe County in the mid–1940s with his second wife, Paulette, they purchased Healing Springs. He was on the medical staff when the new Ashe Memorial Hospital was dedicated October 31, 1971.[12]

Dr. B. Everette Reeves hosted the first "hospital meeting" in his office August 2, 1938. The meeting, sponsored by the community service committee of the Jeffersons Rotary Club, got the ball rolling for building Ashe County Memorial Hospital. He would be among the first elected to serve on the medical staff at the hospital when it opened. But Dr. Reeves efforts to improve community health care extended beyond his home county. He served in the North Carolina General Assembly and was chairman of the committee on public health, affording him a statewide platform from which to pursue his interests in this vital area. For a period of time, he was physician and surgeon for the Norfolk & Western Railway, and he also served as medical examiner for the Ashe County Selective Service board during World War I and immediately prior to World War II.[13]

Benjamin Everette Reeves was born in Lamar in Ashe County, September 21, 1866, the son of Andrew and Mahalia Reeves. Education was important in many mountain families, and even those of modest means, which was almost everybody, willingly sacrificed to provide their children college educations. Dr. Reeves's brother Cicero became a dentist in Alleghany County, and another brother became a Methodist minister, serving in Alleghany and later West Jefferson. B. Everette graduated from the Baltimore College of Medicine and Surgery in 1891.[14]

Dr. Reeves and his wife Pauline Welborn Reeves moved to West Jefferson in 1918 and lived in one of the first brick homes in the area, located at the end of Wilton Avenue, where Anne and Haskell McGuire live now. Prior to open-ing his office in downtown West Jefferson, Reeves maintained an office in his house. Before that the doctor was known for traveling into the rural areas of the region on horseback, carrying his medical supplies in his saddlebags, and stopping at houses to see if his services were needed. Emmett Barker recalls Doc Reeves maintained an ongoing arrange-ment with a local blacksmith to make shoes for his horse for eight dollars a month, because his horse went through so many shoes on the rough roads of the county.[15] When Dr. Reeves moved his office to downtown West Jefferson, his office was located in the back of Graybeal's Drug Store, established by Carl and Ruth Graybeal, and Dr. J. K. Hunter, a den-tist, had an office upstairs.[16] A large man, slightly gruff in manner, Dr. Reeves was known to help out people in need. "He gave me money to buy a little travel trailer to live in," recalls Calvin Miller of the tough times of his youth.[17] Lib McRimmon relates Dr. Reeves was their family doctor. "Every time we

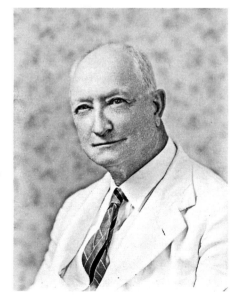

Before Dr. B. Everette Reeves (1866–1944) opened his office in his house at the end of Wilton Avenue in West Jefferson, he regularly traveled to his patients on horseback (courtesy John Reeves).

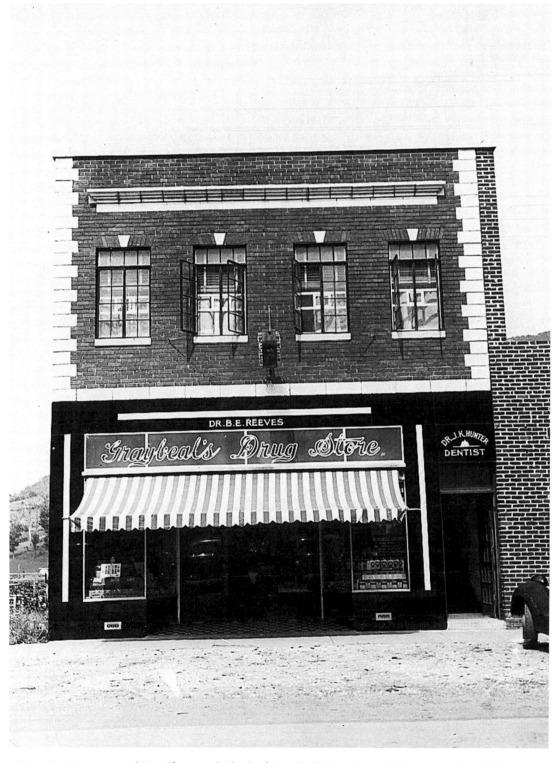

Later Dr. Reeves moved his office into the back of Graybeal's Drug Store in downtown West Jefferson (courtesy Ashe County Historical Society).

were sick, he came out to the house and gave us a pink pill and then sat on the porch and talked to my granddaddy for a while." She speculates the doctor was glad to be away from the hubbub of his practice, sitting someplace peaceful and quiet.[18]

John K. Reeves, great-nephew of Dr. Reeves, relates a story he heard growing up about a pamphlet Dr. Reeves wrote to give out to expectant mothers. At the end of the helpful prenatal care tips, the pamphlet included a caution to patients, something to the effect: "At the time of delivery, I expect full payment in the amount of fifteen dollars. You have had nine months to save up."[19] Ashe County native Clifford Miller remembers Dr. Reeves treated him for St. Vitas Dance, the treatment prescribed—drink all the molasses you can. Since St. Vitas Dance is an affliction characterized by anemia, and molasses is rich in iron, this treatment is probably not as strange as it sounds.[20] Dr. Reeves continued his practice in Ashe County until his death August 31, 1944.[21]

Dr. Joseph Robinson followed a familiar path for many "not from around here," perhaps first visiting Ashe County while vacationing. He practiced medicine under Dr. Stoffel in the Creston community and married Ashe County native Julia Sutherland. The couple settled in Creston, where Dr. Robinson set up his office in their home and served his adopted community from 1905 to 1955. His practice extended to parts of Lansing and Pond Mountain, Todd, Warrensville, Riverview, Sutherland, Pottertown, as well as Creston, covering most of western Ashe County.[22]

Joseph was born in Carter County, Tennessee, September 20, 1879, the oldest son of a physician, and trained with his father until age 19, when he joined Dr. James Butler in Mountain City. He worked to earn his way to the Medical School of the University of Tennessee in Knoxville and then the Medical University of Kansas City, Missouri, where he graduated in 1904. Later he did postgraduate work at the University of Chicago.[23]

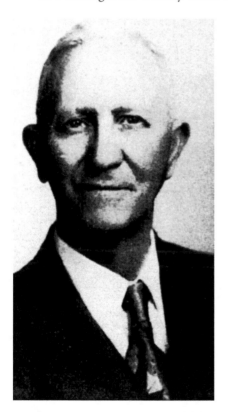

Dr. W. Joseph Robinson, a native of Tennessee, practiced in his adopted home of Ashe County from 1905 to 1955. According to hospital records, he first was elected to serve on the medical staff at Ashe County Memorial Hospital on January 31, 1942 (courtesy Ashe County Historical Society).

Dr. Robinson left his office unlocked—his way of saying he was always available to his patients, and he treated them regardless of ability to pay, accepting barter or trade. People sometimes worked on his farm in lieu of monetary compensation. When his patients could not get to his office, he traveled to them, often on horseback and assisted by his children. Before telephones came to Creston, if a family needed the doctor's services, they hung a lantern outside and put a sheet over it, so that when he passed on his way to other house calls, he was alerted to their need.[24] Like Dr. Bud Jones, he did whatever kind of doctoring was required, from delivering babies to pulling teeth. He reportedly delivered his first baby when he was 18 years old. And once, when he went out to deliver a baby, and the creek had overflowed, he swam his horse across to get to his patient.[25] Doris Oliver recalls Dr. Robinson had "Sunday hours," for the benefit of his patients. He was her parents' doctor, and when her mother had a strangulated hernia, a dangerous situation before there were antibiotics, Dr. Robinson accompanied her father to drive her mother to Bristol, Tennessee, for the needed surgery.[26]

Physicians were often the most educated people in a community, so it is not surprising that some served their communities in political office as well. Robinson was elected to the North Carolina Senate for one term in 1921 and was instrumental in getting Highway 88 completed through Ashe County. Nobody appreciates the need for good roads more than a country doctor making house calls, and Robinson's office was located off Highway 88. He also supported legislation to address the issue of spousal abuse, a problem he was in a position to witness firsthand on some of his house calls.[27] Fortunately, it would be Dr. Elam Kurtz, another outsider, who would take over Dr. Robinson's practice in Creston at his death. Kurtz shared many of the same traits as his caring and competent predecessor, when it came to looking after his patients.[28]

Dr. Lester Lee Long served Ashe and Alleghany counties from around 1919 to 1960 and was elected to the medical staff of Ashe County Memorial Hospital in the first years of its operation. In March 2015, I interview Long's daughter, Lucy Long Miller, who relates

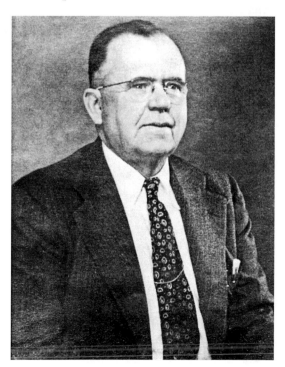

Born in Alleghany County, Dr. Lester Long served Ashe and Alleghany counties from around 1919 to 1960. Many of his medical tools and equipment are on exhibit at the Museum of Ashe County History in Jefferson (courtesy Lucy Long Miller).

the doctor met his wife Lillie Mae Tucker when he made a house call to her parents' home to treat a young Lillie for blood poisoning in her finger. Lillie must have made an impression, because sometime later, at a local baptizing, Dr. Long arrived at the gathering on horseback, showing off a little for Lillie, or so the story goes. His mount took exception to the horsing around and let fly a swift kick at his rider on the dismount. Lillie loved telling this story, despite the horseshoe shaped scar her husband bore as testament to its truthfulness. Dr. Long and Lillie first made their home on a farm in Laurel Springs in Ashe County, and Dr. Long had an office in a separate building nearby. He also owned a general store there with his brother-in-law, although he was too busy with his medical practice to participate in its operation. The family moved from Laurel Springs to West Jefferson in 1939 and lived near the West Jefferson United Methodist Church, which they attended regularly.

In the early years of his career, Dr. Long made his rounds on horseback and was known to personally transport his patients to the hospital in Wilkesboro, when he deemed that level of care was required. In a time when communication was still problematic, he had four telephones installed in his house in Laurel Springs; each line had a distinct ring and was dedicated to a different section of Ashe County. When he moved the family to West Jefferson, he closed the office in Laurel Springs and opened one in downtown West Jefferson, over Roberts Drug Store, near where the town hall is now. Dentist Dr. Edgar Jones shared the upstairs with him.[29]

Lucy Long Miller is one of Dr. and Lillie Long's six children and a twin and lives in West Jefferson, where she grew up. Although Dr. Long's practice was busy and his waiting room always full, Lucy confides her father never sent out bills for his services. He told Lucy "If they can pay me, they will pay me." Sometimes that payment took the form of a pound of butter or eggs or some other barter. "When he died, there were thousands of dollars on the books," adds Lucy's husband Clifford Miller. "It was just thrown away," probably as Dr. Long would have wanted. At least the doctor's overhead was minimal. As was the case with most physicians of his era, there was no assisting nurse or receptionist. "He simply went to the door of the waiting room and said 'next.'" Lucy remembers people coming to the door of their house after office hours to fetch the doctor. Many in the county did not have telephones, and this was the only way to get word to the doctor that his services were needed. He continued to make house calls until his retirement. Toward the last part of his career, his son-in-law Clifford Miller drove him to make his calls on the weekends. Clifford recalls parking the car on the side of the highway in Laurel Springs and watching as Dr. Long crossed over a fence and disappeared on foot into the landscape beyond, hiking in to see a patient who lived a long way from any road. Sometimes the doctor stayed overnight when he made a house call, if he was needed, but usually he was back with his family in the evenings. Lucy remembers their mother was the disciplinarian, as their father was too exhausted from his work to be doling out spankings when he got home. He preferred to have his children sitting in his lap, relating to him their adventures and trials of the day.

Dr. Lester Lee Long was born December 10, 1884, in Alleghany County and received his medical degree from Lincoln Memorial University in Cumberland Gap, Tennessee, in June, 1916. His license to practice medicine was approved the following month by the Tennessee State Board of Medical Examiners, and later the same year, he was licensed to practice in North Carolina. He practiced medicine in Tennessee until 1919, when he returned to Alleghany County.[30] Throughout his career he continued his practice in Ashe and Alleghany, with occasional forays across the state line into Tennessee. Included in his practice was the treatment of prisoners at the Ashe Prison Camp. Only once did he give consideration to moving his practice elsewhere. He travelled to Charleston, South Carolina, in response to an offer to enter into practice with his nephew there. He returned home with the announcement that he was moving the family to Charleston. Lillie, a confirmed country girl, said nothing doing; Charleston was too "big city" for her, and that was the end of that, says Lucy.

It was on that two week sojourn of her father to Charleston that Lucy got sick, and her mother said she was going to take her to see Dr. Ray. He prescribed a medication which

Lucy refused to take, because, "he was not my daddy." With six children, Dr. Long had plenty of doctoring to do at home. Lucy recalls a "yucky" black stuff her father used to paint her sore throat. "My twin, Louise, had pink eye, and she got dark glasses to wear, and I was jealous because I didn't get dark glasses," she laughs at the memory. The children got their shots at home, and "if he was boiling water, we knew we were in for it."

Dr. Long died August 13, 1962, at Ashe County Memorial Hospital, where he had delivered so many babies. He is buried in the Cranberry Cemetery in Laurel Springs, along with his brother Dr. W. Floyd Long (1869–1896), a physician who died young of pneumonia in Pond Mountain, North Carolina.[31] Lucy remembers her father Lester as "a calm, quiet man. I never heard a bad word out of his mouth; he just wanted to help people." An exhibit on the medical history of Ashe County, slated for the Museum of Ashe County History in Jefferson, includes Dr. Long's doctor bag and other medical tools and equipment, artifacts of the legacy of community health care in Appalachia.

Dr. Ritz Clyde Ray, Sr., born September 10, 1888, in Beaver Creek in Ashe County, practiced general medicine in the area for more than fifty years and was elected to the medical staff at Ashe County Memorial Hospital in the first years of its operation. Ray worked in the coal mines in West Virginia to earn money to finance his medical schooling, receiving his M.D. degree from the Medical College of Virginia. In 1916, he began his medical career in Ashe County in a small building near his parents' home. He moved his office to West Jefferson in 1921, where he and his brother Clifford, a pharmacist, established Ray's Drug Store, one of the first drugstores in Ashe County, next to the C. O. Parsons building, in

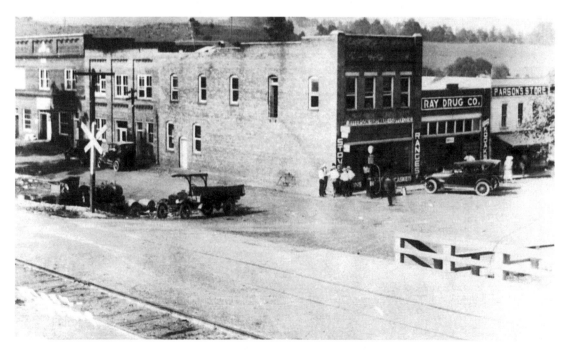

Dr. Ritz Clyde Ray, Sr., and his brother Clifford, a pharmacist, established Ray Drug Company, one of the first drugstores in Ashe County. Dr. Ray's office was located in the back of the pharmacy (courtesy Ashe County Historical Society).

the part of the building W. J. Hardware occupies now. Dr. Ray's office was located in the back of the pharmacy. Later the drugstore, along with Dr. Ray's office, moved to Jefferson Avenue in West Jefferson. Over his long medical career, Dr. Ray, Sr., delivered more than 3,000 babies, served on the examining board in Ashe County during World War I, was a captain in the United States Army Reserve, director and vice president of First National Bank of West Jefferson, and a farmer. Ray died January 16, 1967. His son, Dr. Ritz Clyde Ray, Jr., followed in his father's footsteps, graduating from Duke University School of Medicine, serving as a medical officer in the United Stated Navy, and practicing medicine in Winston-Salem until his retirement.[32]

Dr. Carlton "Carl" Reeves Eller was born in Ashe County August 4, 1890, the oldest of five children of Albert Sidney J. and Laura Etta McMillan Eller. He attended Boone Training School for Teachers and trained in medicine under Dr. Ulysses Jones, before attending Medical College in Richmond, Virginia. Eller practiced in Ashe County for 50 years, maintaining a small office behind where Black Jack's restaurant is now for the last 35 years. In 1915, he married Grace Pauline Sturgill of Nathans Creek in Ashe County. Dr. Eller died December 24, 1965.[33]

Dr. Cameron Eugene (C. E.) "John" Miller (1921–2011) was credited with the best bedside manner of any doctor around, says Ruby Lum.[34] "He was a wonderful diagnostician, because he listened" adds his brother Calvin Miller. "He took time to get to know his patients. People trusted him." Nowadays, his approach would be called "holistic." He was the son of Thurman Greene "T. G." Miller, Sr., and Beulah "Mabel" Nichols of Purlear in Wilkes County. His father dubbed his son "John," and that was the name that stuck. He graduated from Bowman Gray School of Medicine at Wake Forest College and married local girl Melba Gambill. The couple resided in West Jefferson, and Dr. Johnny, as his patients called him, became a prominent and much loved general practitioner in the medical community of his home county, working closely with Dr. Dean Jones, Sr., in both the old Ashe Memorial Hospital and the new, visiting his patients there and delivering babies.[35]

In an interview with me October 2014, Calvin Miller describes to me the tough times in which he and his siblings grew up. Their father lost everything during the Depression, and faced with supporting a wife and children, he made the

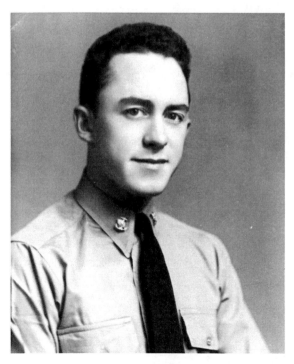

Dr. C. E. "Johnny" Miller was a medical officer in the Fleet Marines during the Korean War. He worked closely with Dr. Dean Jones, Sr., in both the old hospital and the new (photograph, circa 1945, courtesy Calvin Miller).

difficult decision to leave his family for a job with the Civilian Conservation Corps, a public works relief program operating from 1933 to 1942. His older sons, John and T. G., Jr., were sent to live with his mother in Idlewild, North Carolina. His wife Mabel, the two daughters Virginia and Louise and the youngest boy, two-year-old Calvin, settled with Mabel's parents in Purlear. T. G. Sr. was able to return and reunite the family a year later. Exhibiting the kind of pioneer and can-do spirit that brought people through those bad times, T. G. came up with the idea to cut down his old Chevrolet sedan, fashion it into a pickup, and haul slabs from a sawmill to sell as kindling for wood stoves. He made enough from this enterprise to move on to other mercantile ventures.

The influence of his hard working and conscientious parents is reflected in the way Dr. Johnny Miller went about his life and his career. Another strong influence in his life, says Calvin, was A. D. Goodman, a teacher at Fleetwood, who Johnny maintained was responsible for his going to medical school. Johnny started out going to Wake Forest College for two years. He was part of the Navy V12 program, which paid his expenses while at Wake Forest Medical School, but with the end of World War II, he had a year left to go, and he financed that last year on his own. He did his internship at Rex Hospital in Raleigh, married Melba after graduating from medical school, and moved back to Ashe County, where he built an office on the corner of the main intersection in Jefferson. He and Melba lived in an apartment over the office. He was in the Navy Reserves at the time, and he was called to active service in Korea. The county could not afford to lose a doctor and petitioned his release from active duty. The petition was successful, but later Dr. Johnny was called back again for active duty in Japan. He served as a Fleet Marines doctor on a ship transporting Marines to occupied Japan.

When Dr. Johnny returned to Ashe County, Calvin, ten years younger than his brother, remembers going with him on house calls, sometimes driving their vehicle through fields to reach a patient or deliver a baby. The practice grew, and Dr. Johnny and Melba lived in a house they built in Baldwin. Later they acquired the big house at the end of Wilton Avenue in West Jefferson, formerly owned by Dr. Reeves and now owned by Haskell and Anne McGuire. They lived there for several years but eventually moved back to the Baldwin house. After the new hospital opened, Miller moved his practice to the office building behind Ashe Memorial Hospital.

Like other country doctors in Appalachia, Dr. Johnny's schedule was grueling. "He almost had to get out of the county to get any rest," says Calvin. For what leisure time he managed to squeeze into his busy schedule, Miller enjoyed golf and painting. He and Melba painted with well known Blue Ridge artist Florence Thomas, and many of the couple's paintings are on display in Melba's home in Baldwin, along with some of Florence Thomas's work.

For the last four or five years of his life, Miller suffered from chronic pain, the source of which could not be determined, either by the doctor himself or the colleagues whose opinion he sought. He died at age 90, leaving a country doctor's legacy of selflessness and caring. Two sons followed him into the medical profession—Doug is a physical therapist in Charleston, South Carolina, and Cameron "Chuck" is a nurse in Valdese, North Carolina. Melba continues to live at the couple's home in Baldwin, with her daughter, Connie Gambill "Johnnie" Miller.

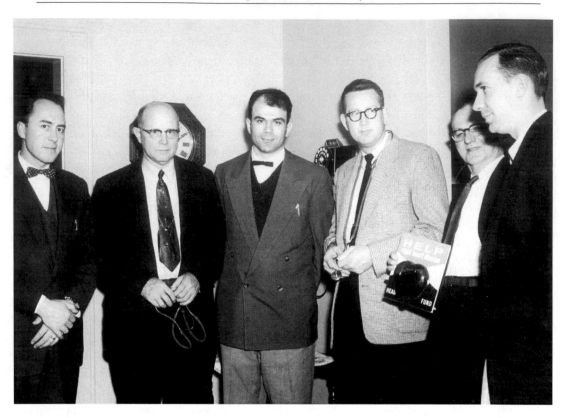

Ashe County doctors gathered for a meeting at Ashe County Memorial Hospital, are, left to right: Dr. C. E. "Johnny" Miller; Dr. Dean Jones, Sr.; Dr. Elam Kurtz; Dr. Roy O. Freeman; Dr. Ritz Clyde Ray and Dr. Carson Keys (courtesy Evelyn Jones).

During the big snow in 1960, relates Doris Oliver, word got to those determined to come to the rescue that a patient needed medical attention somewhere in the back country, and the National Guard stepped up to transport Dr. Carson Keys by helicopter from Ashe County Memorial Hospital to the property of the patient's family. Nurse Betty Ball was tapped for the dubious honor of accompanying the doctor on this expedition of mercy. There was no means of communication available to let the family know there was help on the way, much less that it was coming by air, so the first thing Dr. Keys saw when he stepped off the noisy helicopter was a man running to the barn to fetch his gun and a woman dropping to the ground in the front yard to pray. Keys reportedly quipped that would be the last time he would be the first one off a helicopter.[36]

Carson Meade Keys was born in 1926 at the Long Hospital in Statesville, North Carolina, the son of William Carson Keys, a civil engineer, and Anna Dell Hart Keys, a school teacher from Nathans Creek, North Carolina. He began his education at Nathans Creek School and graduated from both Pharmacy School and Medical School at the Medical College of Virginia, now known as Virginia Commonwealth University, in Richmond. He served his internship in Pontiac, Michigan, and returned to Ashe County in 1953, practicing medicine there until 1965. A likeable and competent physician, Keys may be best known for the many babies he delivered, says Calvin Miller. Keys was married to Elaine Horton, and they had four children. The family moved to California, where Keys practiced internal medicine, with an emphasis on cardiac care. The family returned to North Carolina in 1981, and Keys practiced in Ashe County from 1984 until he retired from his medical practice in 1992 and worked part-time as a pharmacist in People's Drug Store.[37]

I interviewed Dr. Edward James "E. J." Miller, a general practitioner (no kin to Dr. "Johnny" Miller), in July 2014. The doctor is one of the region's home-grown physicians, and he has been affiliated with the AMH since September 8, 1965, the longest of anyone still there—50 years. He started about two years after Doc Jones and considers him to have been one of his best friends. They did not fish together, but they did play bridge together for many years.

Miller was born in Nathans Creek in Ashe County, delivered at home by Dr. Long, and now lives about a half mile from where he was born. After a stint in the U.S. Air Force, making captain, he received his medical degree from UNC School of Medicine at Chapel Hill in 1962 and did a rotating internship and an internal medicine residency at Mid State Baptist Hospital in Nashville, Tennessee.[38] Like many other physicians who were born and raised in Ashe County, he never gave serious thought to going anywhere else to practice medicine.

In a small town, physicians end up wearing a lot of hats, and E. J. Miller is a good example. He worked with the health department, where he instituted a variety of improvements, including prenatal, family planning, and obstetrics clinics. A patient introduced him to the Lamaze method of delivery, and he began to offer this option routinely, before it was widely accepted elsewhere in the state. "We are not always behind the times here," he jokes. His resume also includes an appointment as medical examiner in 1972, election as coroner multiple times, chief of staff and head of the ER at Ashe Memorial Hospital, and president of the Ashe-Alleghany Medical Society. He is now medical director for Margate Nursing Home and Forest Ridge Assisted Living.[39]

In the early days Miller did make some house calls, but usually they were as a follow-up to a hospital stay. There was an advantage to making house calls, he points out—it gave the doctor a good feel for what the home situation was like, which you don't get now. "It used to be you and your bag," he reflects; "now so many tests are routine, it is not practical to handle cases with house calls." When his father had typhoid fever, Miller remembers Dr. Long came every day from his office in Laurel Springs to see him. One of the hardest things about house calls in those early days was finding out where people lived. One rainy November day, Miller headed all the way up to Rock Creek to find a patient, where Highway 88 winds into Tennessee. As it turned out, she just wanted her blood pressure checked.

Miller remembers when nurses from the health department came to Nathans Creek Post Office to give typhoid fever injections. He credits immunizations as making the most difference in health care. "All my children got vaccinations at the health department." Early on, immunizations were about the only preventive medicine. "Now you can nip things in the bud. You have more tools at your disposal, but there is more bureaucracy dictating what you can do. Doctors used to diagnose by family history and examination; now all these tests are done. And many times, 'You've got what's going around,' is still the right diagnosis, despite all the tests. In the early days, we had more people dying young. People put off being seen when no hospital was close by. By the time they sought help, their illness was so far advanced, they could not be helped." Medical record keeping is another area that has seen a lot of change. "I liked Dr. Dean Jones, Sr.'s records," Miller reflects. "They were so simple. Senior's records showed what the patient came in for and what he did for it. Now you have six pages of stuff that documents everything the patient doesn't have wrong with him."

Dr. Miller is well known as a founding organizer of the Ashe Central Little League baseball program, coach for many years, and organizer of the Ashe County Minor League Division. Having delivered so many Ashe Countians and coached so many of them in Little League, he is understandably proud of his "young'uns."[40]

Dr. Jacqueline DuSold and her late husband Dr. William "Bill" DuSold came to Ashe County in 1977 to get away from the rat race and escalating medical insurance rates of Los Angeles, California. In our interview August of 2014, Jacqueline DuSold explained they saw an ad in a pharmaceutical magazine for physicians and general surgeons needed in the Blue Ridge Mountains and decided to explore the area. The couple looked at several places, including Asheville, but when they got to Statesville, the people there told them they would love to have them, but they knew if they were going to look at Ashe County, they would not be back to Statesville. That proved to be the case. The couple went home to California, sold their house, and relocated with their four children to the High Country. "Tom Cockerham took us around. He was Mr. Personality," laughs Dr. DuSold. Dr. Jones, Sr., had just retired, so for the most part, the doctors DuSold worked with Dean C., Jr., Betty Ball, Nancy Edwards, and Sue Hampton at the hospital, and of course Henry and Ruby Lum. Dr. Bill DuSold worked closely with Ruby Lum, as she was an operating room nurse. "He thought the world of her," recalls Jacqueline. "She would work all night and never complain." Bill and Dean C. were the only two surgeons in the county and rotated being on call at the hospital. Dr. Bill put in pacemakers, and performed colonoscopies, endoscopies, bronchoscopies, and tracheostomies.

Both husband and wife were born and raised in Chicago and trained there. Dr. Jacqueline DuSold was in general medicine, and her husband was a surgeon, specializing in vascular and general surgery. The couple came to Ashe County to stay. "We never regretted it," says Jacqueline. "It was the best decision we ever made." Dr. DuSold was the first female doctor in the area, but this distinction did not present any problems for her, and she felt welcomed by the community.

DuSold acknowledges there were differences in big city doctoring and what she found in Ashe County. "There were not enough physicians." Some of the medical personnel had to come in from Wilkes Hospital. The radiologist was an example. He travelled around from one hospital to another, reading x-rays. But advancements were being made. "When the helicopter pad was put in at Ashe Memorial, we thought we were moving up the ladder."

The couple located their practice in the Professional Building behind the hospital. There were a few adjustments, of course, like the snow. The DuSolds built their home in Laurel Springs, and the heavy snows made getting to work a challenge. Jack McClure and Rob Black, from the hospital's maintenance department, were charged with scraping the long drive at the DuSold home to Big Peak Creek Road. Then there was a little bit of a language problem, until the DuSolds grew accustomed to the Ashe County brogue and local euphemisms. "I thought when I could understand Rob Black, I had learned a new language," says the doctor, laughing. DuSold immersed herself in the health care scene in Ashe County, serving on the board of the county health department and the Ashe Services for Aging board of directors. "I think the community has done a wonderful job of building up health care," says DuSold, "particularly organizations, like home health care, something relatively new in health care services. Home health personnel can follow a patient after surgery and report to the doctor, cutting down on the need for follow-up doctor visits."

Dr. DuSold retired from general practice in 1990. Reflecting on her career in her adopted home, she offers an interesting observation. "The people of Ashe County have a high regard for each other and are very caring of one another. I found that out right away, and I liked it. They take care of their family, and it is not simply out of a sense of duty, it is love."

A full professor at the University of Cincinnati, long before he ever made it to Ashe County, pediatrician Dr. Lawrence Kautz saw significant change in his field of medicine, as well. When he started his career, polio was on the way out, relegated to the ranks of smallpox and diphtheria. But cancer, AIDS, and psychiatric disorders were there to take its place. In his thirty years of practicing medicine, perhaps the biggest change he saw was the dramatic rise in emotional problems in children.[41]

Vaccinations represent another development impacting health care, especially for the young. Many of the diseases which cut short lives of children years ago have become a thing of the past. German measles and mumps are seldom seen now, and there is a vaccine for meningitis, as well as polio, diphtheria, tetanus, and hepatitis. The smallpox vaccine is no longer given, as cases have not been seen in decades. When Kautz was growing up in Cincinnati, Ohio, children received check-ups before starting school, but few vaccines. Now children receive several sets of shots before they are allowed to set foot in school. Kautz was a founding board member of the Ashe School Based Health Center, located at Ashe Middle School, and served as school physician. The center stays busy, with approximately 2,000 visits every year. The health behaviors of thousands of children have been impacted by this program since the year 2000. The most critical needs for children Kautz saw toward the end of his career were dental care and emotional health.[42]

Kautz attended medical school in Cincinnati, served in the Korean Conflict as an infantryman and combat medic, and then completed medical school, serving an internship in Miami, Florida, and a residency in Chicago at Children's Memorial Hospital. Prior to coming to Ashe County, he was in private practice in Cincinnati and taught medicine for 20 years at Children's Hospital Medical Center, one of the largest pediatric hospitals in the United States. He met and married his wife Nancy in Miami, where she was an emergency room nurse when he was doing his internship. The two decided to move to Ashe County in 1988.[43]

In July 2014, I interviewed Dr. Kevin J. Kurtz, the youngest of Dr. Elam and Orpah Kurtz's four children. Born in 1964 at Ashe County Memorial Hospital, five years after his parents moved to the county, today he is one of the doctors at Ashe Memorial Hospital who specialize in family medicine. He received his undergraduate degree from UNC at

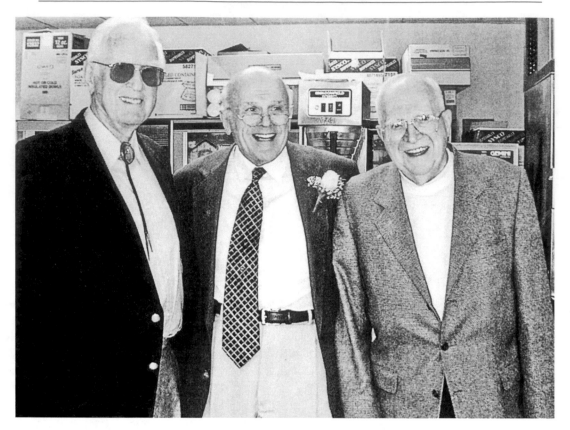

Among the Ashe County doctors credited by Dr. Dean Jones, Sr., with helping to make the hospital a success were, left to right: Dr. Roy O. Freeman, Dr. Elam Kurtz and Dr. Dean C. Jones, Jr. (photograph, circa 2003, courtesy Evelyn Jones).

Chapel Hill and his medical degree from East Carolina University. He met Dr. Leigh Bradley, daughter-in-law of Doc and Evelyn, during his residency in family practice at the Mountain Area Health Education Center (MAHEC) in Asheville, North Carolina, and she joined him at High Country Family Medicine in Ashe County, shortly after its founding in 1994.

Kurtz did not know he wanted to be a family physician at the start of his medical studies, although his father Elam was his role model for his initial pursuit of a career in medicine. He found he liked a little of everything in his field of study and that seemed to match up with his ultimate choice to enter family practice. He misses the close bond formed with a family when he was in the business of delivering babies in Asheville. It kept the practice younger and afforded an opportunity to build on the patient-doctor connection from birth into adulthood, but the liability and the restrictions on lifestyle which come with caring for expectant mothers, prone to deliver at all hours of the day and night, guided his choice to give up the obstetrics side of his doctoring, a reflection of the change in times since his father's early days in Ashe County.

13

Health Care in Ashe County Evolves

One of the many things that impresses me about this part of North Carolina is the willingness of people to take care of their own. So often in these days where families are flung all over the country, and nobody is left within a day's drive of the homeplace and aging parents, folks of a certain age are shuttled off to some form of institutional care, when all they need is a place to live where somebody cares if they are getting three meals a day, taking their medicine, and not falling down. Unfortunately, there comes a time for many of us, when something more is required than can be provided in the most caring and attentive modern day family settings. Before state and federal guidelines detailed the distinct levels of care we have now, from independent living, to assisted living, and finally to skilled nursing, rest homes provided the main alternative to a long term hospital stay for those no longer able to live on their own or with family. In June 1958, *The Skyland Post* proclaimed the opening of "northwest North Carolina's newest and finest rest home, Grand View, located between Jefferson and West Jefferson." The facility was built by James and Bill Badger, with a 25 to 30 bed capacity and semiprivate and private rooms for both men and women. Edith Conklin Badger, a former lab technician at Ashe County Memorial Hospital, was in charge of operations at the new rest home, situated on a hilltop between Jefferson and West Jefferson. Not far from Ashe County Memorial Hospital on McConnell Street, the new rest home shared the "grand view" of Mount Jefferson and Phoenix Mountain.[1] When I interview Bill Badger in July 2015, he recalls the facility underwent at least two additions, increasing the number of beds to about 76. Eventually they ran out of space and built a second, smaller facility on property the Badgers owned nearby. Grand View Number Two had about 26 beds and was managed by Bill's wife, Martha Badger. Roy Badger, Bill's father, lived there in the last years of his life. Both facilities were sold awhile back and are closed now, although the structures still stand, waiting, like the old hospital, for their next purpose.

Not far from the two Grand View facilities, the Ashe Services for the Aging started out in the old Ashe County Memorial Hospital building, the hospital having moved to its new campus by then. Ashe Services for the Aging has expanded its offerings since its founding in 1977 and now sits on a large tract of land off Ray Taylor Road in West Jefferson. The modern facility offers a wide variety of activities and programs for the elderly, the disabled, children, and children with special needs. Services include home care aides, home

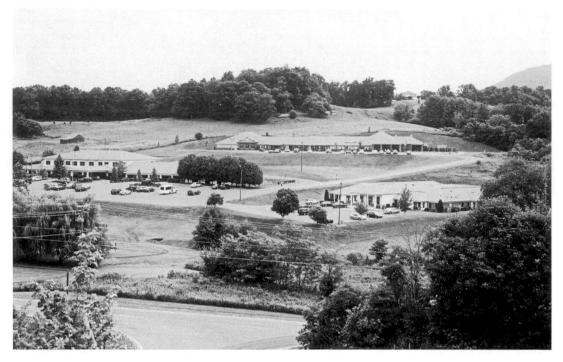

Ashe Services for Aging started out in the old Ashe County Memorial Hospital, occupying the space from 1977 to 1997, when they moved into their current facility on Chattyrob Lane in West Jefferson. Today, in addition to its main building (lower left), Ashe Services for Aging includes two residential facilities—Ashe Assisted Living and Memory Care, the building at the top, and Ashe Senior Village, lower right (photograph, circa 2015, courtesy Ashe Services for Aging).

delivered meals, health screenings and hearing tests, Senior Games, educational classes, quilting, basket weaving, painting, entertainment, and exercise. An innovative and popular intergenerational day care program, called "Generations," is offered on the campus, where both children and the elderly participate together in activities. Housing for the elderly is also available in Ashe Senior Village, HUD approved apartments for the elderly, and Ashe Assisted Living and Memory Care, the most recently constructed building on the hill behind the main complex. Other nursing home and assisted living options are now also available in the county, as well.[2]

By 1983, changes in the Medicare payment system had resulted in acute care hospitals, like AMH, having to limit the patients' length of stay in order for the hospital to survive financially. To be able to place patients in the appropriate level of care, explains former CEO R. D. Williams II, AMH gained approval from the state to add a designated number of long term beds. Fifty years after the dedication of the original Ashe County Memorial Hospital, AMH broke ground May 1, 1991, for the AMH Segraves Care Center, a 60-bed, long term care facility, adjacent to Ashe Memorial Hospital. The center was made possible, in part, through a generous bequest from the estate of James Lester and Lillie A. Segraves. J. L. Segraves was an Ashe County native, and his wife was born in Watauga County.[3] The center started admitting patients May 25, 1992, supported by AMH meal service, pharmacy, physical therapy and administrative functions. Segraves thrived and became the facility of choice in the area, with long waiting lists for beds. But when AMH converted to Critical Access status in 2007 to help address its financial troubles, the Medicare reimbursement model was changed, and AMH was in serious financial jeopardy. The tough decision was made to transfer the beds approved for Segraves to Margate Health and Rehabilitation Center, another long term provider in the county, so that the county would not lose the beds altogether. Along with other offices, the physical therapy department was relocated to the Segraves space and expanded.[4] The PT services, first put in place by Dr. Don and Ann McNeill in the summer of 1975, with a wheelchair, a few walkers, crutches, and exercise weights, initially focused on educating the nursing staff on post-stroke care and rehabilitation and post-hip and knee replacement care. For several years Ann McNeill provided physical therapy services every Thursday, including PT evaluations and care, mainly for inpatients and a few outpatients, until the hospital hired a full-time physical therapist in the late 1970s.[5] The PT program soon grew to department status, and with the additional space afforded by the move into the former Segraves Center, the department now offers a full range of services, not only maximizing utilization of the space, but helping to preserve the legacy left to the community by the Segraves family.[6]

Emergency services in the region also evolved over the years. Although some joked it was a conflict of interest, there was a time when local funeral homes provided the ambulance service in Appalachia and much of the rest of the country. Badgers' Funeral Home and Reins-Sturdivant Funeral Home both provided ambulance services for Ashe County.[7] The funeral homes served as the ambulance service for Ashe County Memorial Hospital, as well. Doris Oliver remembers when the ambulance driver and his helper had to trudge a mile from the road to retrieve a patient, hauling a stretcher the whole way. The hospital released the patient rather than keep him overnight, and the ambulance crew had to carry the patient all the way from the road back to his home. The driver got a quarter for his trouble.[8]

Bill Badger says Badgers' Funeral Home used a "combination," a separate vehicle from the standard hearse, a 1953 Pontiac, which could be used as a hearse or an ambulance, with a few quick modifications. Although the ambulances were not "tricked out" like ambulances today, with life saving medical contraptions, they did have sirens and emergency lights. The funeral homes provided transportation only—strictly pick-up and delivery of the patient to and from a hospital or "throw and run," as it was referred to in the trade. There were no emergency medical technicians (EMTs) to administer to the patient. There was a fold up seat where a family member could ride with the patient, explains Badger, but often it was only the driver and the patient in the vehicle. Mother Nature, however, did not always respect the limitations of the ambulance service, and at least one baby was known to be delivered by James Badger. Bill Badger, who drove the ambulance for the funeral home, along with his brother James and his cousin G. T., tells of one case where Dr. Dean called from the hospital and said he had a little boy who needed transport to Baptist Hospital in Winston-Salem. The child's situation was dire, and Dr. Dean said he probably only had two hours left to live without the treatment he needed at Baptist. Bill Badger could see the mother praying in his rear view mirror. He was not sure if she was praying for her child, or because he was driving so fast. He made the trip to Winston in an hour and a half. The staff was waiting for the boy when Badger pulled in at Baptist. A couple of days later, the boy's

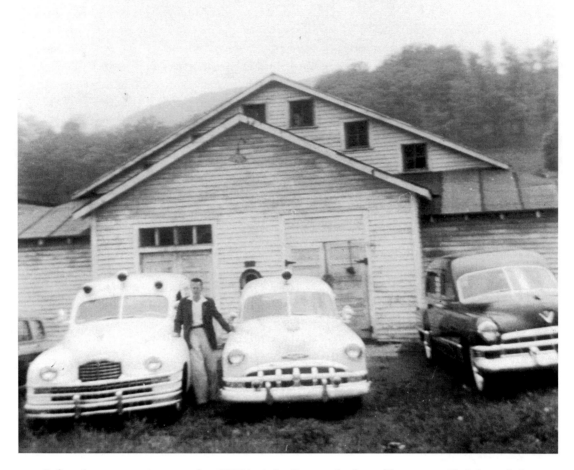

Before there was a rescue squad or EMS in Ashe County, the funeral homes provided the ambulance service. The two white vehicles are the Badgers' Funeral Home ambulances; the black one is a hearse. G. T. Badger, one of the drivers, stands between the two ambulances, parked in front of the West Jefferson School gymnasium. The funeral home, not pictured, would have been to the left in the photograph (courtesy Ashe County Historical Society).

mother brought her son to see Badger and assure him the child had recovered. People in need of an ambulance, placed their call direct to the funeral home, where the telephone was manned 24 hours a day. There was no dispatcher and no line of communication with the hospital. When he was in high school, Bill Badger spent his nights in the funeral home so there would be somebody there to answer the phone, in case of an emergency. Badgers' Funeral Home charged $3 to take someone in the county to Ashe County Memorial Hospital. The charge for transport to the hospital in Winston-Salem was $15. But sometimes it was not a patient in need of transport. On one occasion, Dr. Dean, Sr., called to ask Bill Badger if he was taking anybody to Baptist that particular day, and when Badger said he was, the doctor gave him a biopsy of tissue to deliver to the lab there for testing. Jones kept his patient sedated in the operating room until staff at Baptist called him with the results, and he could proceed accordingly.[9]

The region has come a long way since funeral homes provided the ambulance service. The first rescue squad was chartered in 1962, and John Reeves and Evelyn Jones were in the first EMT training available in the county, a state-operated mobile EMT learning lab that traveled from county to county. Students could get college credit for their participation, and later the program was incorporated into the community college curriculum. Evelyn's participation was part of her volunteer work with the AMH Auxiliary. She had a scanner to keep up with the latest medical crises. John Reeves recalls that Dr. Dean Jones, Sr., faced with periodic shortages of blood at AMH, instituted "blood runs." Jones would call the captain of the rescue squad and tell him the hospital needed blood, and someone would be dispatched to make the run. Members of the rescue squad drove their own cars from Ashe County to hospitals in Raleigh and Durham to pick up the needed blood supply. Bailey Barker and Sherman Myers, both charter members of the rescue squad, often were tapped for this mission, says Reeves.[10]

Larry Lyalls's father was one of the founding members of the Ashe County Rescue Squad, and in our interview April 29, 2015, Larry cited two incidents that stood out in his father's recollections of the early years of the squad, the first being the bridge collapse at Silas Creek in 1966 and the second a plane crash at the local airport. In April 2015, I finally tracked down the driver who survived the bridge collapse, Billy Ray Miller. With the help of his wife Betty, Billy Ray filled me in on some of the details of that Saturday morning, July 9, 1966, when he drove onto the bridge at Silas Creek, which spans the North Fork of the New River. He was 25 at the time, with Betty and their little daughter at home. He gave no thought to the weight of the rig he was driving, with the low boy trailer and bulldozer he was hauling to another work site. He was just doing his job. Riding with him, in the passenger seat, was Harold Bare.

Billy Ray remembers hitting the water as the bridge gave way, but it happened so fast, there was no time to anticipate what would happen next. Propelled by the impact of the collapse, the bulldozer rolled forward into the cab of the truck, the massive blade pinning Billy Ray to the steering wheel. His ribs were crushed; he sustained multiple internal injuries; his face and head were covered with severe lacerations—his nose almost cut off and his mouth sliced across. Bare escaped the blade of the bulldozer and was able to get out of what was left of the cab on his own. The Ashe County Rescue Squad waited for Doc Jones, now on the scene with nurses Edith Blevins and Ruby Lum from Ashe County Memorial Hospital, to assess the victim's injuries and administer a shot of morphine, before they attempted the extraction of the driver from the wreckage. Mercifully, Billy Ray was in and out of consciousness for the three hours it took to accomplish his rescue. A second bulldozer was brought to the site, and a cable was attached to the back of the bulldozer on the low boy, connecting it to the second bulldozer to prevent it from shifting further into the cab.

Rescuers worked as quickly as they could, mindful of the risk the truck could catch on fire. The Rescue Squad credited their ultimate success to two recently purchased pieces of equipment in their arsenal, and Miller was taken to Ashe County Memorial, along with Harold Bare. Bare was released in a day or two; Miller was in the hospital for 13 days. Betty Miller fainted when she saw her husband's injuries. Their three-year-old daughter, Penny, cried and was afraid of her father, not recognizing his disfigured face. Doc sewed up his

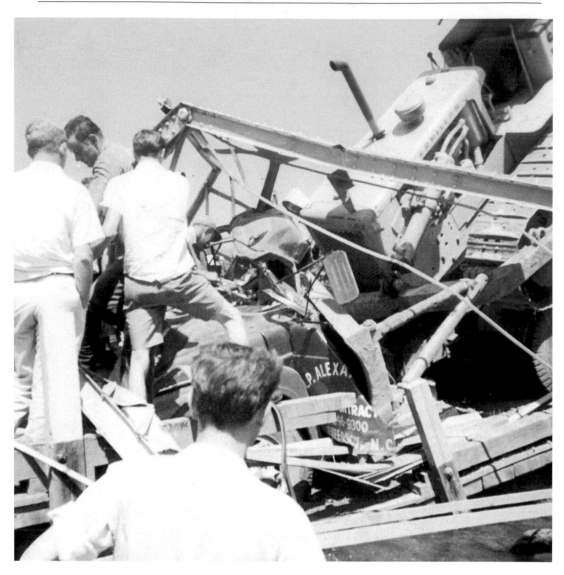

The bridge collapsed at Silas Creek in Ashe County, July 9, 1966. A Ford truck pulling a low boy that was carrying a bulldozer plunged into the river, the bulldozer pinning the driver, Billy Ray Miller, to the steering wheel. Dr. Dean C. Jones, Jr., and nurses Edith Blevins and Ruby Lum waded into the river to help assess and stabilize the victim before his extraction from the wreckage (photograph, circa July 9, 1966, courtesy Billy Ray Miller).

cuts, reattached his nose, treated his internal injuries, and told Betty if her husband had been an inch bigger around, he would have been dead.

"He was just lucky," says Betty, looking over at Billy Ray, sitting across from me. I study his face—there is no evidence of this catastrophe etched in his features, no visible scarring, no clue of the extensive plastic surgery performed in a small community hospital by a surgeon who chose to bring his skills back home to Ashe County. I asked Billy Ray if he had any residual effects from the accident. He said his back hurt some. "I think a lot of the Jones's," he says; "they're good doctors." The July 14, 1966, edition of *The Skyland Post* shows a photo of the Ashe County Rescue Squad, headed by Captain Max Payne, First Lieutenant Sherman Myers, and Second Lieutenant Bailey Barker, carrying Billy Ray Miller through the river on a stretcher, the horrific wreckage in the background. Another photo shows Ruby Lum and Edith Blevins wading out of the water, assisted by rescue workers. Doc Jones is behind them, carrying his medical bag.

Beulah Barker McVey was pregnant with her daughter Renee and hoeing tobacco with her brother Thomas and father Blane Barker in the "holler" just over the mountain from the bridge at Silas Creek, when she heard "the awfullest racket," the prolonged clang and groan of metal against metal, as the bridge broke and crumpled to pieces. People began to scream. The men threw down their hoes and ran to the crest of the hill. "Lord have mercy! The river bridge has fallen in," Beulah's father shouted back to her. The cab was almost filled with water when rescuers broke the glass. Beulah ran to see too, but kept at a distance. "Everybody around went to see. It looked like the army and everything was down there. I saw Dr. Jones in the water and a nurse right with him. Everybody was praying, some silent and some out loud. Nobody thought he (Billy Ray) would make it."[11]

The bridge that collapsed was brought in from Wilkes County after the old bridge was washed out in the 1940 flood. A one-way structure with a six ton limit, it was considered inadequate from the start. It was estimated that the rig driven by Billy Ray Miller was three

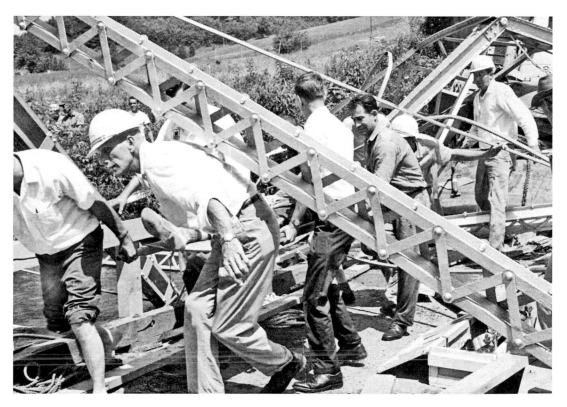

Sherman Myers (second from left, with hardhat) and Harry Lee Miller (fifth from left) help carry critically injured Billy Ray Miller from the wreckage. Bailey Barker is to the far right, with a hardhat. The extraction took over three hours (photograph, July 9, 1966, courtesy Billy Ray Miller).

times the weight capacity of the bridge.[12] The North Carolina Department of Transportation replaced the bridge at Silas Creek in 1967.

The Ashe County Rescue Squad is now a part of the larger Ashe County volunteer emergency medical services (EMS) system. Dr. Leigh Bradley, one of Evelyn Jones's daughters-in-law, is the current medical director and explains that the Ashe County Rescue Squad is the most likely component of the EMS system to have the training to rappel down a mountain to pick up a body. They also are the ones seen on the sidelines at ball games and on the scene of automobile accidents, using the jaws-of-life to free a victim from the wreckage, as was the case at the Silas Creek bridge collapse.[13] The *Ashe Co. Emergency Medical Services, Community Assessment*, released by AMH in March 17, 2015, reports that in addition to the Ashe County Rescue Squad, the Ashe County EMS system currently includes 12 volunteer fire departments and one all-volunteer ambulance service in Helton, providing first responder level care, and a county-subsidized ambulance service, authorized at the EMT-paramedic level. Ashe Medics became the new county-subsidized ambulance service effective July 1, 2014. Eighteen full-time and 13 part-time employees of Ashe Medics are authorized at the paramedic level and receive approximately 150 hours of continuing education per year, surpassing the state requirement of 24 hours of continuing education annually.

When 911 is called, a county EMS unit is dispatched at the same time as the first responders from the fire department are dispatched. First responders are traveling to the site in their own cars, and they each carry an EMT bag in the car. Given the size and terrain of the county, if, for example, a patient lives on the North Carolina/Tennessee border, it might take 45 minutes for the county EMS unit (Ashe Medics) to get there, but, because it is nearby, the Creston volunteer fire department can be there faster. In a case like this, if the first responders know the county EMS unit will take awhile to reach the site because of its location, the closest volunteer fire department's ambulance is dispatched. The EMTs work closely with the county EMS service, and people in the county get the help they need faster and more efficiently.[14]

In our second interview, April 30, 2015, Larry Lyalls recalls being first on the scene when a two-seater Cessna airplane crashed on takeoff at the airport, off Friendship Church Road in Jefferson, in the mid–1980s. He was a paramedic working for the county ambulance service, operated, at the time, by his father, Vernon Lyalls, a veteran of 15 years with the Ashe County Rescue Squad before acquiring the contract for the county ambulance service during that time period. "When we first got the call, we thought it was a drill," says Larry. But the team quickly realized the situation was real. Because the crash site was not accessible by ambulance, Vernon drove his own vehicle close enough to carry the victims to the ambulance. It was all hands on deck, with the rescue squad and volunteer fire department participating, alongside the county ambulance service, but both victims died on impact. One

Opposite, top: The rescue squad and other EMS personnel assisted at the scene of a plane crash in the mid–1980s, near the Ashe County airport. From left to right are: Danny Barker, Danny Anderson, Roger Petty, and Jess McMillan. Larry Lyalls is in the foreground, with his head in the cockpit. *Bottom:* Rescue workers remove the victims from the plane crash, using Vernon Lyalls's four-wheel drive vehicle to access the site and transport the victims to the ambulance. There were no survivors. Carrying the stretcher, from left to right are Jess McMillan, Larry Lyalls, and Roger Petty (both photographs, circa mid–1980s, courtesy Larry Lyalls).

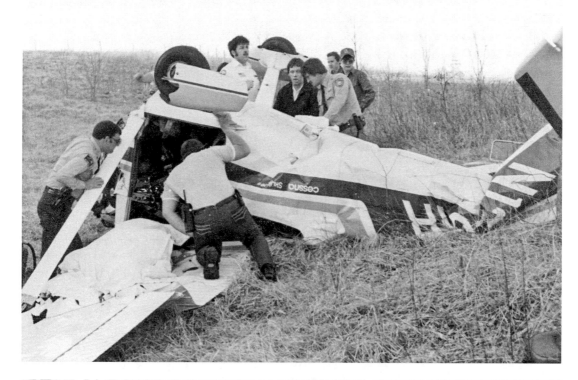

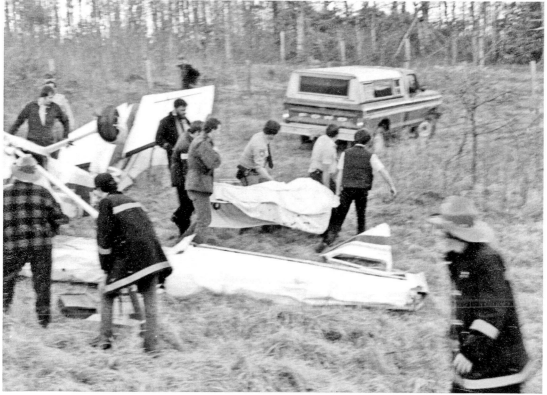

was pulled out onto the plane's wing, without too much trouble, but it took an hour to cut through the wreckage to remove the second man.

No matter which element of the county's EMS system is driving the ambulance, the patient likely is going to Ashe Memorial Hospital. "I have worked in large hospitals, and I've been on the receiving end of medical helicopters," declares Nancy Kautz, "and Ashe Memorial is better than anybody at stabilizing patients. We don't try to do what we can't do well, but we get you the best care until we can get you to the place you need to be." Kautz recalls a patient came into the emergency department at AMH with a ruptured aortic aneurism—a dire situation. Even if a person were to have such an episode in the emergency department's parking lot, the odds of survival would be slim to none. Kautz warned the family of the risk. The emergency department staff stabilized the patient and sent him to Baptist Hospital in Winston-Salem. The patient lived, due in large part to the quick and efficient care he received at AMH.[15]

Evelyn Jones and I first interviewed Nancy Kautz in the AMH cafeteria in January 2015. She was between meetings and sat down to talk with us about her latest projects and how she came to be where she is now, geographically and professionally. "I've been a nurse since I was seventeen years old," Nancy begins. "I graduated from nursing school when I was twenty, and by age twenty-one, I was in charge of the night shift of the ER at Jackson Memorial Hospital in Miami, Florida." Nancy first came to Ashe County with her husband Dr. Lawrence Kautz in 1988. She started off as an emergency room nurse at Ashe Memorial Hospital. "The ER is my passion," she exclaims. "I was one of the nurses called to take care of patients when they had to be transferred to another hospital. I was a certified mobile emergency nurse. I rode ambulances for five years." There were no paramedics for this job at the time, and no county owned and operated ambulance service. The AMH saw to it all their ER nurses were trained as mobile intensive care nurses. When an emergency is called into the hospital, such nurses are able to give orders over the phone direct from the AMH emergency department to the ambulance service taking the call.

14

Ashe County's Model for Community Health Care

"Our hospital is committed to caring for the people of Ashe County, regardless of their ability to pay," declares Nancy Kautz. She describes the county's model for community health care for the uninsured and underinsured, called Ashe County HealthNet, as a three-legged stool, with the Ashe County Health Department, Mountain Family Care Center, and the free clinic as the three legs. The three agencies work together to make health care work for this population.[1]

The Appalachian District Health Department, originally called Ashe-Alleghany-Watauga District Health Department, was first organized in 1938, after a campaign to secure the full-time health department was launched by the community service committee of the Jeffersons Rotary Club.[2] Rotary continued its support of the health department, sponsoring clinics and programs. In April 1939, a clinic sponsored by the Rotary and conducted at the Methodist Church in West Jefferson offered the services of an orthopedic surgeon to fifty "crippled children."[3] Dr. Robert R. King, Sr., was the first district health officer. An article in the May 18, 1939, issue of *The Skyland Post* announced that several typhoid clinics were being held in Ashe County by Mrs. Mary Belle Breece, public health nurse of the health department. The vaccinations were free for everyone and offered in multiple locations in Ashe County, including Scottville, Nathans Creek, Buffalo Baptist Church, Lansing, Glendale Springs and Warrensville. In June 1939, the issue of continued funding for the fledgling health department was scheduled to come before the county commissioners, and *The Skyland Post* argued on its behalf, pointing to the results of an unofficial poll conducted by the newspaper, which found a majority of property owners favoring the health department. "We believe that the Commissioners will meet with the approval of every public-spirited citizen of Ashe, by continuing the Health Department and by so doing, insuring us of our rightful American heritage, the pursuit of happiness along the road of good health." During the year 1940, Ashe County's health department reportedly immunized 3,936 people for contagious diseases, aided in the improvement of sanitary conditions, and examined and treated hundreds of school children, as well as adults. Health officials encouraged communities to make greater use of immunizations against diphtheria, smallpox and typhoid fever, available through the health department. North Carolina ranked second in the United

States in the number of reported cases of diphtheria, and typhoid fever immunizations became even more critical during 1940, when a devastating flood in the region contaminated food and water supplies, increasing the danger of this terrible disease.[4]

In late October 1941, before the official opening of Ashe County Memorial Hospital, the county health department moved its offices from the McNeill store building in Jefferson to space in the basement of the new hospital. Two treatment and examining rooms, an office for Dr. King, a reception area, clerical records office, and supply room were dedicated to the health department. The department was accessible by the left side entrance of the hospital, which entered into the basement.[5] The hospital's "Report of Administration" for 1942 indicates the rent paid by the health department for that year was $81.

After Dr. King, Sr., resigned in 1944, Dr. Robert R. King, Jr., accepted the position in 1946, and Dr. Mary Michal followed in February 1950.[6] Dr. Michal visited county health offices in all three counties, and, at one point, associates joked the doctor was banned from driving on the Blue Ridge Parkway because of her chronic speeding from one far flung assignment to another. My father, an x-ray technician for the State Board of Health's mobile chest x-ray program, was one of those associates and talked about Dr. Michal's stories of

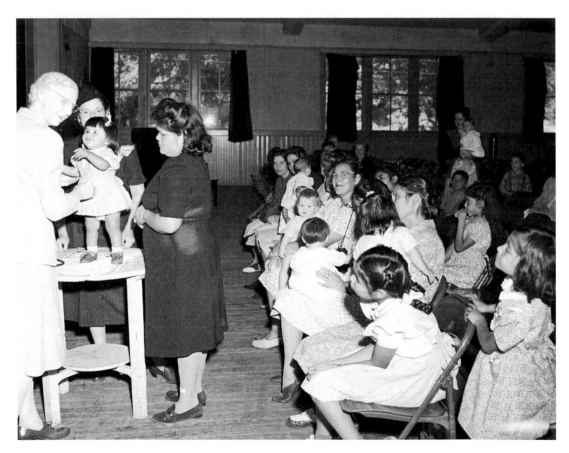

Dr. Mary B. Michal (far left), director of the Appalachian District Health Department, judges a baby contest on the Cherokee Reservation. Dr. Michal was elected as "courtesy staff" to Ashe County Memorial Hospital February 4, 1953 (photograph, circa 1950s, courtesy N.C. Department of Cultural Resources).

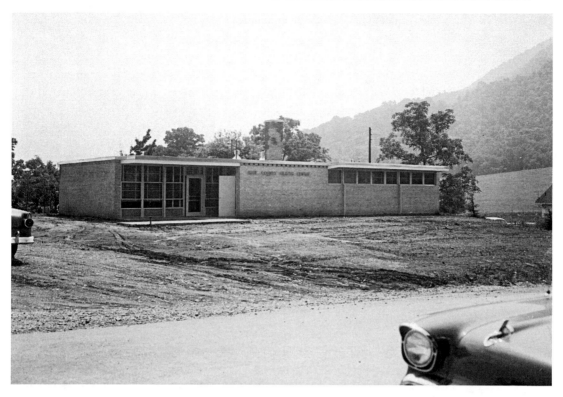

The health department moved into the basement of Ashe County Memorial Hospital before the hospital formally opened in 1941 and was accessible by the left side entrance, which entered into the basement. Dr. Dean Jones, Sr., had limited responsibilities for consultation work with the health department (photograph, circa 1950s, courtesy N.C. Department of Cultural Resources).

her early career in the mountains of North Carolina, when people peered in the windows to see what a lady doctor looked like.

On December 10, 1957, a new health department, across the street from the hospital, was formally dedicated. The land was donated by Mrs. Sallie McConnell, and the building was paid for with a combination of state and federal funds through the North Carolina Medical Care Commission, county funding, and private donations, including a sizable contribution from the West Jefferson Woman's Club. Similar in architecture to the hospital across the street, the original granite façade of the health department disappeared with a major addition that changed the appearance of the exterior to its present, more contemporary style.[7]

After the devastating post–World War II polio epidemic of 1947–1948, the North Carolina General Assembly passed legislation requiring students to be vaccinated against polio as a prerequisite to starting public school, making North Carolina the first state in the country to pass such legislation. The AMH and the health department worked together to accomplish this massive undertaking around the late 1950s. Doris Oliver remembers dropping the vaccine on sugar cubes, as folks lined up to take their medicine one Sunday afternoon in the cafeteria at Beaver Creek High School. Babies got a shot instead, and Doris was relieved she was not assigned to the screaming baby detail.[8]

Over the years, the county health department expanded its hours, its programs, and its services. The fees charged for some programs, like pediatric, maternity and primary care, are based on the size and income of the family, while other programs and services, such as family planning, immunizations, communicable disease, health prevention and promotion, environmental health, home health, and hospice services are available to every citizen of Ashe County. Some services, like immunizations for children, are free.[9] The health department administers the WIC program (Women, Infants and Children), a supplemental food program, and provides physical exams for patients with lower incomes for preschool, day care, Head Start, Special Olympics, 4-H, school sports and the Foster Grandparent Program. In an effort to accommodate the increasing population of seniors, the health department has taken steps to meet nursing care needs through their Ashe Home Health Care program, including physical and speech therapy services.[10]

Throughout its history, the health department staff has worked cooperatively with Ashe Memorial Hospital to provide the best service for the people of the county. Mary Lou Brooks recalls, "We had an orthopedic surgeon from Charlotte, who went to the health department once a month. They sent me over from the hospital to work for him and help with his records. He dictated his notes, and I passed them along to be transcribed. It was a cooperative effort."[11]

The health department contracts with local physicians to help provide clinical services, and many have served in that capacity, including Dr. E. J. Miller and Dr. Lawrence Kautz. Dr. Leigh Bradley and Dr. Kevin Kurtz of High Country Family Medicine in Jefferson served as the health department's doctors early in their practice, as well.[12]

The North Carolina State Health Department targeted other communicable diseases besides polio. The disease known first as phthisis, then consumption, and finally as tuberculosis, had been a serious health problem in North Carolina since Colonial days. Those infected were relegated to sleeping porches to reduce the chance of spreading the infection to family members. In October 2004, I wrote a story for *Our State Magazine* about the efforts of the State Health Department to eradicate this disease in North Carolina. Hand-in-hand with the preventive care initiated from the late 1940s to early 1950s, the Tuberculosis Control Section of the North Carolina State Board of Health deployed mobile x-ray units across the state offering free chest x-rays. The end result was the near eradication of tuberculosis in North Carolina. The silver tractor-trailer rigs were routinely scheduled to work the mountain counties in the warmer months, to take advantage of the cooler temperatures, since this was in the days before air conditioning, and inside the lead-lined trailers could be suffocating.

For some of the most rural counties of the state, the arrival of the caravan of these lumbering giants of the road was a major curiosity. The Highway Patrol usually was called on to escort the seven or eight units into town, and some communities incorporated the caravan into a parade, complete with the high school band. Posters and flyers covered the community, announcing "Get your free chest x-ray." The message was repeated from speakers atop a state-owned carryall, cruising down the main street. Ashe County native John Reeves remembers seeing the big x-ray trailer parked in West Jefferson, below W. J. Hardware, in front of where the music mural is now.

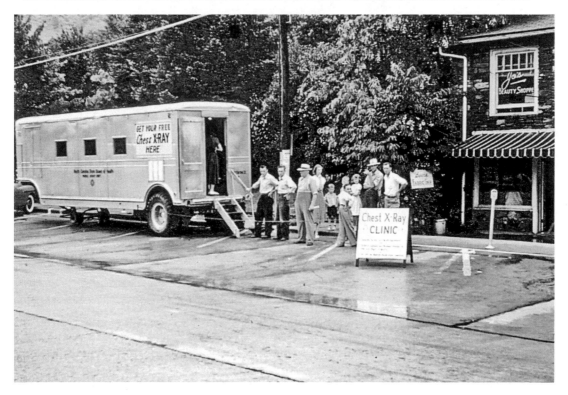

In the late 1940s to 1950s, as part of its campaign to wipe out tuberculosis, the N.C. State Board of Health dispatched mobile units across North Carolina to take free chest x-rays. This unit is parked in Boone, N.C. (photograph, circa 1950s, courtesy N.C. Department of Cultural Resources).

Folks in one Appalachian community reportedly took their blankets, packed picnic lunches, and planted themselves on the side of the mountain to watch the caravan slowly navigate the steep grade. Once when the caravan was moving down a precipitous and winding road from Spruce Pine to their next assignment somewhere downhill, the first tractor-trailer lost its brakes. The Highway Patrol car providing escort raced ahead to warn traffic away from the huge rig gathering speed. The Patrol led the unit into a field at the bottom of the mountain, where, thankfully, it came to a stop in the soft dirt. The other tractor-trailers followed, one by one, and the Highway Patrolman stood counting each one as they pulled into the field, checking to be sure everybody made it down safely.

The survey was manned by a small crew; sometimes one technician drove the 12 to 13 ton tractor and trailer, set the unit up on the street, put up the signs and took the x-rays. Assistance was provided by the local health department and volunteers from the community. Anne Shoemaker McGuire of West Jefferson and her friend Kay worked as clerks on the unit a couple of summers, filling out a card for each person so that the x-ray picture taken could be properly identified.[18]

Bob Ruiz of Swannanoa, North Carolina, was an x-ray technician with the program in the late 1940s until the mid 1950s. I visited him at his home in September of 2014, and we talked about his recollections of working with the program in Ashe County. After the initial survey was done, those x-rays which showed something wrong were flagged for follow-

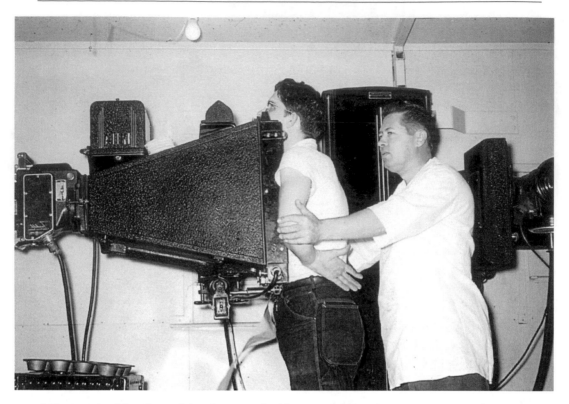

"Chin up, shoulders forward, hands on your hips," instructs technician Tony Hinnant, as he positions a patient for a free chest x-ray in one of the state's mobile x-ray units. The cupcake pan in the lower left was used to keep the metal tags which marked the x-rays (photograph, circa 1950s, courtesy N.C. Department of Cultural Resources).

up, and in 1949, Ruiz did the follow-up work for the survey at Ashe County Memorial Hospital. He used the equipment at the hospital to retake the x-rays, creating larger, 12 × 17 inch images. The follow-up took about a month to complete, and he rented a room at a house in Jefferson, not far from the hospital.

Beulah Barker McVey of Ashe County was working for the Hanes Hosiery Factory in Jefferson, when the mobile chest x-ray unit came to do a survey at the factory. She was called in for a follow-up, because something showed up that looked like it could be TB. Beulah was in a state that she might have exposed her coworkers to the disease. "They wore that machine out x-raying me. I told them I wanted to see that TB." When she was shown the x-ray, Beulah recognized the spot of TB as the life saver she had inadvertently swallowed when the technician instructed, "chin up."[14]

The second element of the Ashe County HealthNet, the Mountain Family Care Center, operated by AMH, offers an alternative for Ashe County residents and visitors in need of non-emergency medical services after normal physician hours. The facility is not meant to be an extension of the hospital's emergency department, but serves as a health and urgent care clinic. The center moved to the AMH campus in January 2011. Its user friendly hours are reminiscent of the days when Dr. Dean saw outpatients until late into the evenings at the old Ashe County Memorial Hospital.[15]

The feasibility of patients' getting in to see a doctor in rural Appalachia is markedly improved with today's better roads and availability of cars. Most people have access to a hospital now if they want it, but affordability of health care continues to be an issue in the area, as it has since the earliest days of the hospital in Ashe County. Minutes from the July 3, 1951, meeting of the executive committee of the Ashe County Memorial Hospital Board of Trustees note: "Ira T. Johnston reported that he had made an investigation of the indigent care problem in the hospital and that he found the matter would require discussion with other county boards if any relief were made available." "Charity care is a huge problem," confirms Dr. Kevin Kurtz. "There are more Medicare and Medicaid eligible people than most areas."[16]

Ashe County Free Medical Clinic, Inc. (ACFMC), the third component of Ashe County HealthNet, serves people who do not qualify for Medicare or Medicaid—the working uninsured and the underinsured. Established in 2005, it is now located on Court Street in Jefferson, behind the Museum of Ashe County History (the old 1904 Courthouse). Although the clinic is not a project of Ashe Memorial Hospital, staff from the hospital volunteer time at the clinic, and ACFMC coordinates with governmental, private and charitable organizations, including AMH, Ashe Services for Aging, Department of Social Services, and the health department.[17]

Dr. Leigh Bradley volunteered at the free clinic for many years and explains the clinic serves as a portal to services needed, such as a surgeon, dermatologist or physical therapist. There is usually a waiting list, since the number of medical professionals available in the region to provide these services on a volunteer basis is limited. "The patients you see have

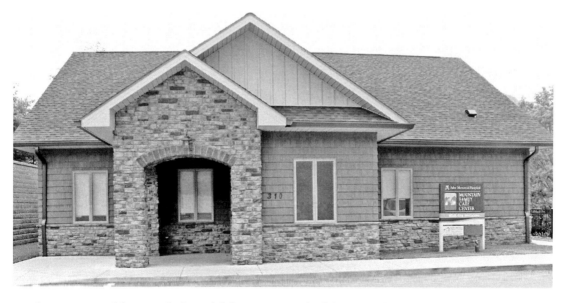

Ashe County HealthNet, today's model for community health care in the county, includes the Ashe County Health Department, the Mountain Family Care Center, and the Ashe County Free Medical Clinic. Mountain Family Care Center, adjacent to AMH, serves as a health and urgent care clinic, providing patients with non-emergency needs, as an alternative to the AMH emergency department (photograph, circa 2015, courtesy AMH).

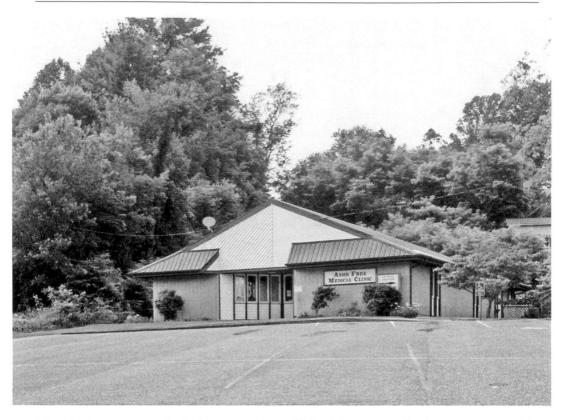

The Ashe County Free Medical Clinic, Inc., is located behind the Museum of Ashe County History (the old courthouse) in Jefferson. The clinic is not a part of AMH, but staff from the hospital volunteer their services (photograph, circa 2015, by the author).

so many more needs than what you can treat—like mental health issues and chronic pain—it can be frustrating," says Bradley. "Unlike private practice, the patients seen at the clinic do not have an established relationship with a doctor." Bradley says her perspective as a medical professional has evolved as she has matured in age. "I find I focus more on the misery I see in patients, and misery is a hard thing to treat." Mental health and dental health continue to be the number one and two needs in the region. After all, the bottom line for community health care is "to help sick people get better and well people stay well."[18]

"When I was growing up," relates Ashe County native Wylene Barker, "you didn't go to the doctor like you do now." Apparently, that was reserved for birthing babies or serious illness or injury—not a check up or a bad cold. "The rural health nurse would come to the Post Office at Silas Creek to give you shots, and your parents would bring you in." Barker remembers the dozen or so five- and six-year-olds from the community lining up at the Post Office for their smallpox vaccine.[19] What constituted rural health care in those days is not what goes by that name today.

The former director of the N.C. Office of Rural Health and Community Care (ORHCC), John Price spent 36 years with the state of North Carolina; that is almost the entire history of ORHCC, created under the administration of Governor Jim Holshouser in 1973 and now housed within the Department of Health and Human Services. I talked with Price by telephone January 21, 2015, and March 11, 2015, to get his reflections on the evolution of Appalachian community health care from the state's perspective.

In the early days of the ORHCC, Price was a primary care systems specialist and worked in the field, assigned to the territory from Burlington to the west, a total of 34 counties. His mission was to help develop rural health centers in underserved communities. His second day on the job, he found himself in Wilkes County, tackling the beginnings of a health center in the community of Hays, northeast of Wilkesboro. The state was to contribute one dollar for every five dollars raised at the local level. "Then you could build a center for less than one hundred thousand dollars," says Price. The centers were often staffed by a single nurse practitioner. The marketing strategy was to get communities to invest in the creation and support of a health center by going door-to-door, soliciting the required local share. "We didn't want one industry to meet the community's share of the project," explains Price. If a person could not afford to contribute when approached via this door-to-door method, at least they became educated as to the nature and importance of the services available through the center. Eventually, four centers were set up in Wilkes County: Clingman, between Elkin and Wilkesboro; West Wilkes in Champion, on U.S. Highway 421; Boomer Medical Center; and Mountain View in Hays. The center in Hays, started in 1977, is a good example of how people in western North Carolina, long credited for their independent thinking, could accomplish a project like this. They knew what they wanted for their community, and they wanted the best. Three of the centers remain open; West Wilkes is closed. Centers do not necessarily close because they fail; more often they close because other resources or providers, such as more doctors or a community hospital, become available to serve the medical needs of the community.

It is important to note that there also were health centers built before ORHCC existed. The Celo Health Center in the Celo community, near Burnsville in Yancey County, has been in operation since 1947, providing primary care in the South Toe Valley. Hot Springs Health Program in Madison County, another especially noteworthy effort, got its start as an Appalachian Regional Commission (ARC) project in the late 1960s to early 1970s, starting off as a health clinic and growing into a county-wide effort with multiple sites.

"It was all about community development," Price reflects. "The state did not prescribe a model but provided general guidelines. We asked communities, 'What do you think you need?' and then helped them to determine a plan and helped them to implement that plan." When Price retired in March 2013, ORHCC had helped start 85 health centers across the state. Meanwhile the mission of the agency had expanded to the recruitment of providers, improving access and cost-effectiveness of health care while still focusing on primary health care. The office assists the uninsured and underserved, spending state, federal and philanthropic funding from a number of sources, and generates hundreds of contracts to support North Carolina communities in their health care endeavors.

As a former outreach coordinator for AMH, Nancy Kautz worked with the ORHCC, the Appalachian Regional Commission (ARC), the State Board of Health, and other health care resources to ensure that the Ashe County community had access to as many health-related services as possible. A current member of the AMH Board of Trustees, she continues to be actively involved in community health care. Retired in name only, Kautz devotes her considerable energies to grant writing, and her efforts continue to make a difference. Her most recent success, announced in June 2015, is a grant for $946,152 from the Golden LEAF Foundation. The award will be used to update and renovate the AMH emergency department. Kautz shared her thoughts on the developments in outreach in our interviews on January 28 and March 27, 2015.

In 1989, Ashe County ranked fourth in the state for cardiovascular disease. Kautz had an idea, pitched it to then Ashe Memorial Hospital CEO Gary Bishop, and he put her in charge of a project that would morph into the establishment of the Mountain Hearts Center for Prevention and Wellness. Dr. Philip Yount was recruited as medical director and pursued and received a state certification in cardiac rehabilitation; Kautz became a cardiac rehab nurse. They put together their program and operated it out of Martin Little's gym on Radio Hill in West Jefferson. Yount and Kautz packed up their gear every morning and were there at six o'clock, ready to roll. Phyllis Jones, Doc and Evelyn Jones's eldest daughter, was one of the first aerobics instructors. The program expanded and moved to space in the Mountain Village Shopping Center, below the hospital. The team explored a grant with the Kate B. Reynolds Foundation and ended up with $250,000 for a new facility, which now sits adjacent to AMH. The track record for the program is impressive. With the implementation of the Mountain Hearts community outreach activities, particularly its strong community education component, Ashe County went from fourth in the state to below the state average in premature cardiac death.

It was this venture into the establishment and coordination of a cardiac rehabilitation program for AMH that inspired Kautz to pursue community outreach work. In her role as Ashe Memorial's outreach coordinator, she wrote and administered grants, and led the way in improving health care delivery systems for Ashe County through programs designed to facilitate the integration of community health and human services. Kautz launched an effort to improve health statistics, marshaling the hospital's resources and financial support in conjunction with community volunteers to create the Ashe County Health Council, A Healthy Carolinians Task Force and an ongoing program to promote a healthier lifestyle for Ashe County residents. A Healthy Carolinians Task Force is made up of several hundred community leaders, working in a collaborative effort to discuss community problems and explore ways to address their resolution. Domestic violence is an example. Council members were shocked to learn from local law enforcement that 90 percent of the calls they answered were related to domestic abuse. The AMH took the lead on pulling people and resources together, getting a grant from Duke Endowment, and the result was A.S.H.E. (A Safe Home for Everyone), a program serving victims of domestic abuse. The Ashe Partnership for Children now maintains this program. The Ashe County Health Department took the lead for the Ashe School Based Health Center, for which Kautz's late husband Dr. Lawrence Kautz served as physician. With the help of local business man Ralph Davis, who designs and fabricates buildings, and the Duke Endowment, a prefabricated building was erected to house the project. Around 1999, the program expanded to include mental health services and is now located at Ashe Middle School. The School Based Health Center has now been serving the community for more than 16 years, helping children to stay well.[20]

Other programs include the Ashe/Alleghany Safe Kids Car Seat project; the Ashe Suicide/Depression Awareness and Prevention (ASAP) Task Force; the Diabetes Education program; and programs for low-cost lipid and free prostate cancer screenings, through the Jeffersons Rotary Club; blood sugar screenings and diabetes awareness programs through the West Jefferson and Riverview Lions Clubs; a breast cancer awareness project coordinated with neighboring counties; and a resource directory of Ashe County health and human services. The mission of the task force is a familiar one to Ashe County initiatives in health care: "To join the hands of the community to address wellness and to involve people in the planning and education necessary to meet their needs."[21]

Nancy Kautz staffed the Ashe County Health Council, A Healthy Carolinians Task Force, and has been credited as the driving force behind the William Anlyan Award for innovative projects to improve health in 1999 and AMH's receipt of the prestigious American Hospital Association 2000 NOVA Award for excellence in community outreach programming. Ashe Memorial was one of five health care facilities in the country to receive the American Hospital Association NOVA Award in 2000. At the time of the NOVA Award, there was a 17 percent reduction in heart disease related deaths in Ashe County from the inception of the task force. Other efforts now underway include maternal, infant or child health care, dental care for children, persons at risk of chronic diseases, and health and human services for the Medicaid-eligible. More recently focus has been placed on access to care for the uninsured and underinsured.[22]

In 2006, the National Rural Health Association (NRHA) recognized the Ashe Memorial Hospital as the Outstanding Rural Health Organization of the Year—that means AMH was recognized as *the* outstanding such organization in the United States. The Hospital's CEO, R. D. Williams II, along with Nancy Kautz, accepted the award for AMH at the NRHA national conference in Reno, Nevada, May 17, 2006. The NRHA is a national non-profit organization dedicated to improving the health of rural Americans and providing leadership on rural health issues. Every year the NRHA recognizes rural health leaders for outstanding contributions and significant achievements in rural health care. The two things that probably most impacted the NRHA recognition, says Williams, were Ashe Memorial's support and participation in the founding and operation of the Ashe County Health Council and the impact of the council on community health care and the 50 percent measured reduction in cardiac mortality in Ashe County, realized over the ten year period since AMH's Mountain Hearts program went into operation.[23]

Kautz maintains health care remains a community business in Ashe County, and local churches play an active role, as they did in the early days of mustering support from the pulpit for the original Ashe County Memorial Hospital. With support from a three-year grant to AMH from the Health Resources and Services Administration of the U.S. Department of Health and Human Services, Kautz relates training is being provided in the community on the use of AEDs (automatic external defibrillators) and CCC/CPR-D (continuous chest compression/cardio-pulmonary resuscitation–defibrillator). Under the program, called "Mission HeartStart," 24 local churches will receive AEDs in 2015, and members of the congregation, young and old, will be trained in its use and in CCC/CPR-D. Each church participating will receive a free AED with a cabinet and a rescue kit.

When I followed up on my initial interview with Nancy Kautz in March 2015, she reported that response to the program was good; 162 people were trained thus far, including Evelyn Jones. "People will know how to respond wherever they are," Kautz comments. The CPR training can help, even if the person is assisting where the AED is not available. The second year of the grant will provide training for 24 hub churches—those in more outlying areas, as opposed to in town. Training is not restricted to the able-bodied. Even if a person is not physically able to perform compressions for CPR or manage the equipment, he or she can instruct somebody else on what to do. When the AED is taken from its cabinet, an alarm automatically rings, alerting others in the church that help is needed. The first order of business, as always, is to call 911. "You are never too young to learn to call 911," advises Kautz.

15

Dr. Charles W. Jones: Fourth Generation of a Family Legacy

Charles W. Jones, M.D., Interviews (January 15 and April 1, 2015)

"This wasn't what I wanted to do," begins Dr. Charles Jones, as we sit down for our first formal interview in January 2015. He is talking about his career as a surgeon, not the interview. His early resistance came despite an eighth grade aptitude test that listed physician or health care as likely career paths. Granted the specified career options also included forest ranger or somebody who worked in the wilderness, but, at that age, who knows where anybody will end up job wise? Charles heard people say to each of his older brothers, "You're going to be the next surgeon." He supposes that had something to do with why he balked at following in the footsteps of his father, grandfather, and great-grandfather. "I didn't want to be a physician or live in Ashe County. It was too small." He graduated from Ashe Central High School in 1982 and entered the University of North Carolina at Chapel Hill. By his second year of college, Charles was starting to turn in the right direction. He was majoring in biology, which he liked, and every career he explored, he found he inadvertently compared to being a surgeon. It was his destiny, he figured, and he stopped trying to run from it. There was no one defining moment for his final career choice, but, he concedes, "I couldn't be anything else." By the time Charles entered medical school at Bowman Gray School of Medicine in Winston-Salem in 1988, he knew he would be a surgeon in Ashe County. Meanwhile, after a five and a half year courtship with Debbie Eller, the couple married in 1988, after Charles finished his first semester of medical school.

Once the decision was made to carry on the family legacy, Charles excelled in his studies. In 1992, he was at the top of his graduating class at Bowman Gray and received the Achievement Award from his classmates for being the student who best personifies the medical profession. He received the Surgical Merit Award for being the outstanding graduate in the field of surgical medicine, based on his participation in surgery during medical school. Jones completed his internship and residency at Carolinas Medical Center (CMC) in Charlotte (1992–1997), the largest hospital system in the state and the third largest in the United States. While there he received the Center's Department of General Surgery award for the

185

highest percentile score in the American Board of Surgery In-Training/Surgical Basic Science Exam in 1993 and 1994. He also was awarded Resident Teacher of the Year in 1997 at CMC.[1] But Charles turned down the opportunity to work at the big hospital in Charlotte; he and Debbie, also with strong ties to Ashe County, chose instead to raise their family at home, in Jefferson.

In looking back at his upbringing, Jones remembers his natural immersion in the family business of Ashe Memorial. Even after his grandparents, Dr. Dean, Sr., and Lettie, built their house behind the hospital on Gentry Street, Dr. Dean continued to take most of his meals at the hospital. "We would go to the hospital for Sunday dinner. My dad and granddad would do their rounds after we ate." Jones realizes now that if the two doctors were going to spend time with their family, they had to integrate them into their work, like Henry and Ruby Lum had done with their children. So Charles and his four siblings sat and played at the nurses' station until the rounds were over. When the children were not sitting quietly and behaving, they were elsewhere, not behaving. The hospital was heated by coal, and the coal was delivered and dumped in the back parking lot. The children delighted in cranking one another up and down in the coal bucket that hung for the purpose of lowering the coal down to the furnace room. This exuberant and noisy play eventually would be interrupted by their father, who would tell them to cease and desist.

Jones's impression of his grandfather was similar to that of others I interviewed. "He didn't speak unless he had something to say. He was a gentleman of the age. And there was no cutting up at Grandfather's house." Charles doesn't recall how his parents prepped their children beforehand, but he declares they were on their best behavior when visiting their grandparents. Maybe, because of their constant exposure to the reverence extended to this local icon by staff and patients, they simply knew to behave.

Family outings were a rare treat with Dr. Dean C., Jr.'s, schedule. There were no pagers or cell phones in those days, and Doc had to leave telephone numbers where he could be reached in an emergency. On one particular outing, Doc got a message he was needed at the scene of a bad car wreck. He was the coroner at the time. He rushed to the scene of the accident, family in tow, parked the car a distance away, and left Evelyn and the five children in the station wagon, the back of which became a makeshift playground, which seemed to grow smaller in the heat of the day. Evelyn struggled to keep the children distracted. Charles was about three years old and didn't understand what a coroner was. His siblings were similarly uninformed. They peppered their mother with endless questions about what their father was doing. "Is Dad going to sew somebody up? Is he going to fix a broken leg?" They did not grasp the possibility that the patient might be dead.

Despite his schedule, Doc always made time for his children, and introduced them to fishing at an early age. "Doc never met a trout he didn't like," says Charles. Doc started them out on a spinner and worms. Dry fly fishing, more of an art form, came later. Charles recalls fishing from his father's back. "He'd say, 'Here you take this for me' and hand the reel to me. 'I think you might have one,' he'd say in a minute, when I'd feel the line jiggle, and I'd catch one while riding on his back." Of course, in retrospect, Charles supposes his father already had the fish on the line when he handed him the reel, but, then, you can't hook a boy on fishing if he doesn't catch a fish.

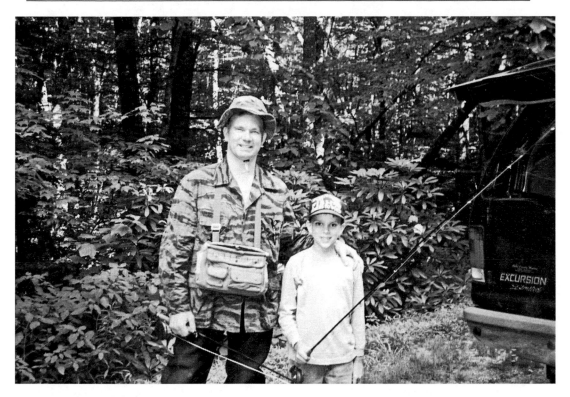

Fishing, like doctoring, is a Jones family tradition, and Dr. Charles Jones and his sons enjoy fishing together, much as Charles and his siblings enjoyed fishing with their dad, Doc Jones. Shown here are Charles and his oldest son, Brandon (photograph, circa 2005, courtesy Dr. Charles and Debbie Jones).

When Charles was six years old, he fell off a slide and broke his hand. The break was so severe his mother, Evelyn, said it looked like a monster's hand. She called her husband at the hospital, "Dean, I'm coming with a broken arm," she warned.[2] "Henry Lum came in to put me to sleep," remembers Charles. "They used gas then. It was interesting, but it was happening to me! As I was going under, I could see my grandfather's house through the window." That was not the only time Charles almost ended any potential of becoming a surgeon. Ruby Lum recalls when Charles and her son Phil were in high school and were using a chain saw out at her homeplace. Charles had the chain saw in hand, and it backed up on him, barely missing critical tendons. Ruby got him to the hospital, and Dr. Bill DuSold worked on him. He made a full recovery.

The Jones family was so closely associated with the hospital that when one of Charles's classmates asked him what his father and grandfather did, he didn't answer they were doctors or surgeons. Instead, he responded, "They run the hospital." To him, as to many, the two surgeons and the hospital were one and the same, their identities were so intertwined with Ashe Memorial.

Both Charles's father and grandfather were big sports fans. The famously taciturn Doc Jones was asked to make a few remarks on the occasion of his induction into the Ashe County Sports Hall of Fame and surprised the audience, with a lengthy and animated account of Ashe County sports history, a subject near and dear to his heart. He included the rivalry between Jefferson and West Jefferson and Major League Baseball player Monte Weaver, from Helton, who pitched for the Washington Senators 1931–1938 and the Boston Red Sox in 1939. People in the audience marveled they had never heard Doc say so much in all the years they had known him. His family laughed and cited his love of sports as the inspiration for his oration.

Both Dr. Dean, Sr., and Doc donated their time as team physicians for the local high schools, a role now assumed by Charles. In the last couple of years, Charles relates, big strides have been made in sports physicals. Ashe County High School has partnered with sponsors Ashe Memorial and Blue Ridge Electric Membership Corporation to include electrocardiograms (EKGs) as part of the sports physicals, an effort to identify heart issues that often go undetected until a player suffers a heart attack during a game or in practice. The free heart screening program, called "Heart of a Husky," is open to upcoming eighth to twelfth grade students involved in high school athletics and students in the JROTC Raiders program. Impact testing is another addition to the sports physical, not yet in place in larger communities. The test, performed on each prospective athlete, provides baseline neurological information in the event of head injury, saving medical personnel valuable time in initiating proper treatment.

Remembering my note from the Lib McRimmon interview, to follow-up with Charles on the subject of wens, I ask Charles if he has ever heard the term. He explains a wen is a pilar cyst or a hair follicle cyst. "It looks a little like a white pearl when it is taken out; trichilemmal is the medical term. I take them off all the time." The old terminology reminds him of some of the adjustments he had to make during his first years back in Ashe County after his big city training. "Your education continues after you get out," he confesses. A nurse came to him and exclaimed, "I've got somebody here that is pieded [pie-ded]!" He had no idea what she was talking about. After finding someone who could explain to him "pieded" simply meant blotchy skin, he realized he still had a lot to learn.

Fortunately, as of June 2015, Dr. Charles is no longer the only surgeon at AMH, and he is grateful Dr. Tammy Thore is back to share the surgical workload. Family time is still a challenge, but, like those

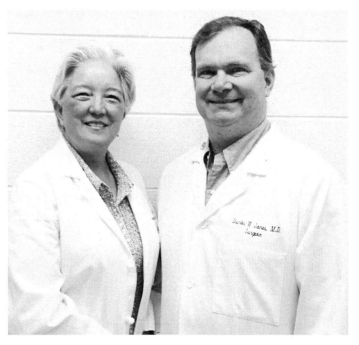

In June 2015, Dr. Charles Jones was joined by Dr. Tammy Thore, daughter of Henry and Ruby Lum, giving Ashe Memorial Hospital two surgeons (courtesy Dr. Charles and Debbie Jones).

who came before them, the family manages to make it work. Most of the credit for this achievement probably goes to the spouses behind those four generations of physicians and surgeons, each remarkable in her own right.

Debra "Debbie" Eller Jones Interview (Jefferson, January 15, 2015)

When it became apparent Debbie Eller and Charles were a forever couple, Debbie received some sage advice from Evelyn Jones, her future mother-in-law—"Never plan on things going as you planned." Evelyn's advice sounds a lot like that given by her mother-in-law, Lettie Jones, when Doc and Evelyn were to marry. "The unexpected is typical, even something simple like a family drive," acknowledges Debbie. The lives of the spouses of those dedicated to the medical profession have changed almost as much as the profession, but Debbie has much in common with the Jones women who preceded her. Like Evelyn, Debbie keeps the home fires burning, makes the many adjustments necessary to accommodate a surgeon's schedule, and is active in church and community. She helps with the food pantry and serves on various committees at Jefferson United Methodist Church, tutors at the school, helping with the reading program, and is involved in the Ashe County Children's Trust Endowment, which raises money to benefit children in the community, providing services ranging from the purchase of cribs for infants to paying for therapy needed by children in abusive homes.

In recent years, Debbie has joined her husband, on a part-time basis, at his office in the Professional Building behind the hospital. The opportunity came to purchase a laser to remove plantar warts and unwanted hair, and to treat veins. Debbie went through the training on the equipment, and, under the supervision of Dr. Charles, offers laser treatments to patients. "I do a complimentary consultation, and we determine if the person is a good candidate for the treatment. It has been rewarding to help people." Debbie's venture reminded me of Fannie Jones working alongside her husband, Dr. Bud, administering the anesthesia for surgery and serving as his nurse. Debbie also assists with the business end of her husband's practice, as Lettie did for Dr. Dean, Sr. "Charles always has those wheels turning," says Debbie, "and I help him jump start some of those new ideas." Doc was fond of saying, "The smartest thing I ever did was marry Evelyn." It seems like marrying smart women is a family tradition too.

Although born in Pennsylvania, Debbie grew up in Ashe County, the daughter of Ashe County natives James Edward Eller and Cora Ruth Miller Eller. She graduated from Beaver Creek High School and received her bachelor's degree in sociology from the University of North Carolina at Charlotte, graduating with honors. She and Charles met when she was a sophomore in high school, and he was a senior. "We started dating the summer before my senior year." Debbie recalls meeting Dr. Dean, Sr., several times, after Lettie died. "He was the most chivalrous gentleman; he would stand up when I came into the room. I was only seventeen." She first met Doc in the summer of 1983. "When I got to know him, I realized we shared a similar sense of humor." The two enjoyed many late nights watching slapstick comedies on television, while Charles and Evelyn dozed.

Phyllis Jones Yount Interview (Raleigh, December 6, 2014)

The eldest of Doc and Evelyn's five children, Phyllis Yount now lives in Raleigh, and one Saturday in December 2014, she spent the better part of an afternoon with me, talking about growing up in the Jones family. Dr. Bud Jones was gone before Phyllis was born, and she has only vague recollections of her great-grandmother Fannie, and those are clearly from a child's vantage point. "I only remember her from the knees down. I remember her black shoes and apron." Since Phyllis was the first grandchild of Dr. Dean, Sr., and Lettie, her early impressions of them were of particular interest to me. What sticks in a child's memory is a fascinating window into the past—the purest of truths. They were loving grandparents, Phyllis attests, although somewhat reserved, by today's standards. "Grandmother was very prim and proper, always well-dressed, with her beads on." Evelyn related her daughter's habit of kissing her grandfather's bald head. "He just loved that." He was not too reserved, then, to appreciate a child's gesture of affection.

Evelyn told me a story about a hair-raising trip one New Year's Day, when she and Doc were still living in Louisburg, North Carolina. She and the children had been visiting with her folks in Grayson County, Virginia, and were on their way back to the home of Dr. Dean, Sr. Struggling with terrible road conditions, Evelyn was determined to get her brood safely back to Jefferson. When she finally neared the hospital and hit the little rise at the turn onto Gentry Street, the snow was piled so high on the sides of the road where it had been plowed, the wheels of her station wagon hung on the rise, and she was stuck. If she let her foot off the brake, the car would slide back into an even more precarious position. She was in trouble, and her children were with her. No one was outside to see her predicament. She could not leave the car for help, because she could not take her foot off the brake. She took the only course of action she could think of and dispatched little Phyllis, still in preschool, to walk the rest of the way to her grandparents' house and fetch help. Evelyn figured her father-in-law would be home watching the ball game, if he wasn't checking on his patients at the hospital. She watched with a mother's fearful anticipation of the worst, as Phyllis's head disappeared behind the snow bank, worried the neighbor's big dog would rush out to greet the child, possibly knocking her down in the snow. The two other children fidgeted in the station wagon, picking up on their mother's concern. Tommy was just a baby and his brother David a toddler. But the adventure had a happy ending, as Dr. Dean, Sr., and Scott McClure, from the hospital staff, quickly came to the rescue.[3]

I ask Phyllis about this early escapade. "I felt like I had to climb and climb and climb," she recalls, pulling together the threads of the childhood memory. "All I could see was white." She doesn't remember anything else about the trek to her grandparents' house, but when she reached their door, she knocked and told her grandfather, "Mama needs some help." Dr. Dean responded, as he always did, immediately and efficiently, with no fanfare or unnecessary conversation.

Phyllis marvels at how her mother ever had the time to do all she did. "She had a big garden, canned and froze. She's a good cook and put healthy meals on the table every day." She always had a hot meal on the table for Doc, no matter what time of day he came home.

Phyllis smiles as she recalls her mother slipping in front of a mirror to straighten her hair and freshen her lipstick, when she heard her husband's car in the driveway. "Mother was very involved in the community too and loved the Girl Scouts; she wanted the girls in the county to have that opportunity."

Phyllis's first recollection of being in the hospital as a patient was when she broke her arm falling off her pony. She was in the fifth grade, playing with her friend Jane Ann, just before school started back from the summer. She was riding with no hands when she fell off. Afraid to tell her parents what happened, for fear they would take the pony away from her, she kept mum about the accident, but Jane Ann blabbed to her mother, who called Evelyn, who talked to Doc, who then pressed his daughter about the injury. She could not hide the broken arm from her father, and Doc took her to the hospital to set the arm. She did not want the shot to numb her arm. "It'll hurt," Doc warned. "I don't want the shot!" Phyllis insisted, more scared of the needle than the pain. Doc set the arm with no anesthesia. "He was right—it did hurt."

The dedication to task shared by Dr. Dean and Doc was accepted by the children as the norm, because it was what they knew. Growing up with a father who was a surgeon meant the children might go what seemed liked weeks without seeing their father. Phyllis's room was situated where she could hear the roar of Doc's car as he came in and out, sometimes more than once, in the course of an evening. "But family was important to him," and that is evident in Phyllis's recollections of her father. "Dad took me to the drive-in to see *Cinderella*, when we lived in Charlotte." Together in the privacy of the car, Doc and his oldest sang "Bibbity Bob" with abandon. Doc always tried to be home when the *Wizard of Oz* aired every year—it was a family tradition to watch the classic. There were camping trips, fishing, hiking and all things outdoors, and trips to the beach, far away from calls and patients. Doc enjoyed these times, especially the beach, even though he regularly got sunburned, despite the precautions available at the time. "He never spanked me," Phyllis confides; his disappointment was a worse punishment and left an everlasting impression. "My dates were terrified of him, because he was so quiet." Once she was late coming home from a date, because the film at the movie theater broke and had to be repaired before the movie could resume. Her father was waiting for her when she arrived. "Your mother's been worried about you," he said. Nothing more was necessary to make his point.

Big sisters often have a different view of childhood shenanigans. For instance, Phyllis does not remember being cranked down the coal chute in a bucket at the old hospital, a tale related to me by her brother Charles. "All that soot and dirt—not my cup of tea." So as not to risk being thought a sissy pants, she does fess up to climbing the hospital's water tower with her friends. On one occasion when she was recruited to babysit her siblings, Tommy and David were roughhousing, and somebody knocked somebody into a shower door, which broke and cut somebody's leg open. Somebody said, "We may need to call Granddaddy." Dr. Dean stitched up somebody, and somebody was none the worse for wear.

Phyllis had a job at Ashe Memorial during her high school years, working in the lab and x-ray, developing film and washing test tubes. Henry Lum and Judy Davis taught her how to do an EKG, and the beginnings of a career path were laid. She knew she wanted to do something in the medical field, but not nursing, because she did not want to give injections. She attended the University of North Carolina at Chapel Hill and earned a two year certificate as a radiologic technologist in 1976. Later she graduated from Appalachian State University with a BS in business. She is now business manager for her husband's practice in Raleigh. Dr. Keith Yount is a specialist in orofacial pain.

Phyllis was working at Ashe Memorial when a patient came in for a follow-up on surgery for a trimalleolar fracture (a three part fracture of the ankle). She studied the x-ray and was impressed with the results of the surgery. She asked the patient where he had the surgery, assuming he had been to a specialist at Baptist in Winston-Salem or some other big city hospital. "Old Doc did it," he replied, referring to her father. Phyllis knew her father especially enjoyed orthopedic surgery, but sometimes you don't realize how extraordinary your loved ones are until you see them through somebody else's eyes, or x-rays.

"When did people start calling you 'Doc'?" Phyllis once asked her father, taking note of the familiar address used by almost everyone she knew. "Since I was in the sixth grade," he chuckled. He always knew he wanted to be a doctor, he explained, and he lived in the hospital. "He gave his heart and soul to the county," reflects Phyllis, and the time came when he had nothing left. "He was worn out." Doc had congestive heart failure. He continued to work for almost a decade with his heart functioning at about 20 percent— about a third of normal. Diabetes cost him part of his foot. He was in and out of the hospital and the Margate Health and Rehabilitation Center. Finally he was at Ashe Memorial, ready to go, waiting. He refused all medications, including Tylenol. The only thing he felt like eating was milkshakes from Hardees. "Well, I've missed it," he said one day when Phyllis was sitting with him. "Missed what?" she asked. "My opportunity to go peacefully."

He showed no fear in dying. He spoke of a bridge. "Where's the bridge; I can't find the bridge." His family reassured him and told him to keep looking. At the end, he wanted to be alone, so Evelyn slept on a stretcher in another room, and the children and grandchildren took turns sitting outside his door, where they could monitor his situation and alert the nurses if he needed anything. Phyllis's son, Nathan, was on hall duty when Doc looked off, as though he saw something or someone at a distance; the last word he spoke was "Mother." Doc had seen his bridge, gifting his family with the assurance he was crossing over with the loving mother, who had walked him to school when he was a little boy in Lansing, a lifetime ago.

Phyllis speaks of the care, love, and compassion extended by the Ashe Memorial staff to her father and the family in those last days. Dying is a hard business, but the people Doc worked with for so many years did everything they could to ease his passing.

David Lee Jones Interview (Jefferson, January 4, 2015)

Phyllis's oldest brother, David Lee Jones, born June 19, 1959, is old enough to remember the family's move from Louisburg to Jefferson after Doc's residency there. David was in the restaurant business in Raleigh for 25 years, but after the sudden death of his wife Robin Barker in 1995, he made his way back to Ashe County and now works in car sales at Empire Dodge in Wilkesboro and shares the house on Gentry Street with his mother, Evelyn.

As we sit at the dining room table in the house his grandparents lived in, I can see the old hospital building across the lawn. David spent most of his growing up years in the home of his parents on Northwest Drive, a short distance away, but he has memories of this house and the old hospital, and, of course, his grandparents, Dr. Dean and Lettie. His grandfather taught him to hunt and fish, although, he clarifies, they didn't shoot much of anything— "it was more like stalking." He describes his grandfather as a good hunter, quiet, reserved and with a very dry sense of humor.

When David and his grandfather went fishing, Lettie often tagged along. "I'll just sit in the car," she would say. Invariably when the two returned to the car from their fishing, Lettie would be gone. They knew they would find her at the nearest house, sitting on the front porch, visiting. One summer day, they were fishing at Three Top. It started to pour down rain, and David ran back to the car to sit with Lettie. They sat and sat—no Granddaddy. Finally the rain stopped, and David headed back out to fish some more. When he returned again to the car, he found his grandfather, with a nice catch, most of which he caught while it was raining. David filed away the fishing tip for future use. Fly fishing was more his father's sport, and they enjoyed many trips together until Doc's health began to fail. Once Doc, David, and a cousin were fishing up around Middle Fork, when a man appeared in the remote area, approached Doc, and, looking hard at his face, asked, "You the man that cut my leg off?" David and his cousin exchanged worried looks. "Yes, I am," Doc replied calmly. Doc and the man exchanged a few pleasantries and when Doc returned to their questioning looks, he explained. Turns out the former patient had been singing Christmas carols with his brother and some others at a holiday function in the back of beyond. It came the brother's turn to sing the lead, and the patient jumped in and started singing the lead. The brother got mad, shouted it was his turn to sing, pulled out a gun, and shot the patient's foot off. When the patient was brought to the hospital for treatment, Doc simply cut off the last little piece of skin that remained and dressed and bandaged the wound. Peace on earth, good will toward men.

Evelyn worked hard to maintain some semblance of routine in the young family, despite Doc's schedule. David remembers father and sons sitting down on the floor every Sunday morning before church to polish their shoes. After church, the family had Sunday dinner at the hospital dining room with Dr. Dean and Lettie. "Then Doc and Granddaddy would do their rounds, and we would do ours," says David. This might entail riding in handy wheelchairs—on two wheels, buzzing by the nurses' stations, or David and Tommy cranking their little brother Charles down the coal chute in a bucket. When the play got too rowdy, a stern look from Doc returned the hospital to a more appropriate noise level.

The family was packed up and ready to leave for the beach, when Doc was called in to the hospital to assist his father with the victims from a bad wreck on Baker Hill. In an hour or so, Doc returned, blood all over his scrubs, but ready to resume the trip. What was it like for the children of a surgeon, with family always at the mercy of the latest catastrophe? "It was never a dull moment," laughs David.

Thomas "Tommy" Mitchell Jones Interview (Jefferson, January 3, 2015)

"When we have a family get together, he is always the first one bleeding," David declares about his younger brother Tommy. Tommy good naturedly admits there is some truth to the claims he is accident prone. "Growing up, I had some kind of injury about every two days." Tommy is the big athlete in the family, participating in every sport available in the local school system. His dad, the team doctor, once set his arm on the football field during a game he was quarterbacking. When Tommy asked his dad why he didn't give him any warning he was getting ready to pop the bone in place, Doc replied, "If I'd have told you, you would have tightened up." Tommy rolls up his sleeves and his pants legs to show off scars from other triage work rendered by his father and grandfather. I decide it is a good thing this man was born into a family of doctors and then, for good measure, married one—family physician, Dr. Leigh Bradley.

"He is always coming to somebody's rescue," says Leigh about her husband. He has a reputation around the county for helping others. And, she claims, "He can fix everything." So I figure it is safe to assume Tommy's tendency to be accident prone might be attributed to his simply doing more things than the average person, thus increasing his odds for calamity proportionately. It was his propensity for caregiving which brought Tommy back to Ashe County from a stint in Raleigh, helping his brother David in his restaurant business. Doc had open heart surgery, and Evelyn had a hip replacement about the same time. He drove them both home from Carolinas Medical in Charlotte. Doc looked bad, pale and weak, exasperated with the state of his health and with his long stay in the hospital, away from his beloved Ashe County. He told his son to pull over at a rest stop on the parkway, just over the Ashe County line. "What's going on?" asked Tommy. "I got to do something," Doc mumbled. Then, still in his bathrobe and slippers, Doc gingerly stepped out of the car, shuffled over to the "Welcome to Ashe County" sign and kissed it. "Dad always maintained there was no prettier place than Ashe County," says Tommy. "He claimed once he thought he saw someplace as pretty, but then realized he was standing in Alleghany County and looking back into Ashe."

Growing up in the Jones household, interrupted family outings and vacations, and late dinners were part of the norm. Sometimes, the car would be loaded for a trip, and the whole enterprise would have to be put on hold while Doc answered a call. His children rarely saw him without his scrubs. When the bridge collapsed in the Silas Creek community in 1966, Evelyn drove near the site, worried her husband might get hurt trying to reach the injured truck driver pinned in the wreckage. Doc made the children promise they would stay in the car and left Evelyn to control the ensuing chaos in the backseat. He returned later, soaked from the waist down from wading out into the river to assess the situation. Later, the boys got a chance to see the cab of the truck. David tried to climb in and recalls, "I couldn't fit between the steering wheel and the seat!" During the blizzard of 1993, the National Guard came to pick up Doc to perform emergency surgery. David was right, there was never a dull moment.

Despite the interruptions in their family time, Tommy enjoyed many fishing trips with his dad, from his childhood on into adulthood. Doc secured his place as his son's hero when on one excursion, he stomped his foot down on a snake which had scared the boy. "He never showed fear," recalls Tommy. At an away game, Doc, serving as team physician, witnessed a bus load of the opposing team's players fast unloading to beat up his quarterback after the game. Doc jumped in his Bronco, headed straight for the ensuing melee, hollered out the window for the quarterback to jump in, and swooped up the player like a one-man army, whisking him to safety. "They don't make 'em like that anymore," smiles Tommy.

Leigh Bradley, M.D., Interview (Jefferson, January 3, 2015)

When Dr. Leigh Bradley, married Tommy Jones, she became a part of the Jones family tradition of doctoring too, and Doc advised her to keep her maiden name as her professional name, claiming there were too many Dr. Joneses for people to keep up with already. But Leigh Bradley fell in love with Ashe County long before she met Tommy. Born in what was then the small town of Monroe in Union County, Leigh got her undergraduate degree at Appalachian State University and while there attended several church retreats at Horse Creek. "I knew I wanted to come here before I knew there was a hospital," she says. After graduating from the North Carolina School of Medicine at Chapel Hill in 1991, she performed her residency in family practice at Mountain Area Health Education Center in Asheville 1991–1994.

One day she was talking to another resident and mentioned she wanted to practice in Ashe County. Her comment was overheard by resident Kevin Kurtz. "Well, I'm from Ashe County," he announced. The two struck up a conversation, and in January 1995 High Country Family Medicine, adjoining Ashe Memorial Hospital, was founded. Meanwhile, as part of her residency training, Leigh worked her three week rural rotation in March 1993 with Kevin's father, Dr. Elam Kurtz, at his office in Lansing. She lived with Elam and his wife Orpah. "Elam Kurtz was amazing," she says, recalling the doctor's dedication to keeping abreast of the latest in medical developments. "When he came home from work, Orpah would have medical magazines laid out for him, and he would read until supper."

At age 29 and single, Leigh Bradley, M.D., moved to Ashe County. Her mother came to help her look for a house. When the realtor asked Leigh what she was looking for, her mother piped up and said, "She needs a house and a husband." As luck would have it, the realtor was Evelyn Jones, who happily supplied everything her client needed. Leigh and Evelyn's son Tommy married in 1998 and now have twin girls, Jayden and Jordan. Leigh juggles her family and practice and coaches her daughters' fifth and sixth grade basketball team and marvels at the memory of Elam Kurtz coming home and reading medical magazines before supper. Like any modern couple, she reflects, there is no time for sitting in a recliner at the Bradley-Jones house.

Leigh is the only one in her family to go into medicine. Her father was a maintenance supervisor at a metal mill, and her mother worked in a florist shop after her children were grown. Leigh doesn't remember when she decided she wanted to be a doctor, but under her name in her high school year book, it says, "I want to be a doctor and practice in a rural area." Are her girls impressed she is a doctor? Leigh responds with a story about her daughters setting up an Instagram account for her. When she read the bio they had posted for her, it described her as the mother of twins and a basketball coach—no mention whatsoever of her being a doctor. The perspective of a child always brings you back to the real priorities of their world.

In the early days of her practice in Ashe County, local doctors took shifts in the emergency department at Ashe Memorial. It took awhile to feel comfortable with the relatively quiet bunch at AMH, but Leigh says, "I knew I had made it when Doc Jones pulled out a joke and showed it to me. Once he took you in, they all thought you were okay." Acknowledging the trust and level of comfort people in the community associated with Doc Jones, Leigh declares all she had to do to win over a reluctant patient was mention that Doc was her father-in-law.

Linda Noel Jones Patterson Interview (Jefferson, March 27, 2015)

All the Jones children played sports, says Evelyn, the girls included. The youngest, Linda Noel, born December 22, 1968, played Little League baseball. She tucked her buffy tails (pig tails) up under her cap, and only her coach, Dr. E. J. Miller, and her teammates knew she was a girl. But Linda's love of the game did not deter her from other pursuits. She took piano and dance lessons, in the dance studio in the basement of the old hospital, and when she was in the fourth grade, she was crowned "Little Miss U.S.A." She took gymnastics too. One evening Doc took her to her gymnastics class in Boone. As was his habit, he waited in the car, going over his patient charts and making notes. During a routine, the promising young gymnast sustained a "career ending injury," dislocating her elbow. She was in extreme pain. Her instructor and the other girls in the class were in a panic, trying to get her arm in a makeshift sling and talking about getting her to the hospital in Boone. It was hard to get her words out, but Linda finally managed to communicate that her father was outside in the car. Now on the scene, Doc treated the injury, quickly reducing the elbow (rotating it back into place) before the muscles and tendons could contract, which would have made treatment much more difficult. With the arm stabilized, he drove her back to Ashe Memorial Hospital, where he put the arm in a cast.

Much to Doc's chagrin, Linda chose to attend North Carolina State University, a bitter pill for the die-hard Carolina alumnus and fan, but Linda wanted to study chemical engineering, making the defection understandable. She now works for a major chemical manufacturer, focusing on environmental work. She is married to Dale Patterson, and the couple lives in Kingsport, Tennessee, with their two sons, Lane and Cameron.

I ask Linda what her favorite thing was about Doc. "I loved his goofiness. He'd wear these goofy hats and ties and go in a patient's room with an arrow stuck through his head. The last week of life, in the hospital, he had a fake arm he used to play tricks on the nurses. He gave the impression to those who didn't know him that he was an introvert, but he was a practical joker." Were her dates afraid of him, I wonder, remembering what her sister Phyllis had said? "No," Linda laughs. "They were afraid of my brothers."

16

Changes in AMH
Management and Services

Over the years, operating a hospital has evolved into a complicated business, with a load of government regulations. In 1981, the Ashe Memorial Hospital Board of Trustees, chaired by J. Gwyn Gambill, made the difficult decision to bring in a professional management company to oversee administration. The contract was awarded to Hospital Corporation of America, which later changed its name to Quorum Health Resources (QHR). While this decision was right for the time, it was not easy to accept—to admit outside help was needed. "We are independent mountain people," reminds Dr. Charles Jones, putting the dilemma into perspective. Under this arrangement, the hospital pays a fee to the company for management and consulting services. The management company hires the CEO for the hospital, who runs the hospital, represents the hospital to the community, as well as statewide and national levels, insures compliance with the Joint Commission on Accreditation of Health Care Organizations and develops the annual budget to present to the board of trustees. The company negotiates on behalf of the hospital with insurance companies to minimize patient out-of-pocket expenses and manages employee benefits. Gary Bishop and Ray Hill were the first two chief executive officers to come on board, and then R. D. Williams II assumed the job in 1994 and stayed 19 years, until the management contract was awarded to Novant Health in 2013.[1]

This change in the way AMH is managed does not change the nonprofit status the hospital has maintained since its first opening in 1941; AMH continues to be owned by the shareholders, and 100 percent of the profits continue to be reinvested in the facility. The cost of a share has gone up from the $10 paid by Dr. E. J. Miller's mother when the shares were first offered, but, as of 2015, anyone can purchase a share for $100. Clairene Cockerham, wife of the late Tom Cockerham, AMH's administrator for 30 years, says, "It is important for people to know you still can buy stock." As originally set up, all shares of the corporation are without par value, which means the shares have no face value to the owner; the only return on the owner's investment is the right to vote for the board of trustees, one vote for each share owned, not to exceed 100 votes per person. The share certificates are non-negotiable, but upon the death of the holder, become the property of his or her heirs.[2]

By the year 2000, the hospital, once so proud of its reputation for operating in the black, was in a decline, struggling to stay afloat financially—the result of a combination of rising medical costs, including drugs, supplies, labor, and insurance, reduced reimbursement for services provided to Medicaid and Medicare beneficiaries, and an economy no longer on the rise. The problems were shared by many nonprofit hospitals across the country. Charity care became more difficult to manage. In one month alone, Trustee Jim Gambill recalls, $250,000 was written off as bad debt—the result of patients unable to pay.[3]

Looking back on the hospital's financial troubles, Gambill reflects, "Things change, and you have to react to them as best you can." The hospital industry was experiencing a move away from inpatient care, explains former CEO R. D. Williams II, a move which put less demand on the number of beds needed in a hospital. Coupled with the declining reimbursement rates for Medicare and Medicaid and the disproportionate number of AMH patients relying on Medicare and Medicaid, the impact on AMH was significant. In the late 1990s, as part of a plan to address the financial crisis, the Board of Trustees, on the advice of their management provider at the time, Quorum Health Resources, and with the agreement and support of the AMH medical staff, voted to pursue designation of AMH as a "Critical Access Hospital" (CAH), as opposed to a general acute care hospital. The CAH program is administered by the North Carolina Department of Health and Human Services through the Office of Rural Health and provides an option for small rural hospitals who may be struggling financially, to maintain access to essential health services for the community in exchange for certain limitations on inpatient services, such as the number of beds and average length of stay for inpatients. When it became a CAH in September 2007, Ashe Memorial reduced its number of beds from 76 to 25. This reduction in the number of beds was not a bad thing, explains Gambill; the beds were not needed. The CAH certification allows the hospital to receive cost-based reimbursement from Medicare and Medicaid for services provided to Medicare and Medicaid patients. Since things are more expensive in a small hospital, because a small hospital lacks the purchase power of a large hospital, allowing reimbursement according to the actual cost involved in treating a patient, instead of reimbursement based on the lower, standard fixed reimbursement rates of Medicare and Medicaid, means the hospital is getting more money for services—closer to their cost.[4]

When the contract for the AMH health management provider was up for renewal, bids were requested, and Novant Health was chosen as the new provider in 2013—that meant a new CEO and a new economic model for the hospital. The ownership of Mountain Hearts was transferred from the hospital to the AMH Foundation; the hospital's cafeteria was contracted out to Morrison Management Specialists, Inc.; the beds for Segraves Care Center went to Margate Health and Rehabilitation Center; and the Segraves space was reconfigured for doctors' offices, administrative offices, and a physical therapy department. An imaging department was added.[5] "The major focus now," says AMH Trustee Bradley McNeill, "is bringing in specialists and family physicians and renovation of the emergency department."[6]

Contracting with Novant Health, explains AMH Trustee Jan Caddell, gives the hospital a tremendous advantage in buying power, because the management provider is buying for all the facilities it owns, as well as Ashe Memorial, which Caddell is quick to point out is still owned by shareholders. The company only manages the hospital, and since Ashe

Memorial is the first nonprofit hospital Novant Health has ever contracted to manage, they have a huge stake in making a success of their involvement.[7] But the financial situation at AMH was not going to be a quick fix. By 2014, the hospital was in such dire straits, the Board of Trustees appealed to the Ashe County Commissioners for help; $500,000 were provided to help support the hospital. The subsidy saved the day, but AMH is not out of the woods yet, although it is certainly on a better financial footing than before the subsidy. A quarter-cent sales tax was passed on the 2014 election ballot, and it is hoped this may provide a short term revenue source for the hospital to increase its quality of care and boost its financial well being, as well as provide support for the public schools.[8]

Laura Lambeth, R.N., B.S.N., Interview (Jefferson, August 13, 2014)

The task of turning things around for Ashe Memorial now rests with the current chief executive officer, Laura Lambeth, R.N., B.S.N. I sit down for our first interview in August 2014. Behind Lambeth's desk hangs Stephen Shoemaker's familiar print of the old Ashe County Memorial Hospital. There is something very fitting about this, I think, reflective of a continuity that is important not to lose. Lambeth, on board since August 2, 2013, is mindful of that importance, and that strikes me as having a lot to do with her success thus far in this daunting job. She is the only person in the hospital employed by Novant Health, a not-for-profit integrated health care system based in Winston-Salem, serving North Carolina, South Carolina, Virginia, and Georgia.

Fortunately, this is not her first rodeo. She started out as a registered nurse and in 2015 had 34 years in health care. She has made a career of turning around troubled institutions. Her goal is to take the hospital out of CAH status, which will allow the replacement of some of the beds forfeited with that designation and the expansion of certain specialized services. The increased cost efficiencies, due in large part to the purchasing clout of the management provider, make the transition from CAH a reasonable goal for the hos-

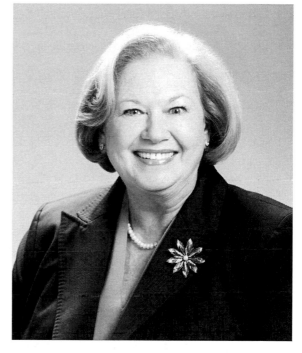

Although AMH continues to be owned by its shareholders, the hospital board now contracts with a professional management company to handle the administration of the hospital. Laura Lambeth started as CEO at AMH in August 2013 and is the only person at the hospital employed by the current management provider Novant Health (photograph, 2015, courtesy AMH).

pital's evolving financial situation. Lambeth's first challenge on the job was a tough one—to start the AMH recovery process without a layoff. But staff stepped up to the challenge and worked with her to make the adjustments needed to economize. "It is very humbling," says Lambeth regarding the staff's support. "This takes a big amount of trust for all parties involved."

Lambeth's strategy for growth includes the recruitment of physicians and specialists and the hospital's own hospitalist program. Previously, local doctors, not employed by the hospital, but with their own private practices, took turns manning the emergency department and providing hospitalist services. Now hospitalists are employed by AMH and work there and only there. Local doctors continue to admit their patients when a hospital stay is required and treat or manage the care of their patients while they are in the hospital. But if a patient comes to the hospital via the emergency department, as opposed to a scheduled surgery, the AMH hospitalist treats the patient. Patients requiring a specialist, such as an orthopedist, used to have to go to Winston-Salem or Boone for treatment. Now various specialists, including pediatric care and ear, nose and throat, come to Ashe Memorial one or two days a week to treat patients. Lambeth reports the specialists are impressed with the hospital and staff, and this bodes well for future expansion of this level of service.

The CEO also was impressed with the quality of care she found at Ashe Memorial. "The nurses take care of patients like they are family." A nurse of the old school, Lambeth believes in this approach. She didn't have to change the culture of care at Ashe Memorial; the best philosophy was already in place. But a hospital needs to run like a business to make it, and that is the challenge.

Other changes at AMH are typical of the health care industry elsewhere in the United States. Today, for instance, patients may be seen by a range of professionals unheard of in the early days of the hospital. A nurse practitioner (N.P.) can diagnose and prescribe medications, while a physician's assistant (P.A.) can provide a diagnosis and prescribe medication, treatment, and lab tests. Both typically have a master's degree, plus a specified number of hours of training with patients while still in school. Technicians perform routine tests, such as drawing blood and running EKGs (electrocardiograms). They are certified by the state, and nowadays many have associate degrees in clinical laboratory science. An E.D. tech is an emergency department technician, and the duties of a certified nursing assistant (C.N.A.) include checking patients' vital signs, monitoring mobility and helping with food and grooming. Ward secretaries process orders and put together necessary paperwork and charts.[9]

Over the years, the dress code for nurses and other hospital personnel has changed too. "We were so proud of our caps," says Evelyn Jones, when we are interviewing Kate Duncan. "They represented the school where we got our training."[10] The traditional nurse's cap was almost a thing of the past by the 1980s, and as more men entered the nursing profession, unisex scrubs became the accepted attire. A dress code implemented by AMH color codes the scrubs worn by each department in the hospital. Nurses, for instance, wear navy blue and white lab coats. The color coding makes it easy to distinguish who is in housekeeping, dietary, radiology, etc. and adds a measure of security—it is obvious when someone is out of place.

What gives Laura Lambeth the confidence her task at AMH is doable? "I think it is the people of Ashe County," she responds. Lambeth is grateful for the support of the hospital Board and the Ashe County Commissioners, who understand the importance of having a hospital in the county, not only because patients do not then have a 30+ minute ambulance ride to get treatment, but because of the distinct advantage a hospital presence gives to the economic development of the region. According to West Jefferson Mayor Dale Baldwin, any business considering locating in the Ashe County area wants to know about the quality of the public schools and the availability of a hospital. Ashe Memorial's role as a major employer in the area is also an important element of the local economy. The hospital continues to provide a welcome first job for many in the county and the only job for some.[11]

Ashe Memorial Hospital has provided jobs and medical care to the people of Ashe County and the surrounding area for more than 75 years, but the hospital that sits atop Hospital Drive in Jefferson is a far different place from the hospital with the pretty stone façade at 410 McConnell Street. This newer Ashe Memorial offers a wide variety of emergency, elective and preventive health services, as well as state-of-the-art labor and delivery services and prenatal and postnatal care on the hospital campus. The Mountain Hearts Center for Prevention and Wellness, formerly Mountain Hearts Cardiac Rehabilitation Center, now owned and operated by the AMH Foundation, has moved beyond cardiac rehabilitation and offers a variety of health and fitness programs for adults, including seniors, and children.[12] The Wilma Vannoy Birthing Center, completed in the fall of 2005, by J. R. Vannoy and Sons Construction Company, Inc., as a major renovation

Right: **Mountain Hearts Center for Prevention and Wellness, now operated by the AMH Foundation, offers a variety of health and fitness programs for adults and children (photograph, 2015, courtesy Louis Pittard).**

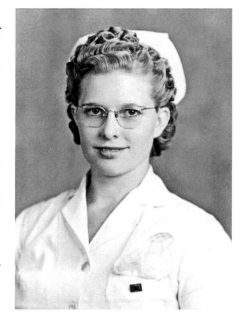

"She looked like a nurse was supposed to look," says Evelyn Jones of Kate Duncan, R.N., a nurse of the old school, like Evelyn. Dress codes have changed markedly from the days of white hose and caps. Now scrubs are color coded according to department (courtesy Nan Robinson).

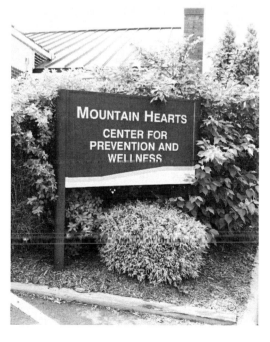

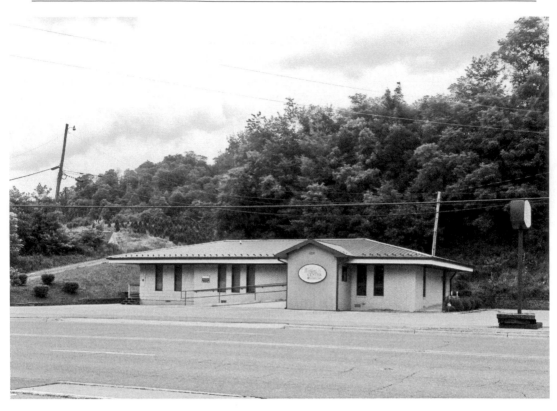

Ashe County Women's Center, located across the street from the West Jefferson Post Office, offers gynecological and obstetrical services for women (photograph, 2015, by the author).

of the AMH obstetrical department, offers a comprehensive approach to maternity care, allowing the mother to stay in the same room during the entire birthing process. The center was made possible through a generous gift from the Vannoy family, in honor of Mrs. "Wilma" Christine Witherspoon Vannoy, who passed away in 2004.[13] The Ashe Women's Center is another AMH initiative, offering a full range of gynecological and obstetrical services to women from adolescence through menopause, with an on-site lab and ultrasound.[14] What would they say about the care and services of today, those midwives and granny women who once presided over the birthing of babies in the backwoods of Appalachia? It was not that long ago that Fannie Jones, wife of Dr. Bud Jones, took a newborn in her arms, while her husband aided the mother on the only bed in a one room cabin, or that mountain women bravely bore child after child in rough circumstances, without the help of any medical professional. Their survival and the survival of their children are a testament to the strength of a people bound to their land and their mountain home, and the loss of those who did not survive is a reminder of how far the region has come in women's health care.

Ashe Memorial does not lag behind larger hospitals when it comes to new technology. In December 2014, the AMH became one of the first two hospitals in the state and one of the first 20 hospitals in the country to use the Fuse endoscope system, a new technology for colonoscopies, enabling better screening for colon cancer. Dr. Charles Jones, who has been performing colonoscopies for two decades, was instrumental in pushing for the purchase of the Fuse system. Colon cancer can be fatal if it is not detected early, Jones explains, but effective screening offers a survival rate between 90 and 95 percent. The improved field of vision offered by the Fuse endoscope is key to lessening the likelihood of missing lesions during the colonoscopy.[15]

Kathy Gilley Lovette, R.T., Interview (Jefferson, April 21, 2015)

In 1972 when Kathy Lovette came home to Ashe County to work at the new AMH, there were only two technicians in the x-ray department. In an interview April 21, 2015, Lovette fills me in on the way things were and the way things are now. Dr. John Bennett from Wilkes Hospital came on Tuesdays and Thursdays to read x-rays and do exams. On Fridays, a technician drove films to Wilkes, so Dr. Bennett would not be so far behind when he arrived at AMH the following Tuesday. Lovette was on call when she was not working her shift and recalls being called back to the hospital 32 times in one day. Fortunately she had taken a room with Theresa Badger, within five minutes of her job. She got paid two dollars a trip, so she made "big money" for the time. AMH has had its own full-time radiologist since the mid–1980s, but that is not the only advancement in imaging. Lovette, who received her initial training in radiology at Wilkes Hospital, is now a radiology technologist

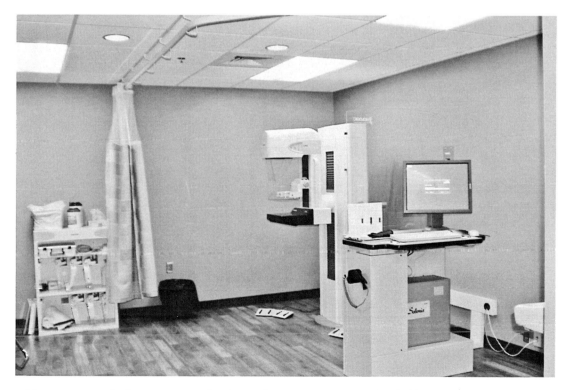

The mammography department at Ashe Memorial was recently renovated and offers the latest equipment (photograph, 2015, courtesy AMH).

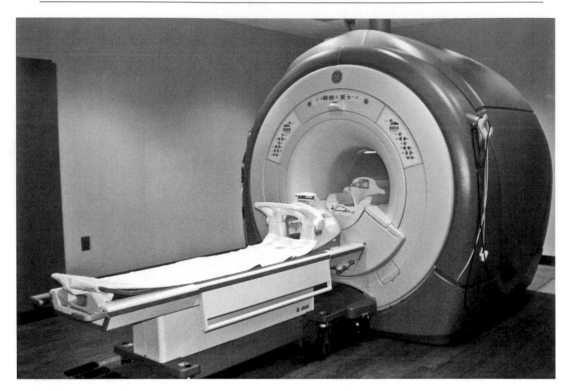

AMH is equipped with an MRI—a big plus for a small hospital (photograph, 2015, courtesy AMH).

(R.T.) and registered in mammography, nuclear medicine and ultrasound. All of these modalities are available at AMH. The hospital is even equipped to do an MRI, a big plus for a small hospital, says Lovette. To better reflect these new technologies available at AMH, the radiology department was renamed the "imaging department."

Jimmy Hendrix Interview (Jefferson, March 27, 2015)

Another significant difference in the operation of the hospital from the early days on McConnell Street is the security. Evelyn Jones says back when there was only one nurse and a few orderlies or aides on duty at the old hospital, one nurse working the night shift kept a "cap buster" or cap pistol under the front desk to scare off any would-be intruders.[16] I was aware of the surveillance cameras and some of the other security measures taken today, but I was surprised to learn that AMH now has its own police department. Its chief, James "Jimmy" Hendrix talked to me about the history when I interviewed him at the hospital on March 27, 2015.

The state legislation allowing a private corporation to have its own police department dates back to the 1800s when North Carolina had mill towns, unincorporated towns which grew up around the textile mills and furniture manufacturers and railroads. These corporations were bringing in huge payrolls, but because the towns were not incorporated, they were not allowed to create a police department to provide protection. More than 125 years later, the "company police law" is still in existence and is the basis for Ashe Memorial Hospital's police as well as other police departments such as the campus police at Appalachian State University. The AMH Board of Trustees made the decision to create the police department in the early 1990s. Jimmy Hendrix and his staff work for AMH and are sworn through the Office of the State Attorney General. Hendrix hires his own staff, and they report to him. They carry weapons and have the power of arrest in their jurisdiction, which includes the physical campus of AMH and all property owned by AMH.

Hospital security, says Hendrix, "is not a place for rookies." And the Ashe Memorial Hospital Police Department does not have any rookies. Hendrix, an Ashe County native, is a veteran of the Gulf War, with 23 years of experience in law enforcement, including about four years with the West Jefferson Police Department. The team of three full-time and four part-time employees is impressive in its background and experience, plus they all have additional special training above and beyond that required for regular law enforcement certification. The biggest challenge for security, Hendrix says, is involuntary commitment of a patient. Medical staff cannot be expected to handle violent patients, and that is where Hendrix and his officers step in to protect the patient, as well as the staff. These kinds of situations tie up a lot of resources. Mental health problems are a significant issue in the High Country; the area's suicide rate is one of the worst in the state. Many problems are self-induced, such as meth abuse and prescription drug abuse. "Our job is to insure patients have a safe and uneventful stay at the hospital," says the chief. The job goes beyond protecting patients—a vulnerable population—and requires the ability to empathize with families and patients facing difficult and sometimes life-altering situations. Hendrix appreciates the delicate balance between protecting and caring. "I really have a heart for people."

Chief Hendrix relates a story which not only demonstrates the enhanced role of security in the hospital's operation, but also the ability of the entire staff to pull together in an emergency. Sometimes the biggest challenge results in the finest hour. Hendrix was working October 15, 2002, when he heard a call go out on his radio just before 2:00 p.m. In a pouring rain, a tour bus of seniors from Charlotte wrecked on Shatley Springs Road. Thirty-two passengers and the driver sustained injuries of varying degrees of severity. One passenger went through the front windshield of the bus. Hendrix immediately alerted AMH administration. It took almost an hour and all of the paramedics from Blue Ridge Medical Transport, Ashe County Rescue Squad, and New River Volunteer Fire Department to get everyone safely off the bus. An Ashe County High School activity bus was commandeered to transport 20 of the injured to Ashe Memorial, while Blue Ridge Medical Transport and Ashe County Rescue Squad took the more serious cases.

Meanwhile, at the hospital, Hendrix was playing the role of Paul Revere, carrying messages, updates and instructions back and forth to every party involved, and that meant everybody at AMH. The external hospital disaster plan was running as intended, aided by the presence of more staff than normal on duty—the result of the required annual in-service training, which was scheduled for the day. AMH employee Rob Black was keeping the parking lot open, so the various emergency vehicles could maneuver. The most critical cases were received in the emergency department, while others were taken to a secondary triage area set up in the hospital cafeteria. Lab and x-ray personnel joined nurses and doctors to insure the necessary treatment was received. Dietary staff prepared food for everyone, and volunteers stayed over. The conference room was converted to a waiting area, and victims were kept updated on the condition of those still receiving treatment and provided telephones so friends and family could be contacted as needed. Dr. Tammy Thore and Dr. Charles Jones were the surgeons on duty and worked with the emergency department staff to stabilize the injured. Dr. Thore recalls one woman was more concerned her new slacks would have to be cut off than she was about the seriousness of her injuries. "I'll never find a pair of pants that fit me this well," she cried, as her clothing was cut away from her leg wound.[17] In general, patients remained reasonably calm in the wake of the calamity, and by 9:00 or 10:00 p.m. the drama was over, and the travelers were on another bus bound for home. "It was amazing," says Hendrix. "Everybody stepped up." The scenario is reflective of what this community has been able to do in hard times, he adds. "That's how Ashe Memorial got started."

While AMH staff continues to handle the common day to day challenges, as well as the not-so-common, everybody needs a little help from their friends now and then, and the goal of the AMH Foundation, established in 1992, is to support the hospital through actions and financial gifts and help to improve the health and wellness services offered. In recent history, the AMH Auxiliary gave money to cover the cost of lighting the helipad at the hospital. The therapeutic swimming pool and whirlpool in the Mountain Hearts Center was the main reason Vita McNeill Blevins joined the board for the foundation. After back surgery for a ruptured disk, her doctor advised that a swimming pool would afford the most productive rehabilitation, and the best way to insure a pool was available for use locally was to help get one built through the foundation. Over the years, hundreds of thousands of dollars have been raised by the foundation to improve the physical plant and operations of Ashe Memorial Hospital, including approximately $150,000 towards the addition of a swimming pool and whirlpool. To help with the foundation's fundraising, the Heritage Club was created in 2000. Membership in the club is for those who have made a commitment in their estate plan for AMH. The funds raised through the Heritage Club are used to build on an endowment account for the hospital, investing the proceeds from interest earned on the account for the future needs of AMH. Blevins has served on the board almost since its inception and is due to rotate off in 2016—time to make room for a younger person, she says.[18]

Much of the money funneled to the AMH Foundation comes from the Gift Nook, a gift shop off the lobby of the hospital, which is operated by the AMH Auxiliary's volunteers. Not so many decades ago, when men dominated the medical profession and most other professions and service clubs, it could be said that behind every good organization was a women's auxiliary. While the AMH Auxiliary was first organized as the Women's Auxiliary for the Ashe County Memorial Hospital in January 1941, its membership now includes both men and women. The original bylaws and constitution followed a plan suggested by the Duke Endowment, so instrumental in providing guidance in all things connected with the hospital project. Mrs. W. B. (Eula Wenonah Neal) Austin was the first chairman of the auxiliary; Mrs. Ira T. (Mary Adalaide Shull) Johnston was elected vice chairman; and Mrs. Robert Barr was elected secretary and treasurer of the group.[19] The group was active in the

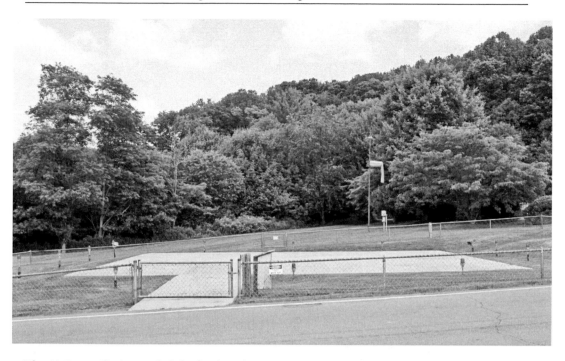

The AMH Auxiliary provided the funding for lighting on the hospital's helicopter pad (photograph, 2015, courtesy AMH).

sale of memberships in the Ashe County Memorial Hospital Association and secured many other donations. Their fundraising efforts took a variety of forms, including teas where guests were invited to bring a gift of linen for the hospital, rummage sales, magazine subscription campaigns, and "tacky" parties, with prizes given for the most outrageous costumes and a variety of other dubious distinctions. The group raised an estimated $300 by the time the hospital opened. Members assumed other responsibilities for the opening of the new hospital, including selecting window shades and curtains for the hospital.[20] The summer before the hospital opened, the auxiliary announced its sponsorship of a plan to collect canned goods from the women of the county for use when the hospital opened. Their slogan for the campaign: "All who can, can for the hospital." More than 200 cans of fruit and vegetables were donated. By the time the hospital opened in November 1941, the auxiliary boasted 146 members.[21]

Lansing native Patricia "Pat" Hudler McNeill remembers her mother, Ruby Carrington Wilcox Hudler, and C. B. Jones's mother making dried apple pies to raise money for the auxiliary. "Mother was a Pink Lady," Pat informs me in our interview. A Pink Lady was an official hospital volunteer. They wore pink coats to identify them as volunteers while they were on duty, and they worked a regular schedule. Their duties were as varied as those of today's AMH volunteers and included wheeling discharged patients out in wheelchairs to whatever transportation awaited them. In years to come, reports from the hospital's administrator indicated the contribution of the Ashe County Memorial Hospital Auxiliary in refurnishing and redecorating the rooms in the hospital, including the doctors' lounge, helping with the control of visiting hours, as well as performing other services.[22]

Assorted local newspaper clippings from the 1950s indicate the wives of prominent local doctors led the way in the establishment of the Women's Auxiliary to the Ashe County Medical Society. The following officers were elected: Mrs. Carson M. Keys, president; Mrs. R. O. Freeman, vice-president and historian; and Mrs. C. E. Miller, secretary and treasurer. Committee appointments included: Mrs. Elam Kurtz; Mrs. Dean C. Jones, Sr.; Mrs. R. C. Ray; and Mrs. (Thomas) Edith Jones. The group took responsibility for the observance of "Doctor's Day," proclaimed as March 30 in 1958 by West Jefferson Mayor Carl B. Graybeal. The purpose was to honor local physicians, both living and deceased, and the hospital they had waited for so long. The special day was designated in memory of Dr. Crawford Williamson Long, reportedly the first doctor to use anesthetic in the area. Posters were placed in drugstore windows proclaiming Doctor's Day, and doctors received red carnations to wear in their lapels. The highlight of the celebration was a donation made to the American Medical Educational Endowment for a scholarship for an Ashe County woman pursuing a career in nursing. Doc Jones made reference at his retirement party roast to the auxiliary sponsored basketball game pitting local doctors against local undertakers to raise the money for the scholarship. Doc quipped, "We buried the undertakers!"

Calvin and Katrina Miller Interviews (Jefferson, October 24, 2014)

Volunteers are the heart of today's AMH Auxiliary, with a total of 64 volunteers in 2014, including those from the auxiliary, and an estimated total volunteer hours of 7,723.[23] I interviewed volunteers Calvin H. Miller, Ed.D., and Katrina Vannoy Walker Miller at their home in Jefferson, October 27, 2014, to get their thoughts on their service in this capacity. The husband and wife are both Ashe County natives with deep roots in the area, and both are continuing the interest of their respective families in Ashe Memorial Hospital. Calvin volunteers in the emergency department, greeting and assisting incoming patients. He also directs families to where they need to go to visit loved ones who have come to the hospital via the emergency department, and he does just about anything else a volunteer can do to help out. In his role as volunteer, Calvin witnesses firsthand the caring spirit of the hospital staff, handed down through the generations. "People are so proud and blessed to have a hospital like this." I ask Calvin what he thinks makes AMH so special. He reflects on this and responds, "The hospital was built by ordinary people, the same people who came to help you get your crops in, drawing on people in powerful positions, like Congressman Doughton, to get the job done."

Calvin is the brother of the late Dr. Johnny Miller. When considering his career path, Calvin thought about going into pharmacy, figuring his brother could write the prescriptions, and he could fill them. But he ended up in the ministry, with his doctorate in education. Calvin is a graduate of Wake Forest College, Southeastern Baptist Theological Seminary, Stetson University, and Virginia Polytechnic Institute and State University in Blacksburg, Virginia.

Katrina puts in most of her volunteer hours at the hospital in the reception area, meeting and greeting visitors, directing them to the patients they are there to see, delivering flowers and wheeling patients out to their cars when they are discharged and in a hurry to go home and don't think they need to ride in a wheelchair. Katrina's mother, Virginia Osborne Vannoy, set the example for her daughter, volunteering her time at both the old and the new Ashe Memorial Hospitals. Katrina's father, Avery Burl Vannoy, the founder of the A. B. Vannoy ham operation, shared his wife's interest in the hospital, reflective of the community-mindedness they instilled in their children. "They were all hard working, creative entrepreneurs, and they all contributed to the hospital," says Katrina of her family. Katrina inherited A. B.'s hospital shares, as well as those of her Uncle Wick G. Vannoy and her Aunt Ruth Vannoy Price. James R. Vannoy served on the board of trustees at Ashe Memorial Hospital and the board of directors of the Northwestern Bank in Jefferson. Katrina's grandfather was Larry Stokes Vannoy, a pioneer in the local lumber business. Katrina has other connections with community health care; her daughter, Kina Walker Jones, is the head nurse in the emergency department at AMH and is married to C. B. Jones, another family with a rich history in community health care in Appalachia. Katrina's granddaughter, Breanne Payne, by her daughter Sandra Gainey, is a nurse at Duke General in Durham, North Carolina.

17

Changes in Appalachian Community Health Care

The changes in health care in Appalachia reflect changes nationwide. To stay in business now, most small hospitals, like Ashe Memorial, partner with large management providers. Nursing has evolved along with other aspects of health care in the region, and Nancy Kautz's trailblazing career is a good example of the variety of directions available for men and women to pursue in this profession. With the opening of the College of Health Sciences at Appalachian State University in 2010 and the development in 2015 of a master of science in nursing degree program in the College's Department of Nursing, there are more opportunities for area nurses and other medical professionals to pursue their education and move into some of the areas pioneered by Kautz.[1]

Doctoring has evolved too. The days when physicians were on call 24 hours a day, seven days a week, are, to some extent, in the past, replaced by a more family-friendly schedule, maybe not quite nine to five, but heading in that direction. Women are not the anomaly they once were in the field of medicine either. Thanks to pioneers like Dr. Mary Martin Sloop and Dr. Mary Michal, women in medicine do not face the level of prejudice and the barriers they did in years past, and their numbers are increasing. Dr. Leigh Bradley reports one half of her class in medical college was female, and of the eight in residency with her, seven were women. Appalachian State University now has a premed program, and Dr. Bradley was in one of the program's first graduating classes. Surgeons remain scarce in much of Appalachia, however, and many small hospitals in the region, like Ashe Memorial, have only one or two surgeons.[2]

The two Ashe memorial hospitals have provided medical care to the people of Ashe County and the surrounding area for 75 years now. But despite a history of growth and modernization, the AMH strives to retain the element of caring instilled long ago by Dr. Dean Jones, Sr., and his wife Lettie and a handful of dedicated staff, determined to make a community's dream of quality health care close to home come true. The proof as to whether or not AMH has succeeded in this regard lies in whether or not those who work there would want to be a patient there. During my interview with Kathy Lovette (Chapter Sixteen), I ask if she would opt for a larger hospital over AMH, given the choice. "I would never go anywhere else for surgery," she declares. Her reason—"the treatment and the personal care—you aren't just a number, here." Certainly things have changed; the AMH is much bigger now; staff can go all day and not see coworkers assigned to another floor. The turnover is higher than in the old days, because that is the way it is with employment today. Some of those in today's AMH family are "not from around here," but, despite the new faces, Ashe County natives continue to make up a significant percentage of the work force. As Trustee Jan Caddell jokes, "The hospital treats you like family, and often you are."[3] And the days when everybody did everything to get the job done are not entirely gone. There are still close ties, still the semblance of a big family, especially if somebody is in trouble. "Then we all pitch in," says Lovette.

Much of the change in Appalachian community health care can be traced through the changes in the patient population over the last four generations. There are still plenty of people who are native to the area and have been served by the Jones family of doctors for their entire lives, but the era when Mary Lou Brooks admitted patients and knew every name in Ashe County is fast disappearing. With the growth of tourism in the High Country and the increase in second homes, the hospital, particularly the emergency department, regularly sees part-time residents, tourists and migrant labor brought in for the Christmas tree business. Health care needs have shifted accordingly, and the hospital is adjusting.[4]

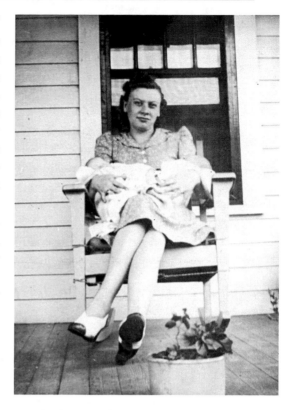

In 1941, the year Ashe County Memorial Hospital opened, a total of 34 patients were reported. By 1942, the total had grown to 492, aided by the birth of the first set of twins to be delivered at the hospital, Janis and Janet Dickson, September 3, 1942, shown here with their mother, Mrs. Bower C. (Iris) Dickson. Although she and her husband, a flight instructor for the military, lived in Camden, South Carolina, Iris was staying with her mother-in-law, Mrs. Charles Dickson, in Jefferson, enjoying the cooler mountain temperatures, at the time of the delivery (photograph, circa 1942, courtesy Evelyn Jones).

Ruby B. Ashley Interview (Warrensville, November 26, 2014)

There are not very many folks left around Ashe County who knew all four generations of Jones family doctors, but Dr. Charles Jones especially wanted me to meet one of his patients who fell into that rarified company—Ruby Ashley, 100 years old at the time. With the help of Ruby's daughter, Barbara McCoy, Evelyn Jones arranged for us to do an interview the day before Thanksgiving in 2014. Barbara met us at the door and ushered us into the front room where Ruby greeted us with a lively smile and eyes that twinkled.

Ruby is an Ashe County native, the daughter of Joseph Cicero (J. C.) and Dema Barker Baldwin. She married Cicero Ashley, a preacher for the Missionary Baptist Church. She has lived in the county her entire life. "There were not very many doctors around," she says of her youth. She remembers: Dr. Waddell in Grassy Creek; Dr. Ray in West Jefferson; Dr. Bud Jones, Charles's great-grandfather, who her mother saw; doctors Tom and Lester Jones, from the Lansing Infirmary; Dr. Manley Blevins, from near Warrensville; and Dr. Ulysses Jones, from the far end of the county, who sometimes went to the Lansing Infirmary to perform surgeries on his patients. Charles's father, Doc Jones, performed the last surgery Ruby needed, and Dr. Dean delivered most of Ruby's six children. Her oldest, Juanita was delivered at home, but the others were delivered at the old Ashe County Memorial Hospital, including Barbara.

Dr. Dean was the family's doctor while he had his office in Lansing, but they lost him when he moved to Ashe County Memorial. "I didn't think we'd ever get used to another doctor." It was Dr. Elam Kurtz who had Dr. Dean's hard act to follow, when he located an office in Lansing. Ruby remembers her son Jack fleeing the doctor's office to avoid a shot. "I had to run all the way down the main street of Lansing to catch him."

When Ruby turned 90 years old, she decided she probably should look into getting a family doctor again, "just in case she was to get sick." She made an appointment with a local physician. He came into the examining room, introduced himself, and asked what the reason was for her visit. She explained she was fine, she just thought she needed a family doctor. "You are ninety years old and you don't have a doctor?" He asked, amazed. "Well, not one who's living!" She retorted.

Until recently, when she was hospitalized and Dr. Charles had to perform surgery, Ruby had not been sick in fifty years. She had typhoid fever twice as a child, and Dr. Tugman from Warrensville came to the house to treat her. "I was real sick," she recalls. Awhile back, she went in for an eye procedure, and when the nurse looked over all the

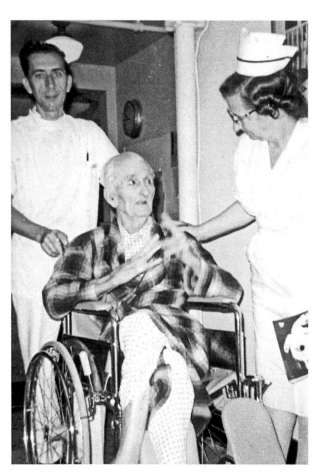

Orderly Lake Barker and Nurse Pauline Barnes assist a patient in the old Ashe County Memorial Hospital (photograph, circa 1966, courtesy Evelyn Jones; published in fundraising campaign brochure for 1966 addition).

forms she and her daughter had filled out, the nurse said Ruby must have misunderstood the instructions, as she had not listed anything under "medications taken." Barbara assured the nurse there was no misunderstanding—her mother took no medicine.

Ruby is fond of Dr. Charles. "He sat on the side of my bed at the hospital and drew a picture and explained all about what was wrong and what he was doing to fix it." Ruby credits Charles and the entire staff at the hospital with giving her excellent care during her stay there. "They sure are good to you there. People can't be thankful enough for the good health programs we have now. I have seen so many changes. We are blessed to have the medical care we have now." Reflecting on her long life, she comments, "I have been blessed every day of my life."

Kada Owen McNeill Interview (Jefferson, January 20, 2015)

It has been said that Kada McNeill is related to half the folks in Ashe County. After talking with her for a couple of hours in January 2015, I find no exaggeration in this claim. "My mother's mother was a Blevins and married a Francis," Kada begins, "and my daddy's mother was a Phipps." The seventh of 12 children herself, Kada's Grandpa William "Billy" Owen had 77 grandchildren, 221 great-grandchildren, and, in 1982, the last published tally, his great-great-grandchildren numbered 367. Evelyn Jones is with me on the occasion of this conversation, and I discover that she and Kada are what Doc referred to as "kin around the corner."

Born in Crumpler in 1919, to Luther and Myrtie Francis Owen, Martha "Kada" was delivered at home by Dr. Carl Eller. Her mother was a midwife, qualified for this calling, Kada speculates, because she bore 12 children of her own. "People would come fetch her when she was needed, and she would stay over if needed." This sometimes resulted in leaving her children in the care of their older siblings. When Kada was 12, she was charged with looking after the five smaller children. One of the boys found a dynamite cap where the new (now the old) Highway 16 was being built nearby. "The little ones were fussing over it. I picked it up and accidentally dropped it on the hot stove." The cap exploded. A neighbor drove her to see Dr. B. Everette Reeves. He cleaned the injury, wrapped it, and sent her to the hospital in Statesville, where the doctor there worked on her for four and a half hours. Kada lost three fingers on her right hand.

Kada married Jones McNeill, and the couple lost their first baby at birth. A second pregnancy followed, and she miscarried one evening. The house had no electricity, and it was hard to see what had happened by lamplight. The next morning her mother-in-law arrived, realized the situation was serious and called Dr. Bud Jones to come to the house. He examined Kada and confirmed she had lost the child, but Kada could still feel movement. Four and a half months later she bore her daughter Vita. Although Dr. Bud did not deliver Vita, he did offer the explanation that Kada had been pregnant with twins, and while one had died in October 1937, the other was delivered at full term and healthy in 1938.

At age five, Vita fell down at school and cut her forehead. "I guess I was running," Vita confesses to me when we talk about the incident. The principal and a teacher took her from

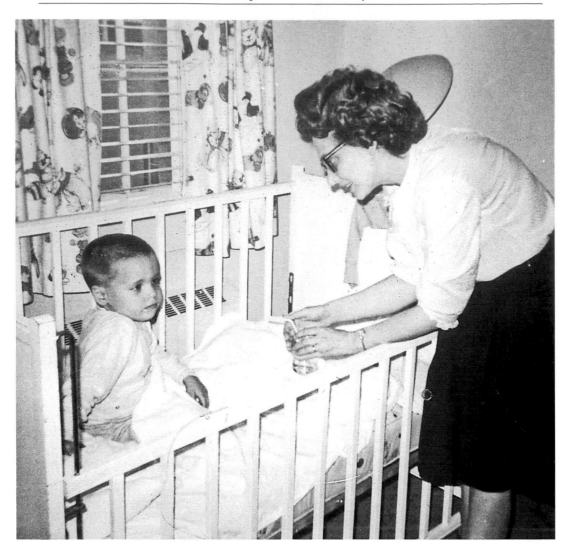

The pediatric ward in the old Ashe County Memorial Hospital was included in one of the additions to the original structure and provided children a more home-like setting for their hospital experience (photograph, circa 1966, courtesy Evelyn Price; published in fundraising campaign brochure for 1966 addition).

the Lansing school to Dr. Bud's office in town, where he used clamps to close the wound, leaving only a faint scar to show for the mishap. "I did not cry," vows Vita, and Dr. Bud sent someone downtown, probably his wife Fannie, to buy coconut marshmallows for a treat, because she had not made a fuss.

It was Dr. C. Pardue Bunch who made the house call when Kada's daughter Edith fell ill. He made an unexpected follow-up visit and found that Kada's mother had come to help with the sick child and had made up an onion poultice to put on Edith's chest and ribs. He got a chuckle out of the home remedy and remarked, "Well, the odor might kill the germs." He advised sending the child to the hospital, but soon after he left, Edith vomited up a vile mess and recovered—thanks, no doubt, to the onion poultice.

Dr. Dean, Sr., was their family doctor later and a friend too. He and Lettie visited with Kada and Jones in their home in Lansing, the doctor and Jones sometimes fishing in the river near the house. Kada tells a story about when one of her younger sisters was working at Ashe County Memorial Hospital, assisting Dr. Dean, Sr., with a delivery. The mother was not married, more of an eyebrow raiser than is the case these days. She was nervous about having the baby and refused to spread her legs so the doctor could get on with his work. Finally time was running out, and Dr. Dean said, "Well, you had to spread them sometime or you wouldn't be here now." Kada relates another tale told by Dr. Dean. A man brought his sick wife in to see the doctor. Dr. Dean stuck a thermometer in her mouth, and after a couple of minutes, the husband pointed to the thermometer and asked, "Where did you get that thing? That's the longest she's not spoken."

Now Kada is seen by Dr. Charles Jones for surgery-related health issues. Comparing the generations of doctors Jones who have treated her and her family, Kada relates, "Dr. Charles talks a little more, but they all knew what they were doing."

Emmett Barker Interview (Jefferson, February 3, 2015)

Emmett Barker, the son of Wil and Pearl Hamby Barker, was only a young boy in 1935 when he rolled off a horse-drawn sled loaded with corn. His fall landed him in the spreads or single trees (the wooden rails attaching the sled to the team). "I broke my arm bad," tells Emmett. The team was unhitched from the sled, and Emmett rode one of the horses into Lansing to Dr. Bud Jones's two-room office, located at the turn to go to the old Lansing School. "There were no automobiles then, and it was getting late in the day," he continues. The bone had splintered, so Dr. Bud had to open up the arm to repair the break. "He had an operating table not bigger than an ironing board. It took him about one and a half hours to fix my arm. If you'd dropped a bomb, it wouldn't hurry him up when he was working, but he knew what he was doing. Dr. Bud was about as good a country doctor as I've ever seen." When the doctor was finished setting the arm, Emmett rode the horse back home; he estimates it was about four miles each way. Before Evelyn Jones and I leave the Barker house that day we interview Emmett and his wife Wylene, Emmett hands me a list he made for me of all Dr. Bud's patients he could remember on Deep Ford Road in Bina, where he grew up. The list, he realizes, includes everybody who lived on Deep Ford Road.

Emmett has been treated by all four generations of the Jones family. "My first operation, for a ruptured appendix, was in the old hospital, which was the new hospital then. Dr. Dean Jones, Sr., looked after me personally. He saw I was in pain and called for a nurse, and three of them showed up right quick." He credits Jones with being the key to getting Ashe County Memorial Hospital built. "I don't know what people would have done without old man Dean." Later it was Doc Jones who tended to Emmett's surgical needs, and most recently, Dr. Charles assumed that responsibility.

Beulah Barker McVey Interviews (Jefferson, May 6 and 7, 2015)

Beulah Barker was 16 years old when Lloyd McVey asked her to marry him. "I'll marry you anywhere they don't make you get a blood test," she stubbornly maintained. Lloyd took her to Ashe County Memorial, where she argued a blue streak with Henry Lum about having her blood drawn. She was so preoccupied with making her point, she missed the point— of the needle that is. Nurse Ruby Lum quietly and efficiently completed the task without Beulah realizing she had been stuck. Lloyd told her to hold her arm up; she said what for; and he broke the news the test was over.

One frigid February day in 1967 when Beulah was ready to deliver her second child, she made another trip to Ashe County Memorial. Lloyd was overseas, so she drove herself. The birth was rough on Beulah, and Dr. Dean had to perform surgery on the young mother. Meanwhile, an ice storm had bent the trees to the ground, and the roads were starting to get bad. Folks were stranded at the hospital. Beulah had things to do at home, including getting back to another little one, left in the care of her mother. "It was time to go!" Beulah relates. She asked an orderly to bring her car around to the ER entrance, bundled up her baby, grabbed her belongings, and headed for her car. A nurse saw her put the baby in the front seat and came over to investigate. Beulah, seeing her escape was about to be thwarted, slid over into the passenger seat with the baby. "My brother's just visiting a friend in the hospital. He'll be right out," she fibbed. When the nurse left, Beulah slid back to the driver's side and made her getaway. It was a long drive home, and the roads had worsened. The bridge at Silas Creek was out, so she had to drive all the way around Lansing, 19 miles, easing the car under the ice laden branches along the way. With perseverance reminiscent of her Ashe County forebears, she made it home safe, her baby not uttering a peep, and Beulah got back to her chores.

Anne Shoemaker McGuire Interview (West Jefferson, July 14, 2014)

Anne Shoemaker McGuire, daughter of Sharpe and Evelyn Brown Shoemaker of West Jefferson, was born in Statesville, just before Ashe County Memorial opened. She was almost five years old when she was taken to Ashe County's hospital to see her new baby brother, Stephen. "I did not like him," she confesses to me, as we sit in her front parlor. "He [Stephen] had dropped into my world. When Daddy took me in to see him, I just screamed and screamed. Grandmother Brown was in the room, and Mrs. (Lettie) Jones was there, and they were trying to calm me down." Anne recovered, as most of us do when siblings are thrust upon us, and, some years later, welcomed her second baby brother, David, with much less drama. She has been treated by three generations of the Jones family doctors, starting with Dr. Dean Jones, Sr. Anne's father was a close friend of Dr. Dean and insisted he wanted Dr. Dean to perform his surgery when he was diagnosed with colon cancer. He did not want to go to Winston-Salem, he declared. But the surgery came too late; the cancer had spread, and his friend could not save him.

Stephen Shoemaker Interview (West Jefferson, September 16, 2014)

In 1998, Anne McGuire's brother, artist Stephen Shoemaker, was reminded of his father's friendship with Dr. Dean and the circumstances of his father's death, when R. D. Williams II, Pat Cooper, and Joe Thore approached him about creating an original painting of the old Ashe County Memorial Hospital. The painting was to hang in the hospital's board room, with prints to be sold as a fundraiser for the AMH Foundation. The painting captures the old hospital as it was during its time, stately and vibrant, full of purpose. But there is something of the artist's painful memories represented in the scene, as well. The car in the foreground of the painting is Stephen's car at the time of his father's death in the hospital. "I wanted to put something in there for me," Shoemaker explains. "My father loved that car as much as I did." The doctor's bag on the hood of the coupe belongs to Dr. Dean, who is the figure standing on the front stoop of the hospital, looking back at the bag. The bag is meant to symbolize the tools needed to save Stephen's father. Those tools were not at hand; figuratively, they were out of reach—the means to save his father's life simply did not exist. He was too far gone. His father's good friend, the doctor, is acknowledging that sad fact when he gazes back at the bag. "He did all he could do," says Stephen of Dr. Jones. "I always thought my father was in good hands." Sharpe Shoemaker was 57 years old when he died; Stephen was 22 at the time.

Stephen had come home on leave from the Army to be with his father in the hospital the night before his surgery. He remembers the kindness of nurse Doris Stoltzfus, who cared for his father. "Her being there made it easier to visit," he said. His father was in the hospital for almost a month after his unsuccessful surgery. At some point during that time, Stephen had to go back to Washington, D.C., where he was stationed. Shortly after his

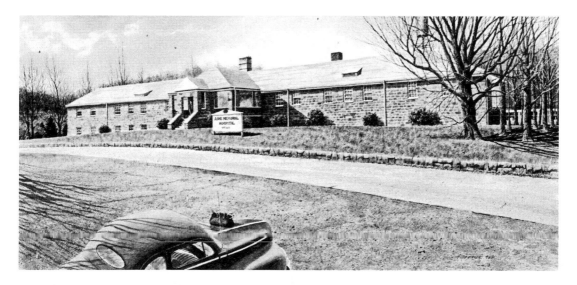

Stephen Shoemaker's print of the old Ashe County Memorial Hospital is a familiar image to many in the Ashe County area. The original was painted by Shoemaker at the request of hospital officials in 1998 (courtesy Stephen Shoemaker).

return to base, he received word his father had taken a turn for the worse. He caught a bus back home, but he was too late to see his father alive. It was a long time before he could come to terms with that—something that just was not meant to be.

Hearing the story behind the painting, I am better able to see the depth of the image portrayed. The hospital is a place of memories, some happy and some sad. It is a place where we are reminded of all the good that one human being can do for another, giving life, saving life, easing pain. And it is a place where we are reminded of our limitations, our inability to fix what is beyond fixing, despite our skill or our caring or our love. This is not a reflection of any shortcoming on our part; it is a reflection of life.

I asked Stephen about his earliest memories of Dr. Dean, whom he held in such high esteem. He painted me a picture with words, as only an artist can do. "When I was little, I was proud when I was told Dr. Jones had delivered me. When I saw him, I always felt I was in the presence of greatness. He was tall and important looking. He was balding, and his head shone. He had that white coat and the stethoscope around his neck; he was so clean, he glistened. His look, his manner, that little smile—he was the whole package—he epitomized greatness in a man." Then Stephen described the hospital, as he would have seen it as a boy. "It was a friendly place. I remember the shiny tile floors, and I remember the old farmers sitting in the lobby in their overalls and muddy boots, such a contrast to the pristine interior of the hospital."

Stephen Shoemaker now serves on the Board of Trustees for Ashe Memorial Hospital. His painting helped raise awareness of the AMH Foundation and its mission, says R. D. Williams II, and the prints are treasured by many in the AMH family.

Betsy Gant Interview (West Jefferson, June 28, 2014)

Betsy Gant is one of the growing number of part-time residents who have had occasion to seek medical help in Ashe County. Betsy was pulling weeds in her garden on Big Tree Road in West Jefferson, when she gave a tug and yanked out a big clump of weeds, disturbing a nest of yellow jackets buried in the ground. The yellow jackets swarmed, Betsy flailed her arms, agitating the insects further, and ended up stung numerous times on her legs. She headed up to the house and sat down to collect herself after the ordeal. "I didn't think much about it at first, but then my throat started to close up, and I called 911." She described her symptoms and explained what had happened, and the dispatcher advised she needed help immediately, and first responders would be on the way. But there was construction equipment partially blocking the road at the house below the Gants, and Betsy was afraid the ambulance could not make the turn to get up the long driveway. Her husband Ed, now on the scene, said he could get her to the hospital faster than the ambulance could get to her, so he hustled Betsy into the car and headed to Jefferson—fast.

By now Betsy was having trouble breathing and looked bad. In the interest of time, Ed dropped her off at the emergency department entrance, while he parked the car. Betsy walked in and started to explain what had happened and what her symptoms were, fumbling in her purse for her medical and insurance cards, but the staff was not waiting for paperwork. Within the few minutes it took Ed to get the car parked and rush into the hospital, Physician's Assistant C. B. Jones and two nurses were working on Betsy.

"I felt very comfortable with Mr. Jones," Betsy confided. "He knew what he was doing; and I was so impressed with his calmness, kindness and gentleness. He reminded me of one of those old fashioned doctors. He explained everything he was doing. The nurses were nice, and nobody was rattled." Betsy survived the incident with no aftereffects, although she now keeps an EpiPen (epinephrine autoinjector) handy.

18

A Legacy

Some members of the fifth generation of the Jones family are old enough to remember when the extended family sat down to Sunday dinner in the hospital dining room with Doc and Evelyn, much like the fourth generation did with Dr. Dean and Lettie. I wanted to understand how this closely knit family had managed to stay so, given the demanding schedules of the surgeons and other professionals who made up their ranks. And I wanted to learn about the aspirations of this latest generation, their thoughts on the family's legacy of doctoring, and how that legacy and their grandparents in particular, influenced their lives.

When you are the first grandchild, you get the honor of coining the nicknames for grandparents. Bryan, Phyllis Jones and Keith Yount's oldest son, born January 10, 1982, was the one who came up with "Nunner" for his grandmother, Evelyn Jones. This was his version of "another mother." Bryan heard people calling his Grandfather Jones "Doc"; he combined that with granddad, and "Grandoc" was the result. "Grandoc, you can't die," his brother, Nathan, born July 14, 1985, announced one day. Grandoc responded he had no intention of dying any time soon, but he asked the reason for Nathan's declaration. "You can't die until you teach me everything you know about fishing!" Nathan must have learned his lessons well, because he is known in the family as an excellent fisherman. Austin Dean, younger brother to Bryan and Nathan, was born December 19, 1987, and is reputed to favor his great-great-grandfather, Dr. Bud, in looks. He takes after Grandoc the most in temperament, though. "He loved his grandchildren," Phyllis smiles, recalling how Grandoc amused his immediate offspring by taking precautions with his grandchildren he never considered with regard to his own children, insisting the fish pond be filled in, because one of his grandchildren might fall in and drown and that the birdbath, clearly a hazard to small children, be removed.[1]

Twins Jayden Laura Jones and Jordan Elizabeth Jones were born to Tommy Jones and Dr. Leigh Bradley October 1, 2003, delivered by Dr. Kevin Kurtz. Their birthdate was the 100th anniversary of great-grandmother Lettie Jones's birthday—that and their red hair especially endeared the twins to Grandoc, a redhead in his youth, like his grandfather, Dr. Bud. It was Grandoc the twins ran to when they had a hurt that needed tending. When their parents explained to them that Grandoc was quitting his medical practice, Jordan expressed immediate concern, "But who will take out my splinters?"[2]

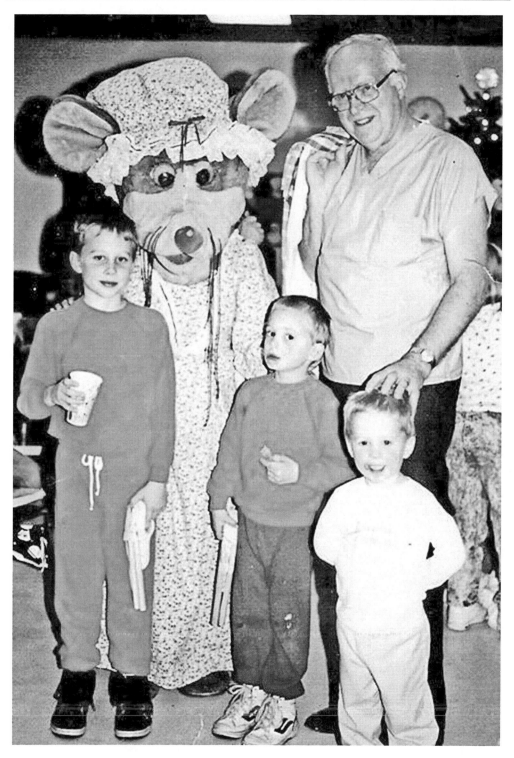

Bryan, Nathan, and Austin Yount enjoy the AMH Christmas party with a very large mouse and their grandfather, Dr. Dean C. Jones, Jr., nicknamed "Grandoc" by his grandchildren (photograph, circa 1989, courtesy Phyllis Jones Yount).

Brandon, eldest son of Dr. Charles and Debbie Jones, got off to a rocky start making his entrance into the world. Born in Charlotte August 5, 1995, at only 26 weeks, he weighed two pounds at birth. The family worried they would never get him out of the hospital, but Brandon was a fighter. His aunt, Dr. Leigh Bradley, calls him "the miracle baby" and recalls Doc asking her what the prognosis would be for a baby born at only 26 weeks. She answered with the grim odds of survival, before she realized he was asking about his own grandson. Fortunately, Brandon defied the odds.[3]

I talk with Brandon January 2, 2015, when he is home on Christmas break from UNC Charlotte. He is in his freshman year in the College of Liberal Arts and Sciences there, studying prebiology. Like most nineteen-year-olds, he is not ready to commit to a major, but he admits, "I've always had being a surgeon in the back of my mind." He has a great love for animals, however, and if graduate study is in his future, veterinary medicine may be a possibility. I ask Brandon if he feels pressure to follow in the footsteps of his father, grandfather, great-grandfather, and great-great-grandfather. "Sometimes I get it from family friends—'Are you going to be the next doctor?' They ask. I don't want to let those people down, but I don't know yet what I want to do."

Whether Brandon eventually chooses a medical related career or not, he does share Grandoc's favorite pastime, fishing, and Grandoc's love of the outdoors, which contributed to a few misadventures. "I've been sewn up numerous times by Grandoc and Dad," Brandon confesses. Once Grandoc set his arm in his dad's office, the result of a poorly executed trip down the sliding board. Later his dad sawed the cast off. "Now that was the scary part." His

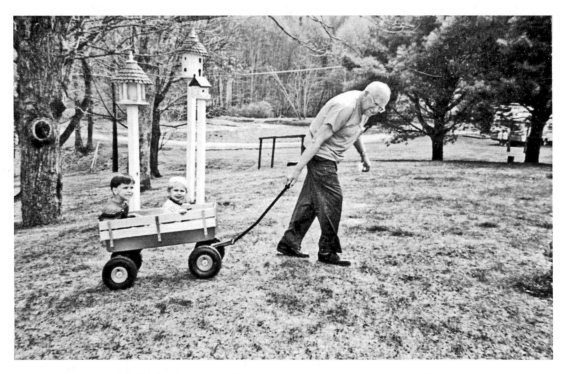

"Go faster Grandoc!" Grandsons Brandon Jones and Lane Patterson catch a ride in Dr. Dean C. Jones and Evelyn's back yard (photograph, circa 2001, courtesy Evelyn Jones).

aunt, Dr. Bradley, is his regular doctor, and although his dad has made some minor repairs over the years, Dr. Charles declares he would not operate on one of his own if he could help it. In years past, when physicians and surgeons were few and far between, that situation would not have been easy to avoid.

Grandoc was a good teacher; he taught by example, which was good says Brandon, "because I don't listen well." "The things I admired most about my grandfather were the things I lack. He taught me the qualities I want to have. He focused on a simple way of life." The example set for Brandon and his siblings and cousins had to do with service and giving back to the community, not just through the medical care provided, but through other philanthropic efforts by the family. Reflecting on the many contributions his grandfather made to his beloved home, Brandon pauses before offering his final thoughts. "I try to have his outlook—he was a very optimistic person. I've always aspired to be like him."

As I set this interview to paper, I ponder how people sometimes wonder why I interview the people I do. Many of those I interview, including Brandon, wonder why I want to interview them. Well, I don't have the privilege to meet and get to know many of the folks I write about—they departed this world long ago, but what better insight could I get into the character of Doc Jones, the third generation of this legacy, than this grandson's testimony?

A couple of weeks after I talk with Brandon, I sit down with his two younger brothers, Connor and Hunter, along with their parents and Nunner. We chat first about what the

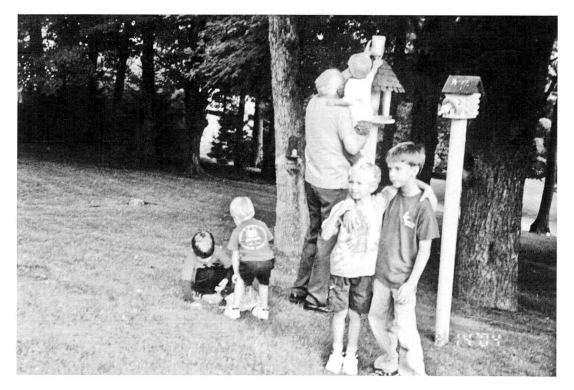

Feeding the birds with Dr. Dean C. Jones are, from left to right: Connor and Hunter; "Grandoc" and Cameron; Lane and Brandon (photograph, circa 2003, courtesy Evelyn Jones).

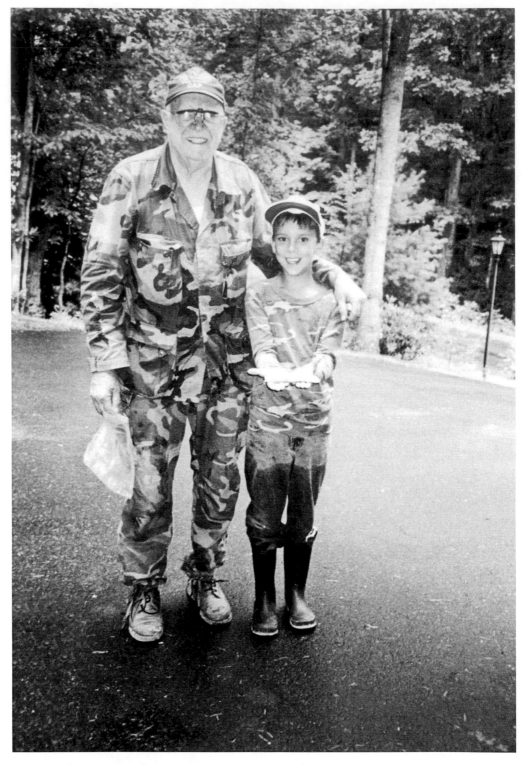

Dr. Dean C. Jones, "Grandoc," and Brandon, son of Dr. Charles and Debbie Jones, show off their catch (photograph, circa 2005, courtesy Evelyn Jones).

two boys have in common with their grandfather. Most family members agree the grandchild most like Grandoc is Dr. Charles and Debbie's second son, Connor Dean, born July 7, 1999, and delivered by Dr. Bradley. Older brother Brandon was the first I heard make the comparison. He was talking about Grandoc's keen powers of observation, when he noted, "Connor is like him in that way. I see him [Connor] sitting there in a group of people just soaking it in." Connor's quiet, methodical nature has earned him the nickname "the professor." He has watched his father perform several surgeries and talks about being a surgeon, but that decision is a long way off.

The first time I met Hunter Jackson Jones, he told me he was going to be a surgeon. Born October 12, 2001, and named for Hunter McGuire Jones, the brother of his great-grandfather Dr. Dean, Sr., he has a few years to change his mind. Hunter invited his father to show and tell at his school, and Dr. Charles took some old medical instruments for the children to examine. The surgical saw generated some excitement, but the big hit was a photograph of a 42 pound tumor Charles had removed from a patient.

I met Lane McKenzie Patterson, born June 8, 1998, the eldest son of Linda Noel Jones and Dale Patterson, one evening when he and his mother stopped to spend the night with Evelyn, during a tour of prospective colleges. He isn't sure what career he wants to pursue either, although engineering has been mentioned. Lane's younger brother, Cameron McCrea, was born February 5, 2001. A good athlete, like his grandfather, Cameron enjoyed feeding

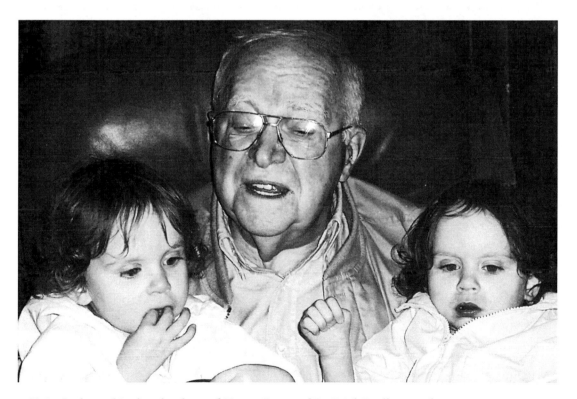

Twins Jayden and Jordan, daughters of Tommy Jones and Dr. Leigh Bradley, were born on Dr. Dean C. Jones' mother Lettie's birthday and had red hair like "Grandoc" and their great-great grandfather Dr. Bud (photograph, circa 2005, courtesy Dr. Leigh Bradley and Tommy Jones).

the birds with Grandoc. I look at the photographs of Doc with his grandchildren, and I am reminded of his wish for a big family. What joy they must have given him.

Taking care of local people locally is important to Dr. Charles Jones, as it was to his father and grandfather and great-grandfather and the community in which they lived, but a legacy can be a burden too. When I am interviewing Charles and his family at Evelyn's house that January afternoon in 2015, I ask Debbie how she and Charles handle the pressures of the family legacy of doctoring where their three sons are concerned. What do they do when folks ask which one is going to be the next doctor or surgeon? "We've heard that ever since Brandon was little," Debbie responds. Will there be a fifth generation doctor or doctors in the Jones family? It is too soon to say what career path the three sons of Dr. Charles and Debbie Jones will pursue, but if there is pressure to join the legacy of doctoring, it will not come from their parents. "We have always told them (the three boys), if your heart's not in it, don't do it," says Debbie. "You don't do it to fulfill a legacy or community expectations." Charles recalls his great-grandfather Dr. Bud's plan to direct the career paths of his two oldest sons by naming one after a famous surgeon and the other after a famous lawyer. It did not work, at least not as he intended. Instead, the destinies of the two boys were reversed, and the son named after the surgeon became a lawyer, while the son named after the lawyer became a surgeon—Charles's grandfather Dr. Dean Cicero Jones, Sr.

Charles is fifty years old now, and he has had time to come to terms with his family's legacy and to embrace it. Behind him are the unsettled times of young adulthood when he felt he must have some purpose, but he had yet to know what it was—he could not grasp the plan. "The older I get the more I realize my life is not my own," says Charles, and that is not a bad thing; it is part of being a grown-up. As for the doctoring he once thought he would not pursue, "I can't imagine not having done this," he concedes. "I know it's what I was put on this earth to do." Moving forward, Charles, like so many before him, is committed to doing his part toward insuring a fully functional community hospital is in place for the generations to come. That means thinking ahead to the next fifty years and setting a course for how to get there, perhaps through the establishment of a savings plan for a new hospital in the future—a legacy fund, to provide for the evolving needs of the community.

As I am wrapping up this family interview with its assortment of generations, whose lives are so intertwined with the hospital that started less than a hundred yards away from where we sit in Evelyn's kitchen, a medical helicopter passes over the house. I watch as each person at the table, Evelyn, Dr. Charles, Debbie, and sons Connor and Hunter, responds in kind—a patient is being airlifted from Ashe Memorial to the hospital in Winston-Salem. Their awareness of the situation is immediate—a whole table of first responders. A quiet prayer goes up. Maybe it is this unity and continuity in caring that is the real legacy of this family and the community where they live.

Gazing at the back of the old Ashe Memorial Hospital, I recall asking Brandon if he ever had been inside the old hospital. Yes, a long time ago, Grandoc and his dad took him and his brothers inside and told them what all the rooms were, while their mother filmed the tour. "Grandoc could remember everything." Did he find the place a little creepy? He laughed, "It probably would still scare me now, but some of the spooky was taken out by being there with Grandoc and Dad and by hearing all the history." Eventually I was able to

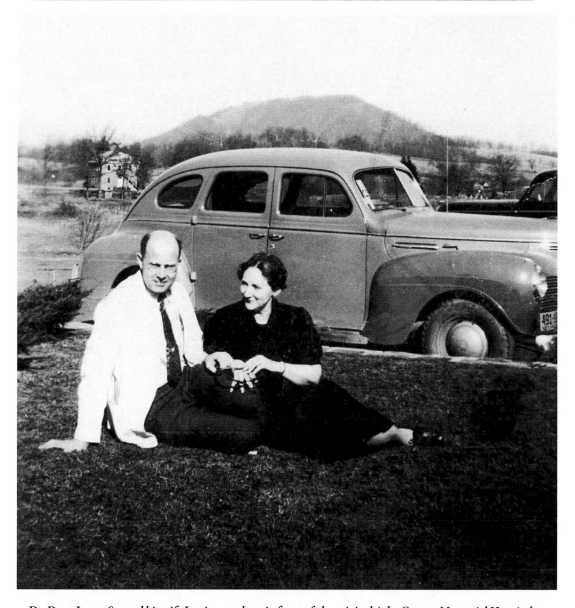

Dr. Dean Jones, Sr., and his wife Lettie, seen here in front of the original Ashe County Memorial Hospital (to the viewer's rear), devoted their lives to the hospital and each other. Dr. Jones's stethoscope is wrapped around their hands, a reminder he was constantly on call, as was she (photograph, circa 1940s, courtesy Evelyn Jones).

view the video of the tour Doc did of the old hospital with Charles, Debbie and their boys. I listened to the voice of this man I had been hearing about for so many months, waiting to hear firsthand some hint of what he was like and how he felt about this place that played such a large role in his life. As Doc shepherded his followers around the outside and then the inside of the building, he pointed out the room where he slept when he first came to live in the hospital at ten years old and the hallway where he first saw Nunner. "She was the prettiest girl I ever saw," he said, smiling fondly at the memory. Then he showed them the

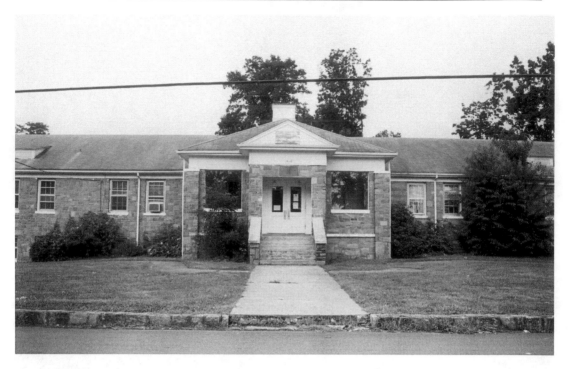

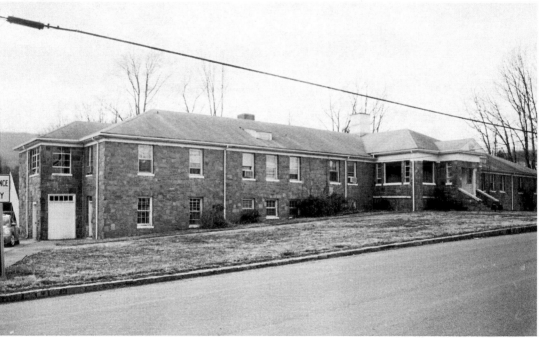

This page and following page: The old Ashe County Memorial Hospital on McConnell Street sits vacant now, waiting for its next purpose to be revealed. These photographs were taken in 2006 as part of the nomination process to place the hospital building on the National Register of Historic Places. The property was listed in the National Register on April 28, 2015. The small one-story addition, attached to the stone façade of the original part of the building, was the emergency room entrance (photographs, circa 2006, courtesy N.C. Department of Cultural Resources).

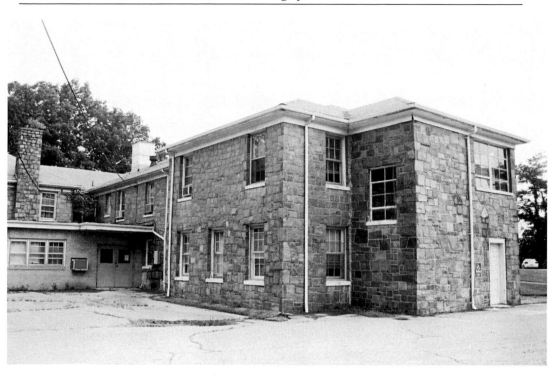

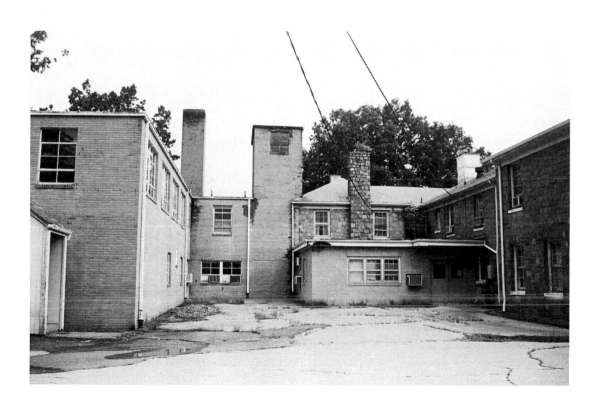

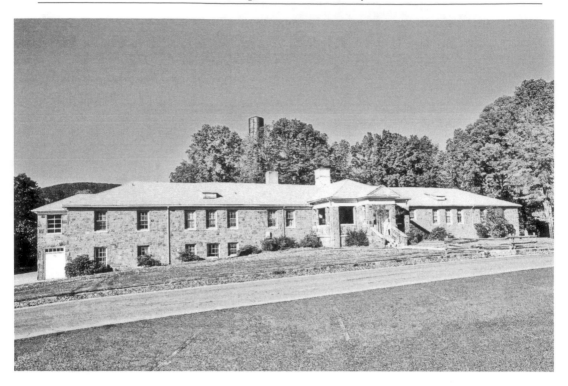

The water tower, visible behind the hospital, was erected sometime after the hospital was built and originally provided the drinking water for the hospital. There was no municipal water system at the time, and when the town of Jefferson put in water lines, the tower was used as backup in case of fire. The tower was demolished in 2001; only the footprint remains (courtesy Ed Reid).

window where Nunner used to wait for him when he drove in behind the hospital. "I didn't know she was watching for me," he chuckled. There it was—the insight I was searching for—this place was not only the realization of a community's dream, it was the unlikely setting of a love story, and more than one—there was Dr. Dean and Lettie, Ruby and Henry Lum, Doc and Evelyn, and Polly and Elliot Osowitt too.

I was lucky. In February 2015, Leigh Derby, who together with his wife Jennie purchased the hospital building and the 2.48 acre lot on which it sits in June 2009, was kind enough to take Evelyn Jones, her son Tommy, and me inside the old hospital to look around. Stonemason Alonzo Baldwin's expertly laid stone columns are obscured now, the entry enclosed to hold back the Ashe County winter winds, but the steps remain. The interior of the original building is laid out along a central hall running the width of the building. The hall linking the addition to the original structure is directly ahead, as we enter the main door, with the nursery at the end. Paneling and dropped ceilings, remnants of the 1970s conversion to county offices, conceal the original finish. The wide doors, built to accommodate gurneys, are still there, but the handsome wood cabinets built by the National Youth Administration that once contained the stuff of hospitals, disappeared sometime after the county vacated the premises. A few features remain, offering a glimpse into the building's past life—the panel outside the operating room where x-rays were displayed, the sink where doctors scrubbed before surgery, and the viewing window for the nursery, minus its glass,

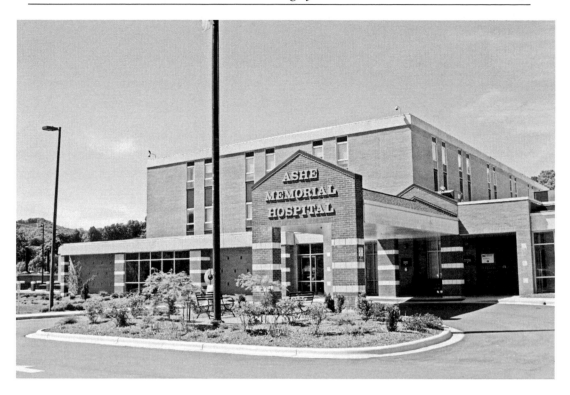

Ashe Memorial Hospital as it stands in 2015, a testament to an Appalachian community's continuing legacy of community health care (photograph, circa 2015, courtesy AMH).

lost to a senseless act of vandalism. We venture into the basement, where the ER was located and where Henry and Ruby Lum lived for a time, and marvel at the size of the room that was central supply, where Evelyn roller skated. Moving back upstairs, Evelyn recognizes the old pediatric ward and the business offices, off the entry. She points out the two small rooms where Dr. Dean and Lettie lived with their son, Dean C., and the nurses' ward across the hall, where Evelyn lived as a nurses' aide. "And this is the room where I gave my first shot," she recalls, stepping into what was once a patient ward. I close my eyes and try to imagine what Evelyn might be seeing—the hubbub of a hospital busy saving lives, bringing new life into the world, and easing the way for those whose time had come. Dr. Dean stops to speak to his life's partner, Lettie, placing a caring arm around her shoulder, before he makes his rounds. Their son, a young man now and home from college, works as an orderly on the halls for the summer, his attention on a pretty nurses' aide, with eyes as blue as an Ashe County sky. If he plays his cards right, and he will, one day she will join him to create the next generation in a legacy he has yet to follow. I look out a window in the back of the building, across the footprint of the water tower, past the day care that was the nurses' quarters, and try to guess the path Dr. Dean took when he walked to the hospital, flashlight in hand, from the brick ranch where Evelyn lives now, to check on patients in the middle of the night. I walk down the steps of the old hospital and into the warm sunshine. The building is much bigger than I expected, and I have a new respect for the limited staff that manned the facility in its earliest days. I also have a better sense of some of the people I am writing about, because I have walked where they walked, in a space that was the essence of their life's work.

An application for nomination of the old Ashe County Memorial Hospital for the National Register of Historic Places was approved in 2015, and there was a plan for converting the property to independent, affordable senior housing, but that has run into problems.[4] Maybe someday the old hospital will have a purpose once again, a new place in the community it served so long. But whether the building finds new life or not, the atmosphere of caring fostered by its founders and its staff continues in the newer, more modern Ashe Memorial, a few miles down the road. And the community which came together to make the dream of a hospital close to home a reality, is still here in the descendants of those who gave of themselves to support this amazing and brave endeavor all those years ago.

I asked some of the people I interviewed if they thought the community today could pull off building a hospital the way their ancestors did 75 years ago. Was it like the Greatest Generation that fought in World War II? Was it an attitude, a philosophy of caring that was lost to history? Or were there others like Dr. Charles Jones, who dared dream of another new hospital, decades in the future, to serve the generations to come? The folks I asked gave this serious thought before they responded, some shook their heads—things have changed too much, they said, but most maintained they still saw tremendous support from the community for health care in the region, akin to the support given to education. Yes, they said, people here in Ashe County have a way of rallying to challenges—never underestimate what a community can do when it sets its collective mind to something, especially here in Appalachia.

Chapter Notes

Introduction

1. Arthur Lloyd Fletcher, *Ashe County: A History,* rev. ed. (Jefferson, N.C.: McFarland & Company, Inc., Publishers, 2006), 24–27.

Chapter 1

1. David C. Hsiung, ed., *Mountaineer in Motion: The Memoir of Dr. Abraham Jobe, 1817–1906* (Knoxville: University of Tennessee Press, 2009), 43.

2. David VanHoy, interview with author, Grassy Creek, Va., February 5, 2015.

3. Ruth Weaver Shepherd and Clarice B. Weaver, eds., *The Heritage of Ashe County North Carolina, Vol. I, 1984* (Winston-Salem, N.C.: The History Division of Hunter Publishing Co., 1984), 203–204.

4. *Ibid.,* 244.

5. Zetta Barker Hamby, *Memoirs of Grassy Creek: Growing Up in the Mountains on the Virginia–North Carolina Line* (Jefferson, N.C.: McFarland & Company, Inc., Publishers, 1998), 145.

6. *Ibid.*; Gayle Winston interview with author, Grassy Creek, N.C., October 14, 2014.

7. VanHoy, interview.

8. *Ibid.*; Kemp Nye, *Jefferson Times,* Vol. 6, No. 48, January 26, 1984; Shepherd and Weaver, eds., *The Heritage of Ashe County, Vol. I,* 486–487.

9. VanHoy, interview; Shepherd and Weaver, eds., *The Heritage of Ashe Co., Vol. I,* 486–487.

10. Shepherd and Weaver, eds., *The Heritage of Ashe Co., Vol. I,* 486–487.

11. Fletcher, *Ashe County: A History*; Betsy Barber Hawkins, "Dr. Joseph Orrin Wilcox" (research paper donated to Museum of Ashe County History, Jefferson, N.C., May 16, 2001, File No. 11.118.03).

12. Ruby Carrington Wilcox Hudler, "Augustus Franklin and Dr. J. O. Wilcox" (research paper contributed to Ashe County Historical Society for publication in *The Heritage of Ashe County North Carolina, Vol. II, 1994,* 300–301).

13. Clarice B. Weaver, ed., *The Heritage of Ashe County, North Carolina, Vol. II, 1994* (copyright Ashe County Historical Society, Delmar Printing Company, Charlotte, N.C.), 300–301.

14. *Ibid.*

15. Fletcher, *Ashe County,* 286.

16. Hawkins, "Dr. J. O. Wilcox," Museum of Ashe County History.

17. Hudler, "Augustus and Dr. J. O. Wilcox," *The Heritage of Ashe Co., Vol. II,* 300–301.

18. Shepherd and Weaver, eds., *The Heritage of Ashe Co., Vol. I,* 169–170; Wylene Barker, interview with author, Jefferson, N.C., February 3, 2015.

19. *The Skyland Post* (West Jefferson, N.C.), December 14, 1939, 1, 4.

20. Sandra Lee Barney, *Authorized to Heal: Gender, Class, and the Transformation of Medicine in Appalachia, 1880–1930* (Chapel Hill: University of North Carolina Press, 2000), 18, 57; Fletcher, *Ashe County,* 286.

21. Hsiung, ed., *Mountaineer in Motion,* 43.

22. *Ibid.,* 44.

23. *Ibid.*

Chapter 2

1. Fletcher, *Ashe County,* 288; Barney, *Authorized to Heal,* 25.

2. Hamby, *Memoirs of Grassy Creek,* 148.

3. *Ibid.,* 149–150.

4. *Ibid.,* 149, 157.

5. *Ibid.,* 149–150, 151–152.

6. Winston, interview.

7. Fletcher, *Ashe County,* 279.

8. Evelyn Jones, interview with author, Jefferson, N.C., October 13, 2014.

9. Fletcher, *Ashe County,* 279.

10. Hamby, *Memoirs of Grassy Creek*, 152–153.

11. *Ibid.*, 158.

12. Calvin Miller, interview with author, Jefferson, N.C., April 2, 2015.

13. Winston, interview.

14. Stephen Shoemaker, interview with author, West Jefferson, N.C., September 16, 2014.

15. Cornetta Price, interview with author, Jefferson, N.C., October 13, 2014.

16. Barney, *Authorized to Heal*, 26.

17. *Ibid.*, 61

18. Anthony Cavender, *Folk Medicine in Southern Appalachia* (Chapel Hill and London: University of North Carolina Press, 2003), 66.

19. Mercer Reeves Hubbard, ed., *The Country Doctor Museum* (Bailey, N.C.: The Compiler, 1971), 13.

20. *The Skyland Post* (West Jefferson, N.C.), December 4, 1941, 2.

21. Sarah Parker Poteete, "By Their Own Agency: A Medical History of Ashe County" (master's thesis, Appalachian State University, 2003), 34.

22. *Ibid.*, 37.

23. *Ibid.*, 30, 36.

24. *The Skyland Post*, August 7, 1941, 8.

25. *Ibid.*, August 28, 1941, 5.

26. Hamby, *Memoirs of Grassy Creek*, 147, 157–158.

27. Anthony Lavender, "A Midwife's Commonplace Book," *Appalachian Journal: A Regional Studies Review* (winter 2005): 184; David VanHoy, interview.

28. Hamby, *Memoirs of Grassy Creek*, 147.

29. Cavender, *Folk Medicine*, 97.

30. Hamby, *Memoirs of Grassy Creek*, 147.

31. Fletcher, *Ashe County*, 295.

32. Calvin Miller, interview, April 2, 2015.

33. Evelyn Jones, interview with author, West Jefferson, N.C., July 28, 2014.

34. Doris Oliver, interview with author, West Jefferson, N.C., July 28, 2014.

35. Cavender, *Folk Medicine*, 33, 35.

36. Barney, *Authorized to Heal*, 27.

37. Cavender, *Folk Medicine*, 69.

38. Hamby, *Memoirs of Grassy Creek*, 146.

39. Cavender, *Folk Medicine*, 74.

40. Winston, interview.

41. Anne McGuire, interview with author, West Jefferson, N.C., July 14, 2014.

42. Hamby, *Memoirs of Grassy Creek*, 146; Cavender, *Folk Medicine*, 71, 96–97; Evelyn Jones interview with author, Warrensville, N.C., November 26, 2014.

43. Cavender, *Folk Medicine*, 71.

44. *The Charlotte Observer*, date unknown, 14; *The Skyland Post,* February 3, 1988.

45. *Jefferson Post,* June 30, 2015, 1, 5.

46. Fletcher, *Ashe County*, 297; *The Charlotte Observer*, date unknown, 14.

Chapter 3

1. *The Skyland Post*, May 22, 1985, 7.

2. *The Jefferson Post*, September 15, 2014.

Chapter 4

1. Mercer Hubbard, ed., *The Country Doctor Museum*, 39.

2. Dr. Charles W. Jones, interview with author, Jefferson, N.C., April 1, 2015.

3. Lonnie C. Jones, interview with author, West Jefferson, N.C., August, 27, 2014.

4. VanHoy, interview.

5. Dr. Charles Jones, interview, April 1, 2015.

6. Evelyn Jones, interview with author, Helton, N.C., July 7, 2014.

7. *Ibid.*

8. *Ibid.*

9. Cornetta Price, interview.

10. Emmett Barker, interview with author, Jefferson, N.C., February 3, 2015.

11. *Ibid.*

12. *Ibid.*

Chapter 5

1. Mary T. Martin Sloop, M.D., with LeGette Blythe, *Miracle in the Hills* (New York: McGraw-Hill Book Company, Inc., 1953), 29–31.

2. Sherree R. Tannen, *Kenneth Killinger: Mountain Missionary* (Lynchburg, Va.: Warwick House Publishing, 2010), 9, 85–86.

3. Evelyn Jones, interview, October 13, 2014.

4. Cornetta Price, interview.

5. Sherree R. Tannen, *Kenneth Killinger*, 86–87.

6. *The Mountain Messenger*, Faith Lutheran Church, Whitetop, Va., summer 1987.

7. *Ibid.*, 91 (reproduction of *Konnarock Echoes,* winter 1945–46).

8. Evelyn Jones, interview, October 13, 2014.

9. Tannen, *Mountain Missionary*, 89.

10. Oliver, interview.

11. Evelyn Jones, interview, July 28, 2014.

12. *The Mountain Messenger*, summer 1987.

13. Tannen, *Mountain Missionary*, 89–90.

Chapter 6

1. Fletcher, *Ashe County*, 281–282.

2. Shepherd and Weaver, eds., *The Heritage of Ashe County, Vol. I*, 317; Fred C. Hubbard, M.D., *Physicians, Medical Practice and Development of*

Hospitals in Wilkes County, 1830 to 1975 (Wilkesboro, N.C.: The Compiler, 1979), 99; *Emory and Henry Alumnus*, spring 1973, Vol. 22, No. 4, 14.

3. Taylor, interview, September 29, 2014; Evelyn Jones interview, September 29, 2014.

4. Emmett Barker, interview.

5. Evelyn Jones interview, September 29, 2014.

6. *Ibid.*; Hubbard, *Development of Hospitals in Wilkes County*, 99.

7. Dr. Jacqueline K. DuSold, interview with author, West Jefferson, August 18, 2014.

8. "Profiles," *Emory and Henry Alumnus*, spring 1973, Vol. 22, No. 44.

9. Nell Jones Taylor, interview with author, Helton, N.C., July 7, 2014.

10. *The Skyland Post*, November 6, 1941, 1.

11. Ruby Lum, interview with author, West Jefferson, N.C., July 1, 2014; Oliver, interview.

12. Evelyn Price, interview with author, Jefferson, N.C., January 5, 2015; Betty Avery, interview with author, Jefferson, N.C., January 5, 2015.

13. McGuire, interview.

14. Lum, interview, July 1, 2014; Oliver interview.

15. Taylor, interview, September 29, 2014; Evelyn Jones, interview, September 29, 2014; Dr. E. J. Miller, interview with author, Jefferson, N.C., July 15, 2014.

16. Evelyn Jones interview, April 1, 2015; Dr. Charles Jones interview, April 1, 2015.

17. Dr. Charles Jones, interview, April 1, 2015.

18. Evelyn Jones, interview, April 1, 2015.

19. Dr. Charles, interview, Jefferson, N.C., September 18, 2014.

20. Evelyn Jones, interview, Jefferson, N.C., September 18, 2014.

21. Geneva Jones Coffey, interview with author, Jefferson, N.C., September 26, 2014.

22. Dr. E. J. Miller, interview.

23. Oliver, interview.

24. Evelyn Jones, interview, West Jefferson, N.C., July 28, 2014.

25. Oliver, interview.

26. VanHoy, interview.

27. Avery, interview.

28. *The Skyland Post*, March 8, 1959.

29. *The Jefferson Times*, November 15, 1984, 1.

30. *The Skyland Post*, June 4, 1978.

31. *The Jefferson Times*, November 15, 1984, 1.

32. Evelyn Jones, interview with author, Helton, N.C., July 7, 2014.

Chapter 7

1. Hubbard, *Development of Hospitals in Wilkes County*, 74, 69.

2. *The Skyland Post*, June 29, 1939, 1, 8.

3. Hubbard, *Development of Hospitals in Wilkes County*, 46–47, 73.

4. Dr. Dean C. Jones, Sr., letter to Dr. Fred C. Hubbard, May 2, 1939, private collection of Evelyn Jones.

5. VanHoy, interview.

6. Dr. E. J. Miller, interview.

7. *Ibid.*

8. "Outstanding Facts About the Proposed Ashe County Hospital," Public Relations Committee, Ashe County Hospital Association; *The Skyland Post*, January 12, 1939, 4.

9. *The Skyland Post*, December 4, 1941, 3, 8.

10. Iris Morphew, telephone interview with author, June 11, 2015; Ashe County High School Journalism Department, *Mountain Arts: Our Heritage*, 2001, 38–40.

11. *The Skyland Post*, October 30, 1941, 1, 3.

12. Fletcher, *Ashe County*, 281–282.

13. *The Skyland Post*, April 6, 1939, 8.

14. Shepherd and Weaver, eds., *The Heritage of Ashe County, Vol. I*, 122.

15. Fletcher, *Ashe County*, 281–282.

16. VanHoy, interview.

17. *The Skyland Post*, October 30, 1941, 2.

18. *Ibid.*, July 4, 1940.

19. Shepherd and Weaver, eds., *The Heritage of Ashe County, Vol. I*, 232–233.

20. Weaver, ed., *The Heritage of Ashe County, Vol. II*, 64; *The Skyland Post*, December 21, 1939.

21. Weaver, ed., *The Heritage of Ashe County, Vol. II*, 64; Mary Gordon Austin Tugman, interviews with author, Jefferson, N.C., August 11, 2014, April 3, 2015.

22. Weaver, ed., *The Heritage of Ashe County, Vol. II*, 64; Tugman, interviews.

23. Tugman, interviews.

24. *Ibid.*; Evelyn Jones, interview with author, Jefferson, N.C., August 11, 2014.

25. Tugman, interviews.

26. Fletcher, *Ashe County*, 282.

27. Cook, interview.

28. VanHoy, interview.

29. *The Skyland Post*, January 19, 1939, 4.

30. *Ibid.*, March 27, 1941, 8; *Ibid.*, April 3, 1941, 5; *Ibid.*, May 1, 1941, 1.

31. *Ibid.*, January 5, 1939.

32. *Ibid.*, October 26, 1939.

33. Fletcher, *Ashe County*, 282.

34. Fletcher, *Ashe County*, 311–312.

35. *The Skyland Post*, January 30, 1941, 5.

36. *Ibid.*, March 13, 1941, 7.

37. Fletcher, *Ashe County*, 313.

38. *The Skyland Post*, October 30, 1941, 1.

39. Fletcher, *Ashe County*, 323–326; Poteete, thesis, 88; Baldwin interview.

40. *The Skyland Post*, October 30, 1941, 2;

Mountain Arts: Our Heritage, 2001, 38, Ashe County High School Journalism Department.

41. *The Skyland Post*, March 9, 1939, 1.

42. *Ibid.,* March 30, 1939, 1.

43. "Outstanding Facts About the Proposed Ashe County Hospital," by the Public Relations Committee of the Jeffersons Rotary; *The Skyland Post*, January 5, 1939.

44. *The Skyland Post*, April 20, 1939.

45. Shepherd and Weaver, eds., *The Heritage of Ashe County, Vol. I*, 472–473.

46. *The Skyland Post*, March 27, 1941, 2.

47. *Ibid.*, October 30, 1941, 1.

48. John Reeves, interview with author, Jefferson, N.C., September 4, 2014.

49. *The Skyland Post*, August 24, 1939, 1.

50. *Ibid.*, January 16, 1941, 5.

51. *Ibid.*, June 6, 1940; Tom Neaves, telephone interview with author, April 26, 2015; *The Skyland Post*, July 10, 1941, 1.

52. *The Skyland Post*, June 27, 1940, 5.

53. *Ibid.*, June 20, 1940, 1.

54. *Ibid.*, June 27, 1940, 1.

55. *Ibid.*, December 21, 1939, 1.

56. *Ibid.*, May 4, 1939, 8.

57. *Ibid.*, April 6, 1939, 1.

58. *Ibid.*, May 11, 1939, 1.

59. *Ibid.*; *The Skyland Post,* September 7, 1939, 1.

60. Mayor Dale Baldwin, interview with author, West Jefferson, N.C., November 24, 2014.

61. Emmett Barker, interview; Leigh Derby, interview with author, West Jefferson and Jefferson, N.C., February 4, 2015.

62. *The Skyland Post*, September 26, 1940, 1, 8.

63. *Ibid.,* September 5, 1940, 4.

64. *Ibid.*, December 19, 1940, 8.

65. *Ibid.*, December 19, 1940, 4, 1.

66. *Ibid.*, January 2, 1941, 1; *ibid.*, January 23, 1941.

67. *Ibid.*, October 16, 1941, 1; *ibid.*, November 6, 1941.

68. Emmett Barker, interview.

69. *The Charlotte Observer*, June 24, 1945.

70. *Ibid.*

71. Mayor Baldwin, interview.

72. *The Charlotte Observer*, June 24, 1945.

Chapter 8

1. *The Skyland Post*, October 30, 1941, 4.

2. *Ibid.*, October 9, 1941, 1, 5.

3. *Ibid.*, November 13, 1941, 2.

4. *Ibid.,* October 30, 1941, 1.

5. *Ibid.*, November 6, 1941, 1; *ibid.*, October 30, 1941, 4.

6. *Ibid.*, March 27, 1941; *ibid.*, October 30, 1941.

7. *Ibid.*, March 20, 1941.

8. *Ibid.*, May 1, 1941; *ibid.*, June 19, 1941.

9. *Ibid.*, April 3, 1941, 1, 4; *ibid.*, April 10, 1941, 5, 8.

10. *Ibid.*, October 30, 1941, 2, 3.

11. *Ibid.*, June 26, 1941, 1.

12. *Ibid.*, June 5, 1941, 3; Doris Oliver, interview, West Jefferson, July 28, 2014.

13. *Ibid.*, July 17, 1941, 3.

14. *Ibid.*, May 29, 1941, 8.

15. *Ibid.*, October 17, 1940; *ibid.*, October 3, 1941, 8.

16. *Ibid.*, October 30, 1941, 2; Fletcher, *Ashe County*, 283.

17. Mary Lou Brooks, interview with author, West Jefferson, August 1, 2014; Fletcher, *Ashe County*, 283.

18. *The Skyland Post*, October 30, 1941, 1, 8; *ibid.*, December 4, 1941, 1; *ibid.*, April 24, 1941.

19. *Ibid.*, November 6, 1941, 1, 8; Cook interview; *The Skyland Post*, December 4, 1941, 1.

20. Fundraising brochure for Ashe County Memorial Hospital Building Fund Campaign, 1966; *Mountain Arts: Our Heritage*, 2001, 40.

21. Fletcher, *Ashe County*, 107–108, 110; Oliver, interview.

22. Mark Vannoy, interview with author, Jefferson, N.C., January 22, 2015.

23. *The Skyland Post*, November 6, 1971.

24. Avery, interview.

25. Oliver, interview.

26. Lum, interview, July 1, 2014.

27. Avery, interview.

Chapter 9

1. *The Skyland Post,* December 14, 1939, 1, 4.

2. *Ibid.,* October 30, 1941, 2.

3. James G. Gambill, Jr., interview with author, Jefferson, N.C., March 31, 2015.

4. Shepherd and Weaver, eds., *The Heritage of Ashe County, Vol. I*, 311.

5. *AMH Monitor*, September 2000.

6. *Ibid.*

7. *AMH Monitor*, Vol. VIII No. 1, summer, 1998; Gambill, interview.

8. Gambill, interview.

9. Shepherd and Weaver, eds., *The Heritage of Ashe County, Vol. I*, 248, 540; James Gambill interview.

10. Weaver, ed., *The Heritage of Ashe County, Vol. II*, 181–182.

11. *Ibid.*

12. *Ibid.*; AMH Foundation publication for 11th Annual Frank M. James Memorial Golf Tournament, 2005, 1.

13. Vannoy, interview.
14. *Ibid.*
15. Shepherd and Weaver, eds., *The Heritage of Ashe County, Vol. I*, 483–484; Vannoy interview.
16. Vannoy, interview.

Chapter 10

1. *The Skyland Post*, June 27, 1940, 8.
2. Fletcher, *Ashe County*, 284.
3. *The Skyland Post*, November 6, 1941, 1; *ibid.*, November 4, 1971.
4. Dr. Tammy Thore, interview with author, Jefferson, N.C., September 19, 2014.
5. Reeves, interview.
6. Oliver, interview.
7. Brooks, interview.
8. Mayor Baldwin, interview.
9. Elam S. Kurtz, M.D., and Michael D. Kurtz, D. Min., *Crossings: Memoirs of a Mountain Medical Doctor*, 15, 5, 16, 85.
10. Kurtz, *Crossings*, 64–65, 11–12, 15.
11. *Ibid.*, 18–20.
12. *Ibid.*, 23–24.
13. *Ibid.*, 86, 15.
14. Weaver, ed., *The Heritage of Ashe County, Vol. II*, 443.
15. Phyllis Jones Yount, interview with author, Raleigh, N.C., December 6, 2014.

Chapter 11

1. Taylor, interview, September 29, 2014.
2. *Ibid.*
3. *Ibid.*
4. Dr. Charles Jones, interview, April 1, 2015.
5. Pat Cooper, interview with author, Glendale Springs, N.C., October 22, 2014.
6. Dr. Don McNeill, interview with author, Jefferson, N.C., October 29, 2014.
7. Ann Brown, interview with author, West Jefferson, N.C., October 21, 2014.
8. Dr. Leigh Bradley, interview with author, Jefferson, N.C., January 3, 2015.
9. David Jones, interview with author, Jefferson, N.C., January 4, 2015.
10. Dr. Bradley, interview.
11. Dr. Charles Jones, interview, April 1, 2015.

Chapter 12

1. *The Skyland Post*, June 6, 1940, 1.
2. Fletcher, *Ashe County*, 285.
3. Calvin Miller, interview, April 2, 2015.
4. *The Skyland Post*, December 4, 1941, 2.

5. Shepherd and Weaver, eds., *The Heritage of Ashe County, Vol. I*, 126–127; Eleanor Baker Reeves, *James Larkin Ballou, Physician and Surgeon ... Ancestral Sketches...*, 10–11.
6. *Ibid.*; Reeves, *James Larkin Ballou, Physician and Surgeon ... Ancestral Sketches*, 62–63, 65–66.
7. *Ibid.*
8. Shepherd and Weaver, eds., *The Heritage of Ashe County, Vol. I*, 126–127.
9. Winston, interview.
10. Cornetta Price, interview.
11. Evelyn Jones, interview, March 27, 2015; Ruby Lum, interview with author, West Jefferson, N.C., March 27, 2015.
12. Shepherd and Weaver, eds., *The Heritage of Ashe County, Vol. I*, 217.
13. Ashe County Historical Society, *Images of America: West Jefferson*, 92–93, 23; *The Skyland Post*, September 4, 1941, 1.
14. Shepherd and Weaver, eds., *The Heritage of Ashe County, Vol. I*, 423.
15. Emmett Barker, interview.
16. Ashe County Historical Society, *Images of America: West Jefferson*, 92–93, 23.
17. Calvin Miller, interview, April 2, 2015.
18. McRimmon, interview.
19. Reeves, interview.
20. Clifford Miller, interview with author, West Jefferson, March 24, 2015.
21. Reeves, interview.
22. Poteete, thesis, 103.
23. *Ibid.*, 94–96.
24. *Ibid.*, 97, 106, 99, 104.
25. Kurtz, *Crossings*, 19–20.
26. Oliver, interview.
27. Poteete, thesis, 102–103.
28. Kurtz, *Crossings*, 19–20.
29. Shepherd and Weaver, eds., *The Heritage of Ashe County, Vol. I*, 349–350.
30. *Ibid.*
31. *Ibid.*
32. *Ibid.*, 420
33. *Ibid.*, 226.
34. Lum, interview, March 27, 2015.
35. Calvin Miller interview with author, October 27, 2014.
36. Oliver, interview.
37. Weaver, ed., *The Heritage of Ashe County, Vol. II*, 191–192.
38. *AMH Monitor*, summer 1990, Vol. III, No. 1.
39. *AMH Annual Report*, 2000, 2.
40. *AMH Monitor*, summer 1990, Vol. III, No. 1.
41. *AMH Monitor*, September 2000 edition, 3.
42. *Ibid.*
43. *Ibid.*

Chapter 13

1. *The Skyland Post*, June 26, 1958, 1–2.
2. Wanda Roten, telephone interview with author, June 25, 2015.
3. *AMH Monitor*, Vol. III, No. 1, spring 1991.
4. R. D. Williams II, telephone interview with author, April 27, 2015.
5. Dr. Donald D. McNeill, telephone interview with author, July 13, 2015.
6. Williams, interview.
7. Kurtz, *Crossings*, 29.
8. Oliver, interview.
9. Bill Badger, interviews with author, Jefferson, N.C., May 27, 2015, July 20, 2015.
10. Reeves, interview.
11. Beulah Barker McVey, interviews with author, Jefferson, N.C., May 6 and May 7, 2015.
12. *The Skyland Post*, July 14, 1966.
13. Dr. Bradley, interview.
14. Nancy Kautz, interview with author, Jefferson, N.C., March 27, 2015.
15. *Ibid.*

Chapter 14

1. *Ibid.*, January 28, 2015.
2. *The Skyland Post*, October 30, 1941, 3.
3. *Ibid.,* April 27, 1939, 1.
4. *Ibid.*, February 6, 1941, 1, 7; *ibid.*, May 29, 1941, 7.
5. *Ibid.*, October 23, 1941, 1.
6. Fletcher, *Ashe County*, 280.
7. *Ibid.*, 278, 280.
8. Oliver, interview.
9. *The Jefferson Post*, May 22, 1990.
10. *Ibid.*, January 12, 1993.
11. Brooks, interview.
12. Dr. Bradley, interview.
13. McGuire, interview.
14. McVey, interview, May 6, 7, 2015.
15. *AMH Medical Directory*, 2005–2006.
16. Kevin Kurtz, interview with author, West Jefferson, N.C., July 13, 2014.
17. Kautz interview, January 28, 2015.
18. Dr. Bradley, interview.
19. Wylene Barker, interview.
20. *AMH Annual Report* 2006, 11; *AMH Medical Directory*, 2007, 11.
21. *AMH Monitor*, September 2000, 1.
22. *AMH Annual Report* 2000, 3.
23. *AMH Annual Report* 2006, 11.

Chapter 15

1. *AMH Monitor*, Vol. VII, No. 2, fall, 1997.
2. Evelyn Jones, interview, January 15, 2015.
3. *Ibid.*, October 13, 2014

Chapter 16

1. Gambill, interview; Dr. Charles Jones, interview, April 1, 2015; *AMH Medical Directory*, 2007, 27.
2. Clairene Cockerham, interview with author, Jefferson, N.C., September 29, 2014.
3. Gambill, interview.
4. *Ibid.*; Williams, interview.
5. Gambill, interview.
6. Bradley McNeill, interview with author, West Jefferson, N.C., January 28, 2015.
7. Jan Caddell, interview with author, West Jefferson, N.C., August 8, 2014.
8. Laura Lambeth, interviews with author, Jefferson, N.C., August 13, 1014, March 27, 2015.
9. Dr. Charles Jones, interview, April 1, 2015; *AMH Annual Report*, 2006, 9.
10. Evelyn Jones, interview, November 17, 2014.
11. Mayor Baldwin, interview.
12. *AMH Monitor*, September 2000 edition, 3.
13. *AMH Medical Directory*, 2005–2006, 22, and 2007, 19.
14. *Ashe Mountain Times*, December 25, 2014.
15. Dr. Charles Jones, interview, April 1, 2015.
16. Evelyn Jones, interview, March 27, 2015.
17. Dr. Thore, interview.
18. Vita M. Blevins, telephone interview with author, April 27, 2015.
19. *The Skyland Post*, January 23, 1941, 1; *ibid.*, October 30, 1941, 1.
20. *Ibid.*, June 12, 1941, 1; *ibid.*, March 21, 1941, 1.
21. *Ibid.*, October 30, 1941, 1, 5.
22. Fletcher, *Ashe County*, 284.
23. Office of the AMH Volunteer Coordinator.

Chapter 17

1. Kautz, interview, March 27, 2015.
2. Dr. Bradley, interview.
3. Caddell, interview.
4. Dr. Charles Jones, interview, April 1, 2015.

Chapter 18

1. Yount, interview.
2. Dr. Bradley, interview; Tommy Jones, interview with author, Jefferson, N.C., January 3, 2015.
3. *Ibid.*
4. Leigh Derby, telephone conversation with author, August 17, 2015.

Bibliography and Sources

Manuscripts

University of North Carolina at Chapel Hill, Wilson Library, Congressman Robert L. Doughton Papers

Published Works

Ashe County High School Journalism Department. *Mountain Heritage, 2000.* Reported by Danessa Pollard.

_____. *Mountain Arts: Our Heritage, 2001.*

Ashe County Historical Society. John Houck, Clarice Weaver, and Carol Williams [editors]. *Images of America: Ashe County.* Charleston, S.C.: Arcadia Publishing, 2000.

_____. *Images of America: Ashe County Revisited.* Charleston, S.C.: Arcadia Publishing, 2002.

_____. *Images of America: West Jefferson.* Charleston, S.C.: Arcadia Publishing, 2014.

Barney, Sandra Lee. *Authorized to Heal: Gender, Class, and the Transformation of Medicine in Appalachia, 1880–1930.* Chapel Hill: University of North Carolina Press, 2000.

Cavender, Anthony. *Folk Medicine in Southern Appalachia.* Chapel Hill: University of North Carolina Press, 2003.

Fletcher, Arthur Lloyd. *Ashe County: A History; A New Edition.* Jefferson, N.C.: McFarland, 2006 (first edition published by Ashe County Research Association in 1963).

Hsiung, David C. *A Mountaineer in Motion: The Memoir of Dr. Abraham Jobe, 1817–1906.* Knoxville: University of Tennessee Press, 2009.

Hubbard, Fred C., M.D. *Physicians, Medical Practice and Development of Hospitals in Wilkes County, 1830 to 1975.* Wilkesboro, N.C.: self published, 1978.

Hubbard, Mercer Reeves, ed. *The Country Doctor Museum.* Bailey, N.C.: Board of Directors, County Doctor Museum, 1971.

Kurtz, Elam S., M.D., and Michael D. Kurtz, D. Min. *Crossings: Memoirs of a Mountain Medical Doctor.* New York: iUniverse, Inc., 2010.

Reeves, Eleanor Baker. *James Larkin Ballou Physician and Surgeon...Ancestral Sketches on Meredith Ballou, Connecting Families and the Ashe County Ballou Genealogy.* Self-published, 1969.

Shepherd, Ruth Weaver, and Clarice B. Weaver, eds. *The Heritage of Ashe County, North Carolina, Volume I, 1984.* Winston-Salem, N.C.: Ashe County Heritage Book Committee in cooperation with the History Division of Hunter Publishing Company, 1984.

Shoemaker, Stephen, and Janet Pittard. *Stephen Shoemaker: The Paintings and Their Stories.* Jefferson, N.C.: McFarland, 2013.

Sloop, Mary T. Martin, M.D., with LeGette Blythe. *Miracle in the Hills.* New York: McGraw-Hill Book Company, Inc., 1953.

Tannen, Sherree R. *Kenneth Killinger, Mountain Missionary.* Lynchburg, Va.: Warwick House Publishing, 2010.

Washburn, Dr. Benjamin Earle. *A Country Doctor in the South Mountains.* Asheville: Stephens Press, 1955.

Weaver, Clarice B., ed., *The Heritage of Ashe County, North Carolina, Volume II, 1994.* Charlotte, NC: Ashe County Historical Society in cooperation with Delmar Printing Company, 1994.

Journal Articles

Lavender, Anthony. "A Midwife's Commonplace Book." *Appalachian Journal, A Regional Studies Review* (winter 2005): 184.

North Carolina Medical Journal, Volume 19, No. 3 (March 1958), p. 112–115, 188.

Newspaper Articles

The Ashe Mountain Times (N.C.), December 18, 2014.

The Charlotte Observer (N.C.), date unknown.

The Jefferson Post (N.C.), May 8, 1992.

The Jefferson Times (N.C.), Kemp Nye on Dr. Waddell, Vol. 6., No. 48 (January 26, 1984).

The Roanoke Times (Va.), March 8, 1954.

The Skyland Post (N.C.), issues from 1938 to 1941 and 1971, as specified in endnotes.

Magazine Articles

Ashe County Guide. Ashe County Chamber of Commerce, fall 2015.

Pittard, Janet. "Dr. Mary Martin Sloop." *Our State,* January, 2008.

Johnston. Ira T. "Things of Interest in Ashe County." *The State Magazine,* April 9, 1949.

Newsletters and Other Published Material

AMH Medical Directory, 2007.

Ashe Memorial Hospital Foundation. Eleventh Annual Frank M. James Memorial Golf Tournament 2005.

AMH Monitor, summer 1990, Volume III, No. 1.

AMH Monitor, fall 1997, Volume VII, No. 2.

Ashe Memorial Hospital, Inc. Program for Dedication Ceremony, October 31, 1971.

The Mountain Messenger, Faith Lutheran Church, Whitetop, Va., summer 1987. Issue dedicated to the memory of Sister Sophia Moeller and Dr. Heinz C. Meyer.

"Profiles," *Emory and Henry Alumnus* Vol. 22, No.4 (spring 1973), 14.

Public Relations Committee, Ashe County Hospital Association. "Outstanding Facts About the Proposed Ashe County Hospital." 1966. (Fundraising brochure for Ashe County Memorial Hospital Building Fund Campaign, 1966.)

Miscellaneous Government Records

Articles of Amendment to the Charter of Ashe County Memorial Hospital, Inc., for purpose of changing name from Ashe County Memorial Hospital, Inc., to Ashe Memorial Hospital, Inc., filed with North Carolina Secretary of State, October 7, 1970.

Theses

Poteete, Sarah Parker. "By Their Own Agency: A Medical History of Ashe County." Master's thesis: 2003 (courtesy of Special Collections, Appalachian State University).

Other Unpublished Sources

Architectural survey for Ashe County Memorial Hospital nomination for National Register of Historic Places, completed in 2006. N.C. Department of Cultural Resources.

Ashe County Memorial Hospital, Inc., original ledger, containing reports and minutes of hospital board meetings and executive committee meetings, December 12, 1939, to early 1950s. Ashe Memorial Hospital archive.

Hawkins, Betsy Barber, "Dr. Joseph Orrin Wilcox." Research completed May 16, 2001, and donated to the Museum of Ashe County History, Jefferson, NC.

Hudler, Ruby Carrington Wilcox. Personal notes for Ashe County Historical Society's *The Heritage of Ashe County, North Carolina, Volume II,* 1994, 300–301.

Letters

Dr. Bud Jones letter to Mr. R. L. Ballou, postmarked in Helton July 12, 1907, private collection of Evelyn Jones.

Dr. Dean C. Jones, Sr., letter to Dr. Fred C. Hubbard, May 2, 1939, private collection of Evelyn Jones.

Tapes/Videos

Dr. Dean C. "Doc" Jones, Jr., Retirement "Quitting" Party, Blue Ridge Dinner Theater, West Jefferson, N.C., May 11, 2007.

_____, Tour of the old Ashe County Memorial Hospital, Jefferson, N.C., summer 2007.

_____. Funeral service, Jefferson, N.C., December 29, 2009.

Interviews and Personal Communications

Ashe Memorial Hospital. Office of Volunteer Coordinator. Email to author, August 6, 2015.

Ashley, Ruby. Interview with author, Warrensville, N.C., November 26, 2014.

Avery, Betty Lou. Interview with author, Jefferson, N.C., January 5, 2015.

Badger, Bill. Interviews with author, Jefferson, N.C., May 27 and July 20, 2015.

Baldwin, Mayor Dale. Interview with author, West Jefferson, N.C., November 24, 2014.

Baldwin, Ella P. Interview with author, West Jefferson, N.C., November 24, 2014.

Ball, Betty. Interview with author, West Jefferson, N.C., August 15, 2014.

Barker, Emmett. Interview with author, Jefferson, N.C., February 3, 2015.

Barker, Wylene. Interview with author, Jefferson, N.C., February 3, 2015.

Barker, Kate Duncan. Interview with author, West Jefferson, N.C., November 17, 2014.

Baucom, Cindy Brooks. Interview with author, West Jefferson, N.C., August 1, 2014.

Black, Robert H. Interview with author, Lansing, N.C., January 7, 2015.

Blevins, Edith B. Interview with author, Lansing, N.C., January 7, 2015.

Blevins, Vita M. Telephone interview with author, April 27, 2015.

Bradley, Dr. Leigh. Interview with author, West Jefferson, N.C., January 3, 2015.

Brooks, Mary Lou. Interview with author, West Jefferson, N.C., August 1, 2014.

Brown, Ann Day. Interview with author, West Jefferson, N.C., October 21, 2014

Burleson, Deeanna. Interview with author, West Jefferson, N.C., April 2, 2015.

Caddell, Jan R. Interview with author, West Jefferson, N.C., August 8, 2014.

Cockerham, Clairene O. Interview with author, Jefferson, N.C., September 29, 2014.

Coffey, Geneva Jones. Interview with author, Jefferson, N.C., September 26, 2014.

Cook, Giona Badger. Interview with author, Jefferson, N.C., August 14, 2014.

Cooper, Pat Bare. Interview with author, Glendale Springs, N.C., October 22, 2014.

Craven, Shirley McClure. Telephone interview with author, April 2015.

Davis, Judy. Interview with author, West Jefferson, N.C., August 7, 2014.

Derby, Leigh. Interview with author, West Jefferson and Jefferson, N.C., February 4, 2015; telephone conversation with author, August 17, 2015.

DuSold, Dr. Jacqueline K. Interview with author, West Jefferson, N.C., August 18, 2014.

Edwards, Nancy P. Interview with author, West Jefferson, N.C., September 17, 2014.

Gambill, James G., Jr. Interview with author, West Jefferson, N.C., March 31, 2015.

Gant, Betsy L. Interview with author, West Jefferson, N.C., June 28, 2014.

Goslen, Mary Ann Miller. Interview with author, West Jefferson, N.C., August 16, 2014.

Hafer, Gene. Interview with author, West Jefferson, N.C., August 6, 2014.

Hampton, Sue. Interview with author, West Jefferson, N.C., September 17, 2014; telephone conversation with author, July 9, 2015.

Hartzog, Toby. Interview with author, West Jefferson, N.C., October 23, 2014.

Hendrix, James. Interview with author, Jefferson, N.C., March 27, 2014.

Jones, Brandon. Interview with author, Jefferson, N.C., January 2, 2015.

Jones, Charles B. "C. B.," Jr. Interview with author, Jefferson, N.C., September 26, 2014.

Jones, Dr. Charles Wade. Interviews with author, Jefferson, N.C., September 18, 2014, January 15, 2015 and April 1, 2015.

Jones, Connor. Interview with author, Jefferson, N.C., January 15, 2015.

Jones, David Lee. Interview with author, Jefferson, N.C., January 4, 2015.

Jones, Debra Eller, "Debbie." Interview with author, Jefferson, N.C., January 15, 2015.

Jones, Evelyn Price. Interviews with author, Jefferson, N.C., July 7, July 28, August 11, September 18, September 29, October 13, November 17, 2014; January 5, January 15, March 27 and April 1, 2015.

Jones, Hunter. Interview with author, Jefferson, N.C., January 15, 2015.

Jones, Lonnie C. Interview with author, West Jefferson, N.C., August 27, 2014.

Jones, Thomas, M. "Tommy." Interview with author, Jefferson, N.C., January 3, 2015.

Kautz, Nancy. Interviews with author, Jefferson, N.C., January 28 and March 27, 2015.

Kurtz, Kevin J. Interview with author, West Jefferson, N.C., July 13, 2014.

Kurtz, Michael D. Interview with author, West Jefferson, N.C., January 16, 2015.

Kurtz, Orpah M. Interview with author, West Jefferson, N.C., July 16, 2014.

Lambeth, Laura. Interviews with author, Jefferson, N.C., August 13, 2014, March 27, 2015.

Little, Betsy Jones. Interview with author, Jefferson, N.C., September 26, 2014.

Little, James Frank. Interview with author, Jefferson, N.C., September 26, 2014.

Long, Donald. Interview with author, Jefferson, N.C., August 30, 2014.

Lovette, Kathy. Interview with author, Jefferson, N.C., April 21, 2015.

Lum, Ruby. Interviews with author, Jefferson, N.C., July 1, 2014, March 27, 2015.

Lyalls, Larry K. Interviews with author, West Jefferson, N.C., April 29 and April 30, 2015.

McClure, Jack. Interview with author, West Jefferson, N.C., August 12, 2014.

McClure, Joy R. Interview with author, West Jefferson, N.C., August 12, 2014.

McCoy, Barbara A. Interview with author, Warrensville, N.C., November 26, 2014.

McGuire, Anne. Interview with author, West Jefferson, N.C., July 14, 2014.

McNeill, Bradley. Interview with author, West Jefferson, N.C., January 28, 2015.

McNeill, Kada Owen. Interview with author, Jefferson, N.C., January 20, 2015.

McNeill, Dr. Donald D. Interview with author, Jefferson, N.C., October 29, 2014; telephone conversation with author, July 13, 2015.

McNeill, Patricia Hudler. Interview with author, West Jefferson, N.C., January 28, 2015.

McRimmon, Elizabeth G. Interview with author, West Jefferson, N.C., September 2, 2014.

McVey, Beulah Barker. Interviews with author, Jefferson, N.C., May 6 and May 7, 2015.

Miller, Betty. Interview with author, Glendale Springs, N.C., April 29, 2015.

Miller, Billy Ray. Interview with author, Glendale Springs, N.C., April 29, 2015.

Miller, Calvin H. Interviews with author, Jefferson, N.C., October 27, 2014, April 2, 2015.

Miller, Clifford. Interview with author, West Jefferson, N.C., March 24, 2015.

Miller, Dr. E. J. Interview with author, Jefferson, N.C., July 15, 2014.

Miller, Katrina V. Interview with author, Jefferson, N.C., October 27, 2014.

Miller, Lucy L. Interview with author, West Jefferson, N.C., March 24, 2015.

Morphew, Iris. Telephone interview with author, June 11, 2015.

Neaves, Tom. Telephone interview with author, April 26, 2015.

Oliver, Doris. Interview with author, West Jefferson, N.C., July 28, 2014.

Osowitt, Elliott. Interview with author, West Jefferson, N.C., October 17, 2014.

Osowitt, Polly. Interview with author, West Jefferson, N.C., October 17, 2014.

Patterson, Linda Noel. Interview with author, Jefferson, N.C., March 27, 2015.

Price, Cornetta. Interview with author, Jefferson, N.C., October 13, 2014.

Price, John. Telephone interviews with author, January 21 and March 11, 2015.

Reeves, John K. Interview with author, Jefferson, N.C., September 4, 2014.

Robinson, Nancy, P. "Nan." Telephone interview with author, November 21, 2014.

Roten, Wanda. Telephone interview with author, June 25, 2015.

Ruiz, Robert. Interview with author, Swannanoa, N.C., September 25, 2014.

Shoemaker, Stephen S. Interview with author, West Jefferson, N.C., September 16, 2014.

Spurlin, Janet Dickson. Telephone interview with author, July 21, 2015.

Taylor, Nell Jones. Interviews with author, Helton, N.C., July 7 and September 29, 2014.

Thompson, Charlotte C. Telephone interview with author, January 19, 2015.

Thore, Joe. Interview with author, Jefferson, N.C., September 16, 2014.

Thore, Dr. Tammy Lum. Interviews with author, Jefferson, N.C., September 16 and 19, 2014.

Tugman, Mary Gordon. Interviews with author, Jefferson, N.C., August 11, 2014, April 3, 2015.

VanHoy, David. Interview with author, Grassy Creek, Va., February 5, 2015.

Vannoy, Mark. Interview with author, Jefferson, N.C., January 22, 2015.

Williams, R. D., II. Telephone interview with author, April 27, 2015.

Winston, Gayle. Interview with author, Grassy Creek, N.C., October 14, 2014.

Worth, June. Interview with author, West Jefferson, N.C., November 25, 2014.

Yount, Phyllis Jones. Interview with author, Raleigh, N.C., December 6, 2014.

Index

Numbers in **bold italics** indicate pages with photographs.